POLAR BEARS AND HUMMING BIRDS

*

A MEDICAL
GUIDE TO
WEIGHT
LOSS

MAINTENANCE AND HEALTH

*

Dr Hendrik v ⌐

MA MBchB BAO(TCD) MRCF

GW00686243

Polar Bears and Humming Birds - A Medical Guide to Weight Loss
Dr Hendrik v Rensburg
Email: weightloss@RxGOFES.com

Published by MDE Publishing

ISBN 0 9775307 0 1

Designed by The Graphic Design Group
Cover design by The Graphic Design Group
Cover photograph by © Frédéric Cirou/PhotoAlto
Author photograph by Gary Peters
Edited by ITPR Marketing Pty Ltd
Printed and bound in Australia by Advance Press

This book is dedicated to Monique, Dominque and Esteé
who were and are my inspiration and life.

I want to thank the following for their direct and indirect assistance in writing this book: all the thousands of wonderful patients I have seen over the years from whom I have learned so much, my parents, Denise Koch, Frances Zampogna, Helen Ruesch, Mary Ciavatta, Ric Yeates, Ian Teasdale, Ian McAlpine, Paul Gordin, David Harrison and David Smith.

CONTENTS

IMPORTANT DISCLAIMER

Any advice taken from *Polar Bears and Humming Birds - A Medical Guide to Weight Loss* and the medical issues raised should always be discussed with your doctor. We are all different. If you decide to follow any part of this book, show the book to your doctor and ask if it is suitable for you in particular.

For fear of too much "self treatment", I have omitted treatment protocols that should only be used under *strict specialised medical supervision*. In spite of this, you will get more than enough to make an enormous difference to your health. *Polar Bears and Humming Birds - A Medical Guide to Weight Loss* will, at the very least, set you on the right course.

INTRODUCTION

INTRODUCTION

"I don't read health books in case there is a misprint"
MARK TWAIN

Not another book on Health, Obesity and Weight?

Bookshop shelves are lined with works on this topic but most have very little practical value. As a doctor, I felt there was a need to approach weight loss from a medical perspective - I didn't want to write "just another book". I wanted something that had meaning and value.

Who is this book for?

This book is for people with a weight problem that they can't control. It is also for the health conscious. I believe that this book discusses health, obesity and weight like never before.

Polar Bears and Humming Birds - A Medical Guide to Weight Loss is based on many years of experience and research in the treatment of obesity, related conditions, and functional health.

My Viewpoint

How a person views a situation depends on whether he is looking down the barrel of a gun or through the sights. This is quite valid in the case of obesity and health. I felt that my views on this subject were diverging from the so-called "main stream". There are so many views out there that clearly aren't based on genuine experience.

However there are many who share my views and as a result we have gained wider acceptance in recent years. Over 25 years ago, when I claimed that obesity was largely genetic and therefore inherited, I was looked on with

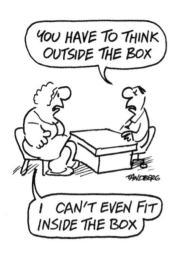

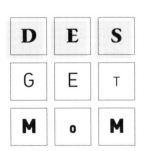

What does the following "puzzle" mean? Can you work it out?

D	**E**	**S**
G	E	T
M	o	**M**

scorn, but in the last few years this view has become more widely accepted. When I suggested that obesity was more than just overeating and lack of physical activity, my claims caused confusion and condemnation in a conditioned mindset. My views were dismissed by many and there was no such thing as rational discussion with some "experts". It reminded me of politics.

The problem of obesity is simple to see, yet can be so confusing, unless you look at it from a bird's eye view.

With obesity and weight loss, those who concentrate too intently on the small details aren't looking at the bigger picture and are missing key elements in treating this condition. The result has been a massive obesity pandemic.

The puzzle on the left contains the "secrets" that explain obesity and unlock its solutions. Most researchers and others working in the field of obesity tend to focus on one or two squares at a time. You will never really control obesity or maintain good health without a full understanding of all the squares as they relate to each other.

This book will help you unlock the enigma of obesity.

So many intellectuals, researchers, gurus and people with a commercial interest in weight loss offer themselves as obesity experts and consultants. They talk about latest studies, hormones and chemicals, and research that shows we watch too much television and eat too much junk food, but they offer little of practical value in providing a solution.

3

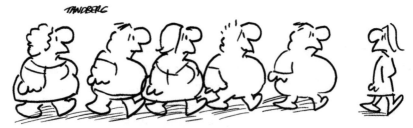

OBESITY INCREASING IN ROUND FIGURES

It's often easier to join the bandwagon and lose us in irrelevant detail than it is to find a solution. There is little to be gained from constantly reminding us that the instance of obesity is on the rise.

In *round figures*, surveys show there are eight million fat people in Australia and 80 million in the USA.

What can be done about it?

In most instances, when you try to get help for your problem, the experts will push their own barrows - gyms will claim you can do it through exercise, dieticians insist that diet is the solution, psychologists will tell you it's all psychological, commercial concerns claim to have all the answers as long as you buy their products, and scammers just prey on your wallet.

Scores of misconceptions need to be addressed and I will deal with them during the course of *Polar Bears and Humming Birds - A Medical Guide to Weight Loss*. I have endeavoured to take the mystique out of obesity and weight problems. There are no secrets. Once we accept that the problem exists, and that it's not as complex as it seems, the solutions will follow.

I can't tell you what you like to hear,
I'll have to tell you what you have to hear.

Weight loss is a funny industry - a diet is never a diet, it's a "meal plan" or "food plan". The fact is, anything that you eat is a part of your diet. Whether it is an Italian diet, an Asian diet, a Palaeolithic diet or a therapeutic deficit diet, it's a diet. A spade should be called a spade when dealing with obesity and health. Let's not pull any punches.

What sort of information and how much detail?

I have come to the conclusion that "over-education" on the subject does not work - *paralysis from analysis.* The only education that does work must be simple and practical with an emphasis on a genuine basic understanding of the subject. For instance, to understand why we eat, shun exercise and get fat in the first place.

This book is not a thesis on health and obesity. It addresses these issues with practical solutions. To be "street wise" is much more successful in controlling obesity than "chic academic talk".

In this way, I hope to reach a wider audience, so that I can put forward techniques and procedures that really work. In some areas I have developed new concepts and terminology and in others I have renamed old concepts to create a new system of awareness.

We need to have an open mind (and a closed mouth!) and a bird's eye view of the subject to be successful.

Repetition

For effect, a certain amount of repetition is used in different guises, expressing concepts in various ways and linking them to others. I have found that people need repetition when it comes to health messages.

I may be criticised for not coming to the point quickly enough, but explaining some concepts requires background information. I hope, you'll find some of this interesting reading. I also use case histories, and sometimes seemingly irrelevant information, to illustrate various concepts. You need patience and persistence to control obesity and acquire good health and this book may test you on one or other of those counts, but I hope it will help change your life for the better.

Certain analogies in *Polar Bears and Humming Birds - A Medical Guide to Weight Loss* are for illustration purposes and should not be taken literally.

Each chapter is a book on its own

Each chapter is a book on its own. With so many "books" in one manuscript, space is an obvious problem. Sometimes this precludes detailed physiological and metabolic explanation, but that is not the purpose of this manuscript.

Leanness and fatness affect our lives on a very broad spectrum and are closely related to what we are as humans. The book is therefore wide ranging. The control of obesity must also be very comprehensive to be successful.

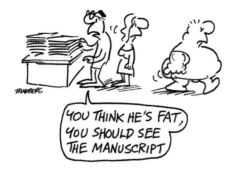

Many references relate to my medical education, my own experience, research and the conclusions I drew from it. You will find some concepts and terminology never published before. Many experts and writers dogmatically state that certain protocols should be followed to treat obesity, but often this lacks a basis in practical experience.

With no gimmicks and frills, some may find this book to be harsh and insensitive, but if you want to be successful in managing your health and controlling obesity, harsh facts needs to be explored and confronted. We live in an age of political correctness. To be "politically correct" and not confront reality is a bit of Alice in Wonderland when it comes to health.

I believe this to be one of the most comprehensive books on health and obesity. It is a practical manual that will enable you to incorporate health principles into your life. *Polar Bears and Humming Birds - A Medical Guide to Weight Loss* is intended to be the first in a series of books on this topic. It will start you on the right track.

I recommend reading the book from cover to cover, since some aspects and concepts will only fit into place when you have the total picture.

Humour

Life... is much too short to be taken seriously.
NICOLAS BENTLEY

This is a manuscript based on personal experience and includes humorous anecdotes told to me by thousands of patients. The use of humour doesn't mean for one second that I am not serious about the subject matter. I hope to make you laugh and cry, but the underlying message is always sincere. Remember, laughing at yourself is therapeutic.

What it is not

Polar Bears and Humming Birds - A Medical Guide to Weight Loss is not a cooking book, but I am planning a recipe-based book as part of the intended series.

A quick start

Experience has taught me that the average overweight person will not read instructions if written on more than one page. I ask you to read the whole book. This may sound paradoxical to you, but since the average obese person is not always successful at managing their problem, more reading is required.

Many computer programs will have a "quick start" section in the instructions. This is usually necessary, since we hate reading the more comprehensive instructions or the facts behind the facts. I've endeavoured to include summaries and shorter sections in this book, but because of the nature of health a "quick start" can gloss over important information that is intended to give you the whole picture. The intended series of follow up books will address more advanced techniques.

You are starting a journey that may be the best investment you will ever make.

Enjoy the trip.

GLOSSARY OF TERMS

BA	Biological age
CA	Chronological age
CZ	Comfort zone
Depalgesic	Appetite suppressant or anorectic
Depalgia	Pain of hunger (POD)
DES	Demand Effort Supply
EC	Environmental challenge
Functional age	The age you function at. See BA
GI	Glycaemic index
GL	Glycaemic load
GOFES	The Genetic over fat environmental syndrome
HR	Host resistance
Hyperadiposis	Excess fat
POD	The Pain of deprivation
POE	The Pleasure or comfort of eating
POEx	The Pain of exercise
SD	"Sin days"

CHAPTER 1

HEALTH

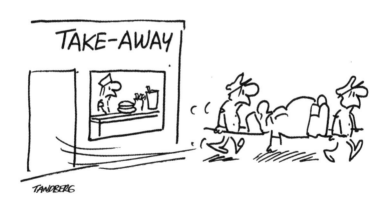

HEALTH

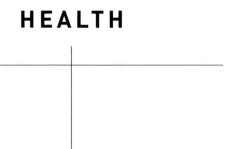

"I am dying with the help of too many physicians"
ALEXANDER THE GREAT

Reported in *The West Australian* newspaper: "More than 18,000 Australians die each year - nine times the national road toll - from medical mistakes made in hospitals".

An American statistic cites some 188,000 people dying in a given year as a result of mistakes made in hospitals across the United States, while in that same year some 45,000 people died on the roads. You may conclude from this that you are safer driving a car than seeing a doctor. This is not quite true, but the figures are alarmingly high.

"You medical people will have more lives to answer for in the other world than even we generals"
NAPOLEON BONAPARTE

Statistics need careful analysis and perspective before drawing conclusions; after all, the medical profession saves a far greater proportion of lives.

"Progress is very difficult without some collateral damage"
ANONYMOUS

There's more to disease than a single disease-causing agent. It's usually a combination of factors operating simultaneously.

A mathematical model of health and disease

The following model demonstrates how health and disease relate to each other in a continuous spectrum. It incorporates various schools of medical practice and thought. In my opinion, *the full spectrum of medical practice needs to be available to the patient for successful treatment of weight problems and maintenance of health.*

Host Resistance (HR) is a person's susceptibility to fall victim to a disease. **Environmental Challenge** (EC) is the strength or virulence of the environment to cause a particular disease.

For the purposes of illustration only, arbitrary numbers and ratios are assigned to these two factors to create a mathematical model of health and disease.

The two extreme scenarios of death and perfect health can be expressed in the following formulae.

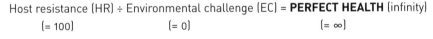

If maximum host resistance (**HR**) = 0 and maximum environmental challenge (**EC**) =100, then the following formula applies:

HR/EC = 0/100 = 0
Host resistance (HR) ÷ Environmental challenge (EC) = **DEATH**
    (= 0)   (= 100)   (= 0)

If maximum host resistance (HR) = 100 and maximum environmental challenge (EC) = 0, then the following formula applies:

HR/EC = 100/0 = ∞
Host resistance (HR) ÷ Environmental challenge (EC) = **PERFECT HEALTH** (infinity)
    (= 100)   (= 0)   (= ∞)

Perfect health (HR/EC = ∞) is not attainable. Every person has some sort of disease process at any one time, even if it is undetectable. We are born to die. Aging is a disease process and so is life itself.

It is easy to understand the two extremes, but the graduations and how they relate are more difficult to appreciate. The interaction between HR and EC symbolises the various states of health and/or disease in the spectrum.

A continuous spectrum

This spectrum can be expressed mathematically by the varying relationship between **HR** and **EC**.

If HR/EC is <1 (less than one) then a disease state exists. The lower the ratio, the more diseased a person is.

Various scenarios can be expressed in diagrammatic form:

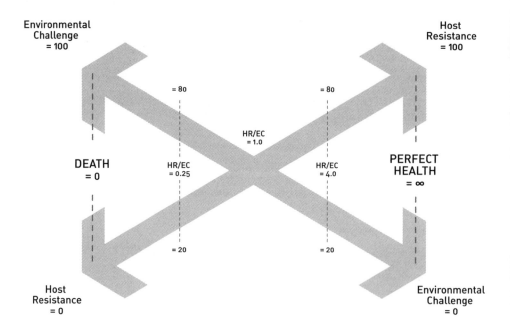

Where disease and health start and end is difficult to determine. Initially medical practice tried to cover the whole spectrum. Then medicine, and especially the field of pharmacology, chose to focus on the <1 disease region of the spectrum, neglecting health.

"Doctor, I'm sick and tired of being sick and tired."

The spectrum of health and disease

This diagram illustrates the point.

Optimum functional health and metabolic fitness

(close to HR/EC = ∞)
This person is as healthy as can be for their age and genetics.

Prospective or Functional Medicine - *health and prevention oriented*

Functional medicine is *proactive*. It is about trying to make patients feel healthier, slowing down aging and *preventing* the move into the conventional part of the spectrum.

Sub-optimum health
(± HR/EC = 4.00)

This person has vague symptoms that won't invite the attention of orthodox medicine unless they progress to the overt illness part of the spectrum.

P R O S P E C T I V E   M E D I C I N E

R E T R O S P E C T I V E   M E D I C I N E

Overt illness or disability
(± HR/EC = 0.25)

Many people have an identifiable disease but can maintain a normal routine, like a man with a skin cancer on his nose.

Retrospective or Conventional Medicine - *disease oriented*

Orthodox or conventional medicine is *reactive*. Only when symptoms appear is this part of the spectrum activated.

Approaching death
(close to HR/EC = 0)

The person is in the Intensive Care Unit due to serious disease or accident.

"There is a limit to health...
disease is always a near neighbour"
AESCHYLUS

"A healthy body is a guest-chamber for the soul...
a sick body is a prison"
FRANCIS BACON

Health Professionals

The life expectancy of the average physician in the USA was only 58 some years back, while their patients' average life expectancy was 70 plus. Doctors are commonly referred to as health professionals, but are they? In fact, medical schools have typically prepared doctors to be "disease professionals" by focusing their training on pathology rather than health.

What we have today is a science of illness (HR/EC = ‹1)
What we need is a science of health (HR/EC = ›1)

Have you ever consulted your doctor to be told they're not sure what's wrong with you? Your instructions are to come back in a week or two if you haven't improved. Your doctor is hoping that whatever is wrong with you will go away during this time, or will develop into something that your doctor can *identify.*

"Ah ha, now I know what is wrong with you and I can treat it."

Usually, only when the arteries to your heart are over 90 per cent blocked will you develop symptoms like angina. Then your doctor will become very interested and start treating you. If these arteries are 40 per cent blocked, with no symptoms, are you diseased or not? Orthodox medicine is more interested in the symptoms, while functional medicine is more interested in a person before the symptoms develop.

If a person is approaching death or has an obvious illness, then retrospective medicine comes into play. Its purpose is to save the patient's life and perhaps treat the disease until there's improvement. To put it in a dramatic way - rescuing a half-drowned person from a freezing river, giving them first aid, drying and warming them, asking if they're comfortable. Once all the symptoms are addressed, toss the hapless individual back into the river.

Knowing all about disease does not necessarily mean you know all about health and vice versa.

At the other end of the spectrum is prospective or "forward-looking" medicine. The idea here is to get a person, as close as possible, to optimum function and health. The philosophy is quite different. The emphasis is on prevention of possible disease before it gets a foothold. This is **Functional Medicine**.

To put it in another way: Planning is bringing the future into the present, so that you can do something about it NOW.

Health funds, private or government, in general only cover orthodox medicine and they are reluctant to sponsor "screening". To achieve optimum function and prevent disease, you need screening and monitoring so that you can act before you get ill or show symptoms of a disease.

Practitioners of functional medicine are quick to acknowledge the value of orthodox medicine where one is more appropriate than the other - for example, if a person has been in an accident it stands to reason that this person should be treated in an orthodox medical establishment such as an emergency department.

But, more typically, the proponents of these two schools of medicine show antagonism towards each other. They should really work together in synergy, each according to their expertise, to the benefit of their patients.

"By medicine life may be prolonged, yet death will seize the doctor too"
SHAKESPEARE

The treatment of obesity and its related diseases requires both orthodox and functional medicine to integrate, ensuring the full spectrum of treatment is available to the patient.

Unfortunately, rivalry and sometimes animosity between the two fields of medicine has in the past led to inadequate long-term management of obesity. On the positive side, doctors today are becoming more aware of health medicine and prevention strategies.

Let me digress with a story about two acquaintances of mine. Andrew had a naturopathic background and Marc was an orthopaedic surgeon. Marc regarded functional medicine as "a lot of alternative rubbish".

I used to pass Marc's house on the way to work. One morning I noticed an ambulance in the driveway. I stopped and was told Marc had suffered a heart attack. He was 44 years old and a bit overweight, but fortunately he survived. A few weeks later, on the way home, I dropped in and we had a bit of a chat. Inevitably the conversation touched on his condition.

I suggested a number of things he could do to prevent further heart trouble. I was surprised how attentively he listened. He changed his lifestyle and lost some of that weight. A few months later he told me: "I feel the best I have in years - this lifestyle and health stuff is powerful. I guess we need *both* approaches".

Why do we wait until it is diet or die?

Turning now to my other acquaintance...

Andrew had a medical science degree, as distinct from being a medical doctor, and trained as a naturopath. He had a large following and was perhaps overly-convinced of the power of his beliefs. He was very anti-drug and of the view that all diseases could be treated with his brand of thinking. I bumped into his wife at a petrol station one day and she told me he was in hospital.

"A hospital - an orthodox medical institution - how could that be?" I asked with tongue-in-cheek. Andrew had developed kidney stones and the pain of the initial attack was so excruciating that he fell off a ladder, breaking his hand in three places.

Ironically, Marc was the orthopaedic surgeon who operated on Andrew's hand.

The most powerful treatment we have in both orthodox and functional medicine today is weight loss, because it achieves so much.

With the treatment of obesity, thousands of metabolic pathways are improved and numerous risk factors are reduced. Your mind, body image and self esteem change for the better. Even the aging process is slowed down. *The treatment of obesity is indeed a complete makeover.*

Bariatric Medicine

Bariatric is derived from the Greek meaning hippopotamus. It is the official name for the branch of medicine specialising in the treatment of obesity and related conditions. Bariatric medicine bridges both orthodox and functional medicine, making use of the full medical spectrum.

It is also the widest field in medicine. What we eat, how we get over-fat from it or not, our culture, philosophies and much more, are all embraced by this field. *That's the reason this book covers so many topics.* Treating obesity successfully demands a comprehensive approach.

What's normal?

If, for instance, a blood test is taken in the community you can determine an average. If you fall outside the average, you're sick.

Do that same test on a diseased population and "normal" is quite different. In most Western countries we are often compared to an already diseased population. The average body fat and cholesterol in Japan is much lower than in the United States for instance. You may think your cholesterol is normal when it's not, because "normal" has been determined from an unhealthy population.

Nick

Nick lost 36 kilograms (79 pounds) when these photos were taken in 1994. Over the next year he stabilised having lost a total of 43 kilograms (95 pounds).

This was more than 10 years ago and he has successfully maintained his weight loss. When Nick was obese, he lacked self confidence with women.

Soon after losing all that weight in 1994 he went with friends to a disco where he saw a girl he'd met when he was obese. He re-introduced himself, but at first she didn't recognise him. The woman of his dreams became his wife - they've been married for eight years and have a four-year-old daughter. Nick is writing a book about his life changing experiences.

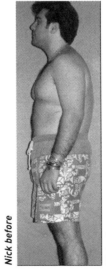
Nick before

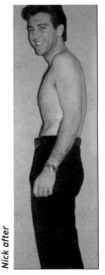
Nick after

Where to from here?

The following three questions need to be addressed before discussing obesity management:

1. What is obesity?
2. What can obesity do to you?
3. What causes obesity?

The next few chapters will deal with these questions.

> **WARNING!** If you decide to follow the knowledge and insights of *Polar Bears and Humming Birds - A Medical Guide to Weight Loss*, it will be life changing.

Synopsis:

1. Obesity cannot be properly managed with only a part of the health spectrum. The patient should be exposed to *proactive* health focused medicine as well as *reactive* disease oriented medicine.

2. The treatment of obesity is the most powerful treatment we have in medicine today, because it achieves so much.

3. "Health is the vital principle of bliss" - JAMES THOMSON.

4. You should avoid getting sick at all costs. Once you become ill, even working together the orthodox and functional arms of medicine can only help *you live ill longer*.

5. When we are well, we all have good advice for those who are ill.

CHAPTER 2

WHAT IS OBESITY?

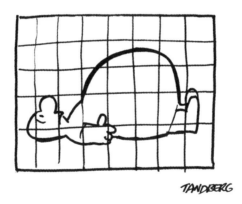

WHAT IS OBESITY?

"Obesity is surplus gone to waist"

The answer to this question is central to the treatment of this menacing and depressing disease now epidemic in the Western world and on the march into Asia. There was a time we had to pay to see the fat lady in the circus. These days it ubiquitous - it is like a free circus out there.

Obesity is a chronic disease that leads to an over-production of fat. Nothing more, nothing less.

Let's look at some of the misconceptions in society when it comes to defining obesity.

Defining obesity

Contrary to popular opinion, obesity is not the equivalent of over-mass. By assessing over-mass the physician does not necessarily determine whether the patient is too fat. It is important for you to understand the difference between obesity and over-mass. The two have never really been successfully differentiated in practice. However, competitive body builders have always distinguished between over-mass and over-fat (obesity).

Your doctor, dietician or health care professional usually wants to know three things about you... your age, height and sex. Next, your details are compared to a chart full of tables and figures. Suddenly, like some magical insight, you get the answer:

"Your ideal weight is 57 kilograms (125lb)."

This is about as accurate as saying a person with their head in an oven and feet in a freezer will on average be comfortable. And, statistics show that 50 per cent of all people getting married at Easter are women (think about it!). The fact is, the average person does not exist. You've just been compared to a statistical average.

According to these statistical tables, a person weighing 25 per cent more than his or her "average" weight for age, is obese. As a medical practitioner, I've seen many a "thin" person with excessive fat rolls and conversely, many a person who "statistically" falls into the overweight or obese range, but are actually quite lean when examined closely.

Some professionals may tell you your Body Mass Index (BMI) is in the "obese" or "overweight" range. While BMI is a better method for calculating obesity, it can still lead to confusion. Forget about this one too... it's of little practical value, other than fulfilling the need of some therapist to classify you in a category that's fashionable at the moment. I will of course be criticised for these radical thoughts, but controlling your weight problem isn't about toeing the party line, it's about finding solutions that work.

Skin fold testing is a more accurate measure, but is heavily reliant on the consistency of the person who conducts the measurements. Allowing for inherent inaccuracies, it more or less gives you your total fat percentage. This brings us closer to defining obesity.

In preference to skin fold testing, bioelectrical impedance testing is easier to perform and can give you more information. It works on the principle that electricity flows faster through muscle and water and much slower through fat. But the results aren't always consistent unless repeated measurements are taken over a period of time. The latest and more expensive equipment is more accurate, but you need to fast - no food or liquids - for three hours and the procedure is best done later in the afternoon.

One accurate way of determining your fat percentage is *hydrostatic weighing* - weighing under water. It is cumbersome and complicated and often impractical for busy people living real lives. There are less cumbersome methods too, but we're talking about expensive equipment found in research facilities and sports institutes - equipment that isn't yet practical for the average person.

With all of this discussion, we're getting closer to defining obesity. It is not your weight or your Body Mass Index, it's not what you eat or your self discipline. It has to do with the *amount of fat* in your body. Composition is the key word, and whether you fall within or outside the normal range for the amount of fat that your body ought to contain.

Normal ranges are between:

	Male	Female
Range	5 - 25%	15 - 30%
"Safe"	20 - 25%	25 - 30%
Ideal	10 - 18%	20 - 25%
Athletic	5 -15%	12 - 20%

Where you fall within these ranges depends on your genetic make up. Asians, for example, can't tolerate the same fat percentages as most Europeans. This also applies to other ethnic groups.

In medical parlance, it is common to find the body *over* or *under* producing an essential product, tissue, substance or hormone. The body tries to keep things within certain limits for good health - it's called homeostasis. It is the metabolism's way of creating conformity within the body. The body has systems in place to keep the metabolism operating in a certain range - neither over nor under. If it creeps outside these normal ranges the body tries to correct this, but if it is unable to do so, a disease is diagnosed.

If insulin is either over or *under-produced*, it leads to disease. If it is absent or under-produced, diabetes type 1 develops. But in diabetes type 2, insulin is usually *over-produced*. All healthy people produce uric acid, but an over-production can cause a painful attack of either gout or kidney stones, or both. And too much stomach acid may cause duodenal or stomach ulcers... and the list goes on.

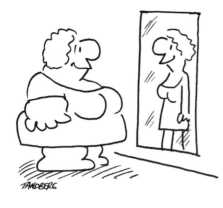

Bobby Sands, the Irish hunger striker who died in H Block in Belfast, Northern Ireland, had lost only 12 kilograms in weight when he died. At post mortem it was thought that he died mainly because he depleted his fat stores. We all need fat in our bodies - it is essential to life. Just as we can have too much or too little insulin causing different types of diabetes, we can have too much fat or too little fat. *Too much* fat is obesity - *too little* fat is malnutrition or some other disease state such as anorexia nervosa.

If your blood sugar is *just* within the diabetic range, you suffer from diabetes. It may be called mild diabetes, but it is diabetes nonetheless. If your blood sugar is very high, you suffer from a serious case of diabetes. While there may be degrees of difference, diabetes is diabetes.

If you suffer from mild form of asthma or severe asthma requiring constant medication, you're still an asthmatic.

If your body *over-produces* fat in significant amounts or small amounts, obesity = obesity = obesity. Full stop!

Obesity has developed a stigma and to make it sound more acceptable, it is usually described as being "overweight". The fact is, it's still obesity - you're still carrying too much fat.

Normal fat versus what we view as normal

In 2,000 BC we worshipped a fat person, while we were thin. In 2,000 AD we are fat and worship thin people.

What we view as normal is normally driven by the latest fashion. As society gets fatter, we tend to move the goalposts. What was seen as "fat" 80 years ago, is now seen as thin. The kids bought me a t-shirt recently and I decided to wear it to a BBQ the next day. My custom is to tuck my shirts in my pants. When the kids noticed it, they protested vigorously - "Dad that's not cool, let it hang loose!"

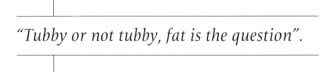

"Tubby or not tubby, fat is the question".

At the trendy BBQ, all the other men had their t-shirts hanging loose. It suddenly dawned on me - the majority of the men had, instead of six packs, beer kegs. In order to hide, or rather, not to make it too obvious, their t-shirts were hanging loose - like the rest of their bodies! Since it is now so common to have a gut, this has become the fashion and the norm. *It is a fashion out of necessity.*

The bell-shaped curve has shifted to the heavier side. The norm is now fatter that ever before. We tend to judge what is normal on what the average person looks like. Fifty to 100 years ago, the average person was much thinner. Today, when a person loses weight, bringing them into the normal fat percentage range, they sometimes stand criticised as being "too thin" by today's "standards".

The big problem is, the body doesn't care for fashion. Even if it may be "normal" to be fatter nowadays, *it is certainly not healthy.*

Even medical equipment is reflecting the increase in size of the population.

Overweight versus obesity

Animals constantly fed by humans thus obtaining an easy and abundant food supply also develop obesity like this temple monkey.

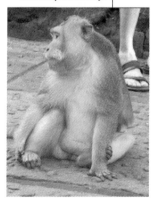

I often hear people say to me "I am a bit over-weight, but I am not obese". Hello! - If you are overweight from being over-fat, you suffer from obesity.

A person can be over-mass (weight) due to:
- muscularity (not obesity)
- adiposity (excess fat - obesity)
- or both (obesity)

Obesity is the production of excess fat. If you are overweight due to excess-fat, you are a victim of obesity. Why would a little bit of excess-fat be called something different to a lot of excess fat? We do like to give different names to different degrees of the same condition.

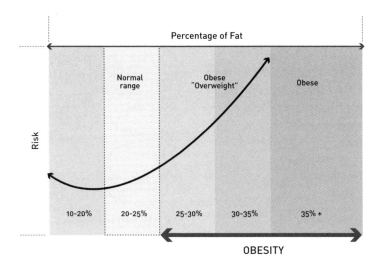

The moment you start putting on excess fat, your body starts to suffer. The tinted line in the graph illustrates the risk. Initially the increased risk is linear, but becomes exponential the fatter you get. Whichever way you look at it, increased fat equals increased risk.

"Overweight" is an attempt to play word semantics and to sound politically correct by not upsetting a person. What does overweight mean? Is the treatment different? Who benefits from this vague category?

Types of obesity

There are two types of obesity. Transparent Obesity can be diagnosed by just looking at a person. The average person and the average doctor do not, sadly, see the second type as obesity. Invisible Obesity is where people weigh within the normal ranges, so it is not obvious that they have excess fat simply by looking at them.

Some health care professionals skirt around the issue. By trying to be "gentle" with the patient, these therapists do the patient a disservice. Telling the truth to the patient in the case of obesity is, for a start, one of the best things than can be done for victims of this miserable disease.

What happens to this excess fat?

Excess fat is stored in places where we do not usually want it to be deposited. In the thighs in the form of saddlebags, sofa buttocks, big upper arms, pot bellies, double chins, and buffalo humps, as the list gets uglier. It is mostly not a pretty sight – and it's not healthy either.

Somatotypes:

Somatotyping is the study of the form of the human body. The following terms illustrate some of the areas where excess fat is commonly deposited. The body shape and where fat is deposited have strong genetic influences, with differing metabolic consequences.

- Hypofeminine
- Hyperfeminine
- Feminine
- Virile Type
- Asexual Intermediate
- Disproportionate Group

Some have a tendency to put excess flab on their upper arms, others on their abdominal area and others on the buttocks. Once these areas are filled, the buffalo hump and saddlebags form. Even the earlobes get bigger. Eventually the skin forms folds that are accentuated by gravity.

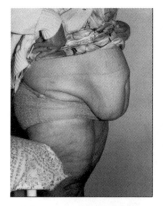

This illustrates what can happen if you yo-yo a number of times with your body's fat percentage and composition. This woman is 28 years old and has already lost 52 kilograms. Her abdomen was much lower before she lost weight, but her hands have not aged beyond what is expected of her age.

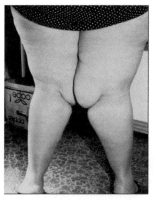

This 25 year old can't bring her ankles together because of the excess fat between her thighs. The poor alignment of her knees has caused severe osteoarthritis and in due course she will need total knee replacements.

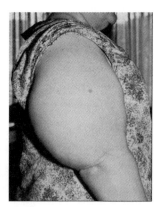

Excessive fat accumulation in upper arm.

All fat is not the same

There are various types of fat performing different functions.

This isn't a medical treatise so I'll confine my comments to main functions and impacts on the body. For example, abdominal fat is more dangerous for your liver and cholesterol than fat distributed in other areas of your body.

Normal structural fat

Ever tried to send porcelain crockery through the post without packing it in foam? Our organs need packaging too. For example, the kidneys are packed in fat, even in quite lean people. This helps suspend the kidneys in their correct position and serves to cushion them in case of trauma, like a kick to the area during a sports game.

We should also have a little pad of fat over our buttocks, just to make sitting comfortable - but we're talking a cushion rather than a sofa! Structural fat also plays an aesthetic role, for example, to give your face form and shape. And it's important that you don't lose that structural fat when you lose weight.

Normal reserve fat

Reserve fat is typically stored around the belly button and between muscles and is constantly being broken down and re-deposited. It's there for when we need it. You don't want to lose this fat either. Unfortunately there are plenty of weight-loss programs that impact on both structural and reserve fat. Apart from being unhealthy, you won't look the best.

Abnormal excess fat - obesity

Structural and reserve fat are normal and essential. You need them, but you only require a certain amount or percentage. If you exceed the limit, the penalty you pay is in excess fat, which is called "obesity".

In a credible weight loss program you should only lose this abnormal excess fat. If you don't have excess fat for your genetic body type, it is medically unwise to attempt to lose weight. Some exceptions can be made for certain athletic goals.

How successful is the treatment of obesity?

"Every time I lose weight, it finds me again."

Some commercial weight loss programs claim 100 per cent success rates. If they are so successful, why is obesity an increasing problem? As they say, buyer beware!

Statistics compiled by universities and credible research organisations reveal a vastly different picture. Research shows that 100 over-fat people put on the best anti-obesity programs will have the following success rates:

- Only 20 will reach their goal weight
- After one year, only five will have maintained their goal weight
- And after five years, only one will have achieved success.

That's a one per cent success rate!

"Isn't it amazing! You hang something in your closet for a while and it shrinks two sizes!"

These statistics have never been disproved. They've been disputed, particularly by purveyors of commercial weight loss programs. It's all about hiding from reality - if I tell you the success rate is higher, you'll be encouraged. As a politician once remarked "let's get the facts first, we can distort them later."

A trip to fat city seldom reverses itself - at least not without enormous dedication and perseverance. Once ugly fat is comfortably sitting around your tummy, your lower back and your hips, it is not easily dislodged.

When I first started treating obesity, my own success rates more or less reflected the above statistics, although I found that between 70 and 80 per cent reached an acceptable goal, and the majority of the remainder still lost some weight. However, the statistics came back to haunt me, and the majority soon regained much of their weight. I was as despondent as my patients!

One day I was discussing with a rheumatologist a patient we both looked after. He lamented that we cannot help the "poor wretched soul" and all we can do is give her analgesia, cortisone and tender loving care. When I hung up, the thought struck me - we have many chronic diseases in medicine and we should not abandon patients simply because the treatment is not yet satisfactory.

Secondly, I made a decision, there and then, to study the successful patients, rather than put all my efforts into the "unsuccessful" ones as I had done to that point. My "successful" patients were leading the way. Like the 20/80 rule, it seemed better to divert most of my attention to the 20 per cent who deliver 80 per cent of the results.

In the years since, I've spent a lot of research, time, money and effort in tracking down the "one per cent" of very successful patients and understanding their success. This research has paid huge and unexpected dividends.

By way of classification, I have grouped my success stories as "gold", the partial successes as "silver" and the unsuccessful as "bronze". I then went for gold. In my view, anyone trying to improve their health, deserves a medal, even if they haven't achieved their goal.

So far, I have isolated more than 15 characteristics in the gold medal winners, characteristics that are shared to a lesser extent with the silver medallists, and to a lesser extent again with the bronze medallists.

I will go as far as saying that if you do not acquire at least twelve of these characteristics, you will not keep the weight off that you lost.

This book addresses many of these characteristics.

The *first characteristic* that I discovered is that gold medallists understand their condition. A better informed patient is a better patient. However, this doesn't mean over-education – just basic hands-on facts. None of my gold medallists suffer from paralysis by analysis.

1st characteristic of successful weight maintainers:
Knowledge and knowhow. Understanding pays off.

The silver medal winners may not be gold medallists, but they did maintain some of their weight loss, with resultant health benefits. The bronze medallists lost some weight and sometimes a lot, but in the main they regained it all. Some even regained more than they had lost, which is the worst possible outcome.

Hot on the heels of the first characteristic I noticed that the gold and silver medallists had a different attitude to their therapy. When a doctor treats a patient's middle ear infection, the patient is a passive recipient. But since a doctor cannot physically lose the excess fat for a patient, the patient needs to become an *active participant*. Unfortunately the bronze medallists chose to be *passive recipients*.

If you intend to be successful with health and weight control, you must make up your mind here and now that the following will apply to you too.

2nd characteristic of successful weight maintainers: The patients were active participants, not merely passive recipients.

Synopsis

1. Obesity is simply an overproduction of fat, no matter what the cause.

2. The long term success rate in treating obesity still leaves a lot to be desired.

3. Because there are so many obese people in today's society, we have come to see fatter people as the norm,

4. Obese people need a balanced understanding of their condition.

5. If you think old soldiers just fade away, try getting into your old Army uniform.

6. Nobody can lose your excess fat for you or stay healthy on your behalf. You need to become an active participant in your treatment regime. Go for gold!

CHAPTER 3

WHAT CAN OBESITY DO TO YOU?

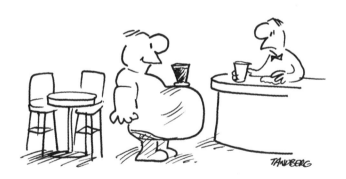

WHAT CAN OBESITY DO TO YOU?

"We are what we eat", as the saying goes. Or are we? I believe "We are what we *cheat."*

We only live on a third of what we eat and the medical profession lives off the other two thirds.

It has been calculated that two thirds of doctors in the Western world spend a vast proportion of their time addressing obesity and its degenerative and metabolic side effects diseases. There is no end in sight. We are getting fatter, bigger and sicker than ever before.

Initially, neither education nor scare tactics about the serious side effects of obesity are effective in motivating the average obese person. They are more likely to be motivated by:

- Cosmetic goals
- Sex
- Career improvement prospects
- Self esteem
- Community attitudes to others who are obese.

But, in the longer term, a working knowledge of obesity and its side effects is effective, and this book is about long term results, so please read on.

Obesity is a serious disease affecting all the systems and organs in your body - it is not just a cosmetic problem. It is the gateway to many chronic illnesses. A fat person's body is running up hill all the time, even if he or she is sleeping. The American Health Department classifies obesity as a "killer disease".

The body is the best debt collector there is. It will always collect, sometimes many years later. For every kilogram (2.2 lb) of excess fat on your body, your body must produce three kilometres (1.9 miles) of extra blood vessels to supply the extra baggage with nutrients and oxygen. That means a person with 20 kilograms (44 lb) of excess fat, forces their heart to pump through an extra 60 kilometres (38 miles) of blood vessels day and night.

In another scenario, increasing your weight from 70 kilograms (154 lb) to 77 kilograms (169.4 lb) is only a 10 per cent increase in weight. Assuming you started with a body fat percentage of 10 per cent at 70 kilograms (154 lb), your seven kilogram (15 lb) weight increase will typically be pure fat, which means you've doubled the amount of fat you carry from seven kilograms (15 lb) to 14 kilograms (30 lb), and have increased your body fat by a massive 90 per cent.

Add to this lean tissue losses that occur as the body ages and percentage fat increases can be even higher.

It's easy to rationalise and say: "it's only seven kilograms (15 lb)", but the bottom line is that even small increases can reflect a massive fat percentage increase. These fat increases, especially in the abdominal area, can cause a myriad of metabolic and health problems.

Seven kilograms (15 lb) is the weight of two babies. At the very least it is extra gravity load on your system that will compromise your athletic performance and health.

Fat is also very oxygen hungry. To pump all the oxygen to those seven kilograms (15 lb) of fat along those extra 21 kilometres (13 miles) of blood vessels is a burden on your body that can only have ghastly consequences on your metabolism.

Traditionally medical schools taught that there are two diseases that effect all the systems in the body, being tuberculosis and syphilis. These two can affect your hair, nails, skin, brain, bones, teeth and organs. In my view they forgot to tell us about the third disease - obesity. Obesity impacts every facet of your body and mind.

Body parts affected by Obesity

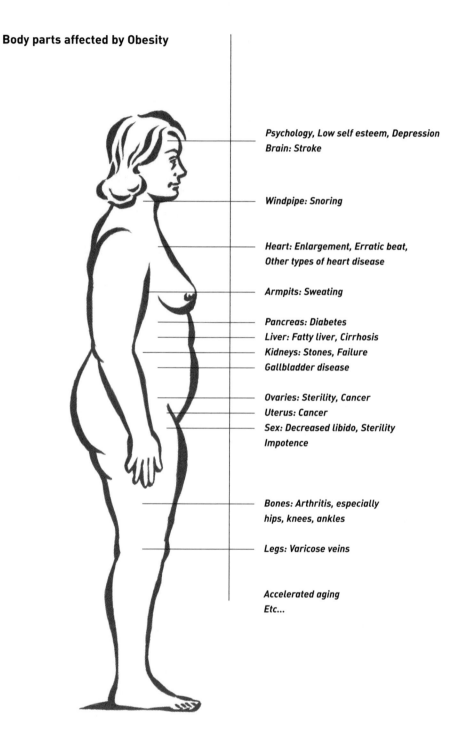

Psychology, Low self esteem, Depression
Brain: Stroke

Windpipe: Snoring

Heart: Enlargement, Erratic beat,
Other types of heart disease

Armpits: Sweating

Pancreas: Diabetes
Liver: Fatty liver, Cirrhosis
Kidneys: Stones, Failure
Gallbladder disease

Ovaries: Sterility, Cancer
Uterus: Cancer
Sex: Decreased libido, Sterility
Impotence

Bones: Arthritis, especially
hips, knees, ankles

Legs: Varicose veins

Accelerated aging
Etc...

Obesity shortens your life

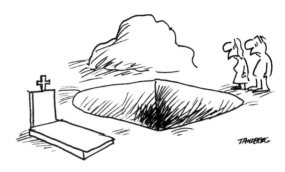

From 1981 to 1992 the mortality rate fell by 3.6 per cent for men and 2.6 per cent for women. An increase in body fat, noted during the 1980's, threatens to reverse these improvements. The current generation of children will have a considerably lower life expectancy than their parents because of this disease.

The more weight you carry, the less time you'll have to carry it.

Obesity kills

Studies show that an additional five kilograms (11 lb) of fat above normal fat percentages will shorten your life expectancy by years.

While some studies have suggested a mild degree of obesity might increase your life span, these studies have been found to be seriously flawed. One of the arguments is that while we are getting fatter, life expectancy is increasing. While we are living longer than people in the Middle Ages, we'd be living even longer *but* for obesity.

Life span is typically increased when body weight is at least 10 per cent below average. Remember, the average nowadays is abnormal. So to be 10 per cent below average is metabolically normal. If we are going to talk averages, we need to compare with a healthy population and not one that is already sick.

As we get fatter, the average weight increases. Sadly, average isn't normal any more. Although an extremely low relative weight, such as that caused by anorexia nervosa, is certainly harmful, very few people in the general population are at an increased risk of death because of excessive leanness.

In the end, obesity kills prematurely. It accelerates aging, bringing the degenerative diseases of the elderly to a much younger age group.

Heart and cardiovascular compromise

Your heart is an amazing organ. Pumping approximately 8,000 litres of blood a day for 70 years or more. In a marathon athlete it can pump as much as 29,000 litres a day, and your heart never rests.

Have you ever tried to put the engine of your lawn mower in your car, expecting it to perform properly? But here's the crunch, your heart is made for a normal size body. Not for an over-fat body with kilometres (miles) of additional blood vessels. Avoiding obesity in the young adult protects against heart disease, according to Dr Hubert of the National Heart, Lung and Blood Institute, Bethesda. Conversely, weight gain, especially after the age of 25, is associated with increased risk of cardiovascular disease.

Arteriosclerosis or "clogging or silting of the arteries" is much more common among those with obesity. While rules are bound to have exceptions, in general, the fatter you become the faster you destroy your arteries.

"Being fat will break your heart." Strange, but true: the wider the waist, the narrower the arteries in the heart.

"You are as old as your arteries." Even if you are only 25 years old, if your arteries are blocked you are in effect an aged person.

Deep Vein Thrombosis is also more common and more dangerous in the obese. Obesity is also linked to heart muscle abnormalities, setting the stage for heart failure.

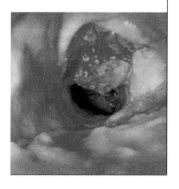

The coronary artery of a 33 year old obese person who died of a heart attack.

Blood pressure (BP)

Normal blood pressure is 120 over 80, but medical evidence shows that those with a lower blood pressure live longer. To achieve any increase in life expectancy you need a blood pressure of 110-100 over 70-60, but 100 over 60 is even better. On the other hand, your blood pressure can't afford to be too low - zero over zero and you're dead!

High blood pressure, or hypertension, is very damaging to your health. It speeds up the ageing process of your cardiovascular system, affecting your brain, heart, blood vessels and kidneys, causing stroke, arteriosclerosis and renal failure. And dementia is more common in people with elevated blood pressure. It even increases your chances of osteoporosis.

What is the *main* cause of hypertension?

Obesity and insulin resistance. It's as simple as that. Being even mildly over - fat is enough to cause hypertension. Sure, there are other causes of hypertension, but obesity is the main culprit.

Popular wisdom blames high blood pressure on stress. Certainly you'll become stressed and your blood pressure will rise if someone holds a gun to your head, but when the threat is removed, your blood pressure should gradually revert to normal. Studies show that people in very stressful jobs fall into two blood pressure groups - hypertensive and normal. And what's the difference between the two groups? Surprise, surprise, the hypertensive mostly suffer from obesity. The majority in the normal fat percentage group have normal blood pressure.

Over time, constant stress can cause hypertension in some individuals, but most will be over-fat too. Stress is over rated as the cause of sustained high blood pressure.

Are you on medication for hypertension? Do you suffer from a degree of obesity? If so, losing that excess fat and keeping the weight off may allow your doctor to introduce you to a drug-free regime. Losing 10 kilograms (± 20 lb) of excess fat can be just as effective as any anti-blood pressure drug. Much safer and cheaper too. At the very least, losing your excess fat should enable your doctor to reduce your medication.

Word of warning: Never make any decisions about your blood pressure without your doctor's advice. Your case may be different.

What is disturbing, however, is that even if your blood pressure is normal because of drug treatment, it may still not do much to improve your mortality. According to studies, an increase in body fatness threatens to reverse improvements in cardiovascular mortality from treating hypertension. *You therefore have no choice but to rid your body of excess body fat.* Why wait until it is diet or die?

Stroke

An obesity sufferer who is lucky enough to have normal blood pressure still has a much higher risk of suffering a stroke.

The Soggy Brain Syndrome

I have often wondered why most over-fat sufferers cannot concentrate for as long as individuals with a normal fat percentage. A Scandinavian study has shown that, as obese people become fatter, they fall victim to a type of "fluid retention" in their brains. This affects thinking ability. It's even been suggested that people with normal fat percentage will benefit from losing a kilogram (2.2 lb) or so before an academic exam or a chess championship. They may improve their thinking by doing this. Students typically do the opposite, over eating and gaining a kilogram (2.2 lb) or two when they become stressed.

The obese also develop a fat pad behind their throats that gradually encroaches, bringing pressure to bear on the throat. A potentially dangerous condition can develop when the weight of these fat pads, while sleeping, constricts breathing - sleep apnoea, sometimes confused with chronic fatigue syndrome. Best treatment for it? Get rid of the excess fat all over your body and this constricting fat pad will disappear too.

Respiratory disease

Just as the heart buckles under the stress caused by excess fat, so do the lungs. In marked cases, Pickwickian Syndrome may develop. This is a medical emergency. Victims can smother to death as the mass of fat around the chest prevents the proper expansion of the lungs.

Kidney stones

An American study found that younger women who had gained 15 kilograms (33 lb) or more since age 21 had an 82 per cent increased risk of developing kidney stones.

Your joints

Your body's weight pushes down on your ankles, knees, hips and spine. When you jog, six times your body weight bears down on these joints.

If you carry just five kilograms of excess fat and you walk one kilometre a day, you are applying an additional 5,000 kilograms (11,000 lb) of stress on your body joints. That's five tonnes a day! Actually, it's proportionally more if you take the smaller surface areas of the relevant joints into account.

None of this is a major worry if you're under 25 - your body still has the ability to repair the damage. But from 25 onwards it's downhill all the way. While the body can still repair some damage, the damage is cumulative and the body remembers your mistreatment - it has an excellent memory, and wear and tear soon sets in.

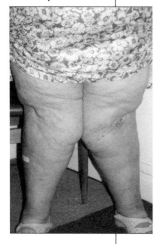

Waiting to have bilateral knee replacements.

Overload your car constantly and you can be sure that the shock absorbers and structure will soon begin to show the signs. Wear and tear on the joints typically leads to osteoarthritis as cartilage is destroyed and bone scrapes on bone - very painful. Losing the excess fat and the accompanying weight loss always improves the situation. Better still, prevent obesity in the first place.

This patient can't even bring her ankles together because of the fat between her thighs. This mal-alignment alone is causing severe damage to her knees, not to mention the excess gravity causing bone and cartilage to grind away at every step.

Diabesity

Attending an obesity conference at Harvard University, I overheard doctors talking about "diabesity". While I understood the meaning, I had never heard the term used in clinical practice and so I asked "why diabesity?" The answer was swift and to the point: "If you suffer from *obesity* and you have a family history of *diabetes*, it is almost a foregone conclusion that you will also acquire diabetes - *diabesity*."

Of the two types of diabetes, type 1 and type 2, the latter is more commonly caused by obesity. With type 1 the sufferer produces none or very little insulin. In type 2, the victim usually produces too much insulin. Two different diseases if you will.

Diabesity has taken on epidemic proportions in industrial countries - such that it threatens to collapse the health systems and budgets in these societies in the next 10 years or so. Estimates put the number of diabetes sufferers at 300 million worldwide and growing - diabetes and obesity are escalating in tandem.

In many ways we never had it so good, but we seem hell-bent on destroying our progress and advancements in many spheres of life by demolishing our health and happiness.

Diabetes is a much more serious disease than the populace, including many victims and doctors, realise. It is the major cause of blindness in the Western world, the major cause of renal failure, amputations and impotence in men over 45. If you have a family history of diabetes and you become obese, you will almost certainly develop type 2 diabetes. Despite a massive medical effort, the incidence of this formidable disease is steadily increasing. Preventable adult-onset diabetes is now the largest cause of blindness and the largest cause of amputations in America.

Diabetes accelerates AGE-ing where AGE stands for Advanced Glycation Endproducts, covered elsewhere in this book. A diabetic's body, cardiovascular system and organs age five or more years in one year.

I often see young, obese men lamenting their lack of sexual performance. Most have high blood sugar levels, typically pre-diabetics... and the combination of constant high blood sugar and high insulin levels due to insulin resistance, affect the blood vessels and nerves supplying the body's organs, including the sexual organs.

In my opinion, the criteria for defining diabetes should be changed. Let me illustrate this.

We don't talk of being pre-asthmatic - you're either asthmatic or you're not, yet at one stage people spoke of being pre-diabetic. That expression then fell from favour, but has since returned to favour. Diabetes is diagnosed as 7.1 mmol/l of fasting blood sugar. At one time, the cut off point was higher. Talk now is of 6.9 mmol/l. Even if there is no glucose tolerance impairment on a glucose tolerance test, if the fasting blood sugar is higher than 5.4, there is something wrong.

This beating around the bush may suit some, but if something is medically *wrong* it is abnormal. It is not optimum health. If your fasting blood sugar is higher than 5.4 it is a *degree* of diabetes and it is not desirable. *Polar Bears and Humming Birds - A Medical Guide to Weight Loss* is written for people with optimum function in mind.

A man lost his left arm and left leg in an accident - he's alright now.

As we age we gradually develop insulin resistance. The latter is a form of diabetes, even if not diagnosed as such, and any point of fasting blood sugar over 5.4 is damaging your body.

In advanced cases of diabetes, the nerves and blood vessels to the legs and toes can be compromised to such a degree that gangrene develops, requiring amputation. Diabesity can also badly affect your kidneys. Finding diabetes in fit, lean athletes is like looking for a needle in a haystack. Therefore diabesity is an entirely preventable disease. What's more, if you already have diabetes type 2, you may be rid of it. Sounds too good to be true?

A patient, Lynn, was on drugs to control her diabesity. Told by her doctor that her condition was deteriorating and that insulin injections were inevitable, she was motivated to do something about the problem. She lost 27 kilograms (59 lb) and I suggested she cease her diabetic drugs and monitor the situation. To her amazement, her blood sugar and insulin levels stayed normal, without drugs. She was ecstatic.

When she proudly told her doctor she was no longer a diabetic, he slammed his fist on the desk and exclaimed: "Once a diabetic - always a diabetic! Here - take your prescription!"

She rebutted: "I'm not a doctor, but I'm not stupid either. Give me a valid reason why I should take these drugs while my blood sugars are persistently normal - every day - without these drugs!"

She was, in effect, cured of diabetes. However if she were to regain the excess fat she had lost, her chances were high of again falling victim to diabesity. While I have numerous patients like Lynn, others have addressed their obesity but are still slightly diabetic, requiring much less medication and in smaller doses. Some long-standing diabetics have at least avoided the need to use insulin. All have benefited from losing excess fat.

The treatment of diabetes = the treatment of obesity

Lynn's doctor has since referred one of his diabesity patients to me, while another has addressed his obesity and his diabetes has completely disappeared such that he no longer requires drugs. I'm told the doctor is now convinced.

"Syndrome X"

Also called "Reaven's Syndrome", the "Deadly Quartet" or the "Metabolic Syndrome", Syndrome X is a combination of obesity - particularly abdominal obesity - insulin resistance, high blood pressure and high blood cholesterol. There is dispute about its diagnosis. Other criteria are added or taken away depending on who is the latest expert.

I do not really get the big deal about Syndrome X. It is only a consequence of being over-fat. It may be a cluster of conditions caused by obesity, but the primary cause is still obesity. While Syndrome X is portrayed as a separate, stand alone disease, in my view the solution lies in addressing obesity.

When your doctor declares: "You suffer from Syndrome X", what have you actually been told?

It sounds dramatic, but it's vague. Should a combination of obesity, sleep apnoea and high blood pressure be called Syndrome Y? Syndrome X is nothing more than a neat way of describing the connection between abdominal obesity and insulin resistance.

We're good at beating about the bush...

Consider a 175cm (5' 9") tall man weighing 75 kilograms (165 lb), of which 15 kilograms (33 lb) is total body fat. His abdominal fat mass is five kilograms (11 lb). If he doubles his abdominal fat mass to 10 kilograms (22 lb) his Body Mass Index changes from 24.6 to 26.1. He's doubled his abdominal fat mass while barely impacting his Body Mass Index - another nail in the coffin for Body Mass Index.

In these circumstances, the patient's metabolic risk factors have risen considerably. Syndrome X is simply a variant of the many *consequences* of obesity and ultimately the management and treatment will be the same, because obesity is the primary culprit.

"Beating about the bush" is part of our ingrained survival instincts. Our psyche doesn't like to confront the reality of obesity.

Without wanting to trivialise, if you suffer from excess fat you are a victim of Syndrome O - obesity. Depending on a person's genetics, the greater the degree and the longer duration that you suffer from obesity, the more likely you will eventually acquire Syndrome X, or any other combination of obesity-related diseases.

If we lump various consequences of over fatness together and call them a syndrome, what have we achieved? It gives the wrong message to sufferers and doctors alike. The message should be clear: obesity is the primary culprit and needs to be addressed first and foremost.

SYNDROME "O" OBESITY

A. MECHANICAL		B. METABOLIC		C. PSYCHOLOGICAL/ SOCIOLOGICAL	
Joint degeneration		Coronary heart disease	Syndrome "H"	Depression	Syndrome "E"
Skin deterioration		Heart failure		Low self esteem	
Stress incontinence		Gout		Body image distortion	
Respiratory diseases	Syndrome "P"	Dislipidaemia	Syndrome "X"	Sex life	Syndrome "L"
Soggy brain syndrome		Hyperglycaemia		Social life	
Sleep apnoea		Hypertension		Discrimination	Syndrome "W"
Hernias		Insulin resistance		Accident prone	
Cellulitis	Syndrome "V"	Type 2 diabetes			
Varicose veins		Kidney stones			
Oedema		Renal disease			
		Gall bladder disease	Syndrome "A"		
		Polycystic ovaries			
		Fatty liver and organs			
		Cataract			
		Breast Cancer	Syndrome "C"		
		Colon cancer			
		Prostate cancer			
		Stroke			
		Menstrual problems	Syndrome "S"		
		Fertility problems			
		Erectile dysfunction			

In the illustration above, I have made up a few extra "syndromes" to make my point.

A person with too much fat will become insulin resistant, especially if unfit. Since the normal amount of insulin is not enough, then the pancreas is under stress to produce more insulin. Higher insulin levels floating around the body have a number of nasty metabolic effects. We now know that insulin is the fat hormone. You need insulin to deposit fat. It is also needed for muscle growth. And insulin is also one of the strongest of all appetite stimulants.

Portion distortion leads to more insulin resistance, more insulin and more fat. You are caught in a vicious cycle in which you are eternally hungry.

Insulin resistance is also implicated as a cause in a number of disease states like stroke, diabetes, hypertension, breast cancer and cardiovascular disease.

And what causes insulin resistance? Obesity. Normal aging also causes some insulin resistance.

A word of caution... for good health and to lose that excess fat loss, insulin levels must be kept low. Avoid spiking *your insulin*. This usually occurs if you consume high glycaemic products on an empty stomach. I'll talk more on this later.

Save your skin

The skin has the tendency to cover what is beneath it. If you are big, your skin needs to grow and stretch to cover. Lose all that excess fat and your skin needs to grow smaller. This is all hard work for the skin. It would rather be left alone and in one place.

Contrary to popular belief, weight loss is good for your skin, but weight gain is bad. Each time your skin is compelled to grow, it suffers damage and your skin never forgets. During repeated weight gains, the skin adds up, as it were, all the gains until a skin collapse occurs. It is exhausted and its elasticity is gone.

A 48 year old patient who lost 70 kilograms was concerned about her loose skin. My response was "not to worry" because she lost weight faster than her skin could tighten. "Give it eight months or so," I confidently advised, "it will tighten."

Eight months later, she informed me, "I don't think my skin is going to tighten."

I could hold her abdominal skin like a towel in front of her. On letting it go the flap hung lower than her knees. Lifting her arms, the loose skin hung from her elbows to her hipbones. She was not short of a sense of humour - as a party joke she would stand in the breeze allowing her loose

This 25 year old patient suffered from an unusual eating disorder. She would starve herself, become skin and bone and require force feeding. Recovered, she would then binge before going into starvation mode again. Her skin is suffering from psoriasis and has an old leathery feel, having been damaged not by her losses, but by her subsequent gains.

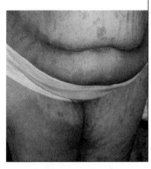

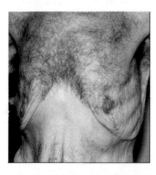

This 46 year old lost 50 kilograms on four separate occasions. The 200 kilograms of cumulative gains caused his skin to collapse.

skin to flutter like flags. When taking a bath the floppy skin drifted "like seaweed" next to her, she told me.

She had to tuck in the flaccid skin of her buttocks as you would a long shirt into pants.

This was the fifth time she had lost more or less the same amount of weight in her life. At that time I did not realise how weight gain causes premature ageing of the skin, sapping its elastin and collagen, leading in this case to a collapse. She needed nine operations to remove the surplus skin.

At one stage I was only aware of two causes for skin ageing. There's the normal aging process. Hair, nails and skin never stop growing. Facial cartilage also keeps on growing. Have a look at your grandfather in his eighties compared with his youthful days. His nose and ears are much bigger. His features have coarsened with wrinkly, loose skin.

A patient, Tina, was quite shocked when bending over she caught her reflection in the vanity mirror to see her loose facial skin hanging down. It wasn't so noticeable when she stood normally.

Tina was only 46. She told me when she and her husband made love, she liked to be on top. She decided there and then that it would be the last time she was on top. She asked to be referred for a face lift, but I felt it was a little premature.

People clip their hair and nails all their lives. Some decide it is time to clip their skin. There's nothing wrong with a face lift, it can do wonders for self-esteem, like a good haircut. There is only two weeks' difference between a good and a bad haircut, as the saying goes, but not a bad face lift.

The second cause of skin aging is over-exposure to ultra-violet rays from the sun. The normal aging process of the skin can be accelerated many times over by exposure to the sun's rays. For example, the skin of an average 25 year old Australian female is typically like that of an average 40 to 60 year old European female... not to mention the increased cancer risk.

Smoking also plays havoc with your skin in the premature aging department.

It is only in the last few years that we have come to recognise that accelerated skin aging can also be caused by weight gains due to obesity.

This 28 year old experienced a sudden fat loss of 48 kilograms, but his skin has tightened rapidly and well because this was his first weight loss.

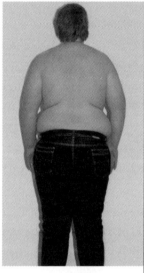

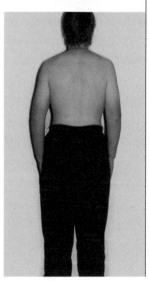

All of these factors explain why models go to great lengths to stay out of the sun, keep their fat percentage normal and stable - the best protection you can give your skin - and abstain from smoking.

Incidentally, weight gains do not affect the skin around the ankles and hands.

Message: Lose weight only once. Save your skin. Keep a normal fat percentage. Do not smoke.

Maintain what you have lost. Any gain will double or triple the ageing acceleration of your skin. If you are serious with your skin, lose weight and keep it off!

Be kind to your gallbladder

Gallstone formation is increased with obesity. Losing excess fat also causes an increased risk of gallstones, but you are better off losing the excess fat than being worried about the slightly increased risk of gallstones. And it's relatively easy to deal with gallstones medically.

Fatty infiltration of organs

In some countries ducks and geese are force-fed to deliberately produce a fatty liver (foie gras). Foie means liver in French and gras is when an animal is fat. Their livers cannot cope with this amount of food and the liver turns into fat and is a delicacy in gourmet circles.

The duck is slaughtered just days before it dies from its condition, with a four to five kilogram duck producing up to a kilogram of fatty liver.

Humans do not need to be force-fed. We do it ourselves and end up with fatty livers too. Medically it's called hepatic steatosis and is a much more dangerous condition than many in the medical profession realise. Latest studies confirm an increasing incidence of fatty livers and insulin resistance in children and teenagers.

While hepatic steatosis can develop due to chemical injury to the liver, such as alcohol and pesticides, over-consumption is now a more common cause of fatty liver than alcohol. The liver is infiltrated with fat, causing inflammation and scar tissue. The end-result is always cirrhosis if it is not reversed in time. The medical fraternity is already noting an increase in liver transplants due to over-eating and obesity.

It is not a pleasant condition and can be fatal.

Cattle are over-fed and confined to produce market-ready meat in record time. Their muscle becomes interspersed with fat or marbleised. Up to 80 per cent of the calories in a piece of meat can come from fat in marbleised steak.

Fatty muscle may be juicy and tender, but it is not good for the animal and in humans, where the condition is known as myo or sarco-steatosis, it's not good for you either.

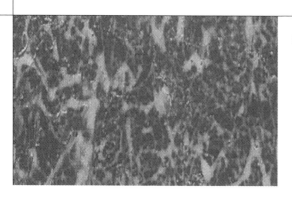

Marbleised meat

Fatty infiltration does not stop here. It affects other organs too, like the pancreas where it damages the beta cells influencing insulin production, and infiltrates the walls of blood vessels.

It never ceases to amaze me the increasing number of fatty livers that I come across. Treated prior to the point of no return, you can only get rid of obesity-induced fatty liver and muscle by:

LOSING YOUR EXCESS FAT AND GETTING FITTER.

You must treat the cause. There is no other way.

Footnote: In the region of France where foie gras is produced and eaten, the coronary heart disease risk is half the national average. Fatty liver from birds is a mono-unsaturated fat. Conversely, fatty marbleised beef is primarily saturated fat and is implicated in vascular heart disease.

Avoid cancer

Most forms of cancer are more common in the obese, including breast cancer, prostate and colon cancer. According to the Journal of Gerontology, most forms of cancer are avoidable. Obesity, along with the associated intake of poor quality food, can be attributed to 48 per cent of all avoidable cancers. Meanwhile, smoking can be attributed to between 30 and 33 per cent of cancer. Losing all your excess fat, leading the life style to keep it off and not smoking is like decreasing your avoidable cancer risk by some 80 per cent.

Cancer cells love sugar. There are about 15 times more insulin receptors on a cancer cell than ordinary, healthy cells. Obesity leads to increased insulin levels, increasing the risk for cancer initiation and cancer progression.

Infertility

Scores of patients decide to lose weight after failing to conceive in spite of undertaking IVF treatment. Many patients are surprised when they conceive naturally after losing their excess fat. Your reproductive organs and associated hormonal system, like your heart, are made for a normal sized body - they can't compensate for obesity.

As you lose that excess fat, you become more fertile whether you are male or female. I always warn young women undergoing my treatment program, that if they don't want to fall pregnant they should consider contraception.

In spite of my warning, every so often some fall pregnant. Nothing to do with the clinic of course!

One of my patients, Jacky, informed me she felt nauseous in the mornings.

"Could you be pregnant?" I enquired.

"Definitely not!" she replied.

Jacky was convinced it was the vitamin tablets I'd recommended. Finally she conceded to a pregnancy test - surprise, surprise, it was positive.

"My boyfriend and I have been together for five years. We were sure either or both of us were infertile."

"Jacky, you lost 31 kilograms (73 lb). Your body works differently now."

It all ended well. Jacky got married and when little Claire was eight weeks old she came to visit. That photo of me holding the baby is one of my proud possessions.

There may be other reasons why a couple cannot have children. A lady told me once that the heavy apron of fat hanging almost to her knees made sex impossible. She and her husband tried elevating one end of the bed, but she nearly suffocated. It may sound amusing or bizarre, but it is actually very sad.

The three ED's - more serious than you think
Endothelial Damage (ED) in the penis leads to Erectile Dysfunction (ED). The latter is usually an early warning sign that the person is clogging up their arteries in his heart as well. If this happens the person will end up in the Emergency Department (ED). Thus Erectile Dysfunction (ED) is seen to be an early warning signal for a heart attack.

Lifestyle changes and weight loss can successfully treat men with erectile dysfunction. According to a study reported in the Journal of the American Medical Association, as little as a 10 per cent weight loss can have a marked effect.

Gynaecological and obstetric problems
Over-fatness is bad for both mother and baby. Not only does excess fat change the birth canal, but almost every complication during pregnancy is more severe and common in women carrying excess fat.

Complications during and after surgery
We never know when we will need emergency surgery. In order to save a life, surgeons will operate on any person, obese or not. However, for routine operations they are very reluctant to operate on the obese. They know how dangerous it can be. The bigger and longer the operation, the higher the risk.

I regularly receive referrals from surgeons for obesity treatment. They sometimes refuse to operate unless the patient loses weight. Even smaller operations, such as circumcisions, result in referrals to me if a patient has significant excess fat.

Accidents

Accidents, including car accidents, are more common among the obese. Have you seen a successful obese racing car driver? The incidence of accidents was originally attributed to clumsiness, but further studies have revealed that the reason is not that simple and the exact cause remains a mystery. However, we know that the loss of excess fat can diminish accident proneness. Perhaps the "soggy brain syndrome" has something to do with it?

Discrimination

For years we have been conditioned not to discriminate against others, yet when it comes to the obese, we certainly discriminate.

Promotion at work is often reserved for the thinner applicants. Scores of my patients searched in vain for employment until they lost weight. There are token laws to protect the obese, but studies have shown if there are two people in court for the same offence, the fat person is more likely to be found guilty. If both are found guilty, the fat person is more likely to receive a heavier sentence.

I confess to discriminating once on this basis. We advertised for a new nurse. When I opened the door there was a large girl standing with a folder under her arm. I thought she was a patient, but she introduced herself and said she'd come for her interview. In hindsight, I wasn't tactful when I told her: "You must be mistaken. This is an obesity clinic and we cannot employ fat people like you."

The next day she phoned: "I will lose weight with the patients. I really want this job."

To cut a long story short, I found out she was the daughter of a colleague and offered her the job. She turned out to be one of the best people that ever worked for me.

Patients would come to the clinic and be a little surprised to see her working there, but she quickly put their minds at ease: "I work here, but I'm also a patient... I'm losing weight with you."

Gail lost 54 kilograms (119 lb) and a year later became engaged. Sadly, her father and my colleague died the day after her engagement. She worked for a while after she got married, but her husband was transferred. We kept in touch for another eight years and she still kept her weight off.

Psychological health

A person at a party told me he had just lost an ugly heap of fat.

"How did you do it? I enquired.

"I divorced my wife," was the reply.

Being obese affects more than just your body. And it's not just a cosmetic problem. I have come across very few obesity victims with self-esteem. It is obvious why - their excess flab.

The obese are well aware of the cultural condemnation, the medical disapproval and the moralistic view that "slimness is next to Godliness". Being overweight in mid-age dramatically increases the risk of subsequent dementia, up to 74 percent.

Few are happy to endure the derogatory jokes that are aimed at the obese. A famous jockey came to see me once with his fat wife. He had flaming red hair and was a chain smoker. His wife, 22 years old and about 25cm taller than him, trailed behind him as they walked into the clinic.

"Don't make my wife too thin now, doc," he instructed half wittingly. "It's very useful to have a fat wife, she keeps you warm in winter and in summer you can sit in her shade," and then followed a few belly laughs.

Out of courtesy I chuckled too, but I could see his wife had heard the joke before and felt denigrated by it.

Patients send me fat jokes all the time and I have collected hundreds of them. I was once contemplating writing the "Fat Joke Book". I changed my mind when I observed how disturbed the jockey's wife was.

Where can I hide?

During the 1920s, the only doctor in a small country town saw his first patient of the day.

"Doctor, I can't see the use of living anymore. I am so down. My life has no meaning. I am in a mess."

In those days there was no medication for depression - all a doctor could do was give patients a pep talk and hope for the best.

"When you came to our town, you must have noticed the circus on the outskirts," the doctor said.

"Last night I took my wife and three little daughters there. We had a ball. We enjoyed the clown. We couldn't stop laughing.

"This morning the children dressed in some of my wife's clothing, pretending to be the clown. We laughed all over again.

"In fact, we are seriously thinking of going to see the clown again tonight. If you are still in town, why don't you go and see this clown. I am sure he will cheer you up. It will be the best medicine for you. You'll see life in a different light."

Said the patient: "But doctor, I am that clown."

Many obesity sufferers feel like this clown. Most over-fat suffers try to compensate by being jolly in an attempt to gain acceptance. When I see them in a clinical environment there is great sadness in them. And when they have lost their excess fat, friends have remarked that they're not as jolly as when they were fat.

Once you've lost weight, you can be yourself. You don't have to be artificially overly-friendly to gain acceptance.

A successful businessman lost 46 kilograms (101 lb) at the clinic. One day on the maintenance program he mentioned he had an 11 year old boy who also suffered from obesity. He wanted to know if I could help him too.

At our first appointment, 11 year old Jimmy gave me a firm handshake, made strong eye contact and said: "Doctor, I am glad to have met you at last. Congratulations on what you have done for my dad. Maybe you can do the same for me too?"

While he seemed outwardly confident, during our consultation he burst into tears because people at school called him "fatty". All his insecurities surfaced. He wouldn't swim with the other children unless he could keep his t-shirt on.

But then a new teacher took over and insisted he took his t-shirt off while swimming. A scuffle broke out and Jimmy ran off in the street. His dad had to be phoned to pick him up. After that, he refused to go back to school. It is a wonder that some of these children grow up to be normal after being humiliated at such a tender age.

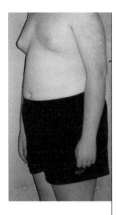

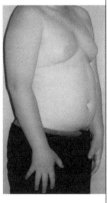

These boys were brought to my clinic to lose weight. Both were teased endlessly about their breasts - their gynaecomastia. Typical comments included: "Where's your bra today? Couldn't you find your sister's?" Others would run up, squeeze their "boobs", and run off giggling, often leaving bruises.

Most obese people are painfully aware of the need for rigorous personal hygiene. The underlying skin cannot breathe and can become irritated and harbour odour-causing fungi and bacteria.

One lady contacted me by phone requesting a house call and sounded rather disappointed when I explained that she would need to visit the clinic. When she did make an appointment, she needed to turn side-on to walk through the door, and needed two chairs to sit on - one for each cheek.

"Doctor you have to help me. I cannot keep on living like this. If I go to the toilet my stool comes through all the layers of fat like and everything gets dirty. My husband built me a special toilet shed in the garden. I clean myself with a garden hose... I never do any shopping anymore or leave the house."

The expression, "opening the bowels", comes from when a person squats and the "cheeks" part, "opening the bowels".

Obesity also impacts on intimacy. I have stopped counting the number of obese women who tell me they've stopped undressing in front of their husbands.

Another patient in tears, pleaded with me: "Please help me doctor. My husband has just left me... I am devastated. When I married him at 18 my weight was normal, now after three children I'm like this."

This lady was only 25 years old.

I phoned her husband and reminded him he married for "better or worse".

He was very pleasant: "Doctor, I'm glad you phoned. Maybe it's my fault. I knew about your clinic three years ago and I should have brought her to you then, but I found someone else. I can't make love to a blob of fat any more. She can't even clean herself properly."

She lost all her excess fat, always wearing her wedding ring in the hope that he was coming back. To my knowledge, he never did.

If you live in a damp, dark, cold house in winter with small windows and in a rundown neighbourhood, you'll have low morale. If you live in a nice clean, warm house with big windows, you'll be in a much better *state of mind*.

The operative phrase here is *state of mind*. All that changed were your circumstances.

A man was looking at the cover of a magazine displaying a gorgeous girl in a skimpy swimsuit. Said his wife: "That's shameful. If I looked like that I wouldn't leave the house." Said the husband: "If you looked like that, neither would I."

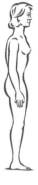

Here you see a young woman in her slim state and the same woman in a state of obesity. To improve her state of mind, she changed her circumstances. With the stigma attached to obesity, the sarcastic jokes and the intolerance, it's little wonder that the obese suffer psychologically as well as physically.

Do you still think fat is jolly?

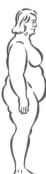

Very few physicians seem aware of the latest discoveries linking obesity with hypertension, insulin resistance and heart disease, and the explosive knowledge that you cannot treat any one of these diseases successfully without treating *all of them*.

For example, the doctor who gives an over-fat patient blood pressure medication and sends that person home is being negligent, leaving the patient at risk of heart attack.

Bruce

I got a call many years ago from a woman begging me to come and see her son. The urgency and anxiety in her voice was conspicuous.

When I got there, I was taken aback. The odour in the house was quite unpleasant. Bruce was lying on a double mattress, filling it with his body. Six months prior, a dentist came to the house and wired his teeth together so that he could not eat as much, but he still found a way to squeeze the food in.

Typically he'd blend together all of the food and soft drink imaginable and would suck it through a straw. Bruce was drinking a dozen or more litres of soft drink a day, and when the wires were removed from his teeth, there was no stopping him. He couldn't even leave the room to go to the toilet.

To get Bruce to hospital for treatment, a wall of the house had to be demolished and he had to be removed by crane.

In hospital he lay across two mattresses, you couldn't even see his individual toes and everything was covered in layers of fat. Every half hour his legs had to be moved by the nurses to assist his circulation. He looked close to death. The hospital system was hopelessly inadequate to cater for a person his size.

He was placed on oxygen, drips, protein powders though a nasal gastric tube, and various medications. For the first week he was on assisted breathing. How he had survived this long was a miracle, but after two weeks he began to make dramatic progress. The occupational and physiotherapists took an interest in him and he became partially mobile within a month, but it was five months before he was discharged home even though he was still grossly over-fat.

Bruce soon regained all of his lost weight and spent a further six months in hospital.

Within a month of returning home for the second time, his mother died and Bruce used his inheritance to ultimately eat himself to death.

This may have been an exceptional case, but many of us seem to dig our graves with our teeth, never mind with our knives and forks. Obesity, unmasked by an abundant and corrupted food supply, can be devastating to our wellbeing even to relatively mild degrees. What we do to ourselves is in many ways just as gross as what Bruce did.

Are you convinced that obesity is a disease and a very serious one? The intention of this chapter was to give you the incentive, based on credible research, to lose excess fat, and to get fit and healthy. Getting rid of the complications of obesity serves as a powerful motivation to keep excess fat at bay.

"Hypochondria is the only disease I don't have."

Synopsis:
1. We are getting fatter, bigger and sicker. Obesity is not just a minor cosmetic problem; it is a very serious disease that can hurt more than just your looks.

2. Losing your excess fat, keeping it off and quitting smoking are the best cancer preventing strategies there are.

3. Obesity makes you age faster.

4. Obesity can destroy your love life.

5. If you are over-fat, you will break your heart - in more ways than one.

6. The best way of preventing and treating diabetes type 2 and high blood pressure is simply to prevent or lose excess fat and improve your fitness.

7. It's not so much Syndrome X, Y or Z that you need to worry about - you need to address the basic problem which is *Syndrome Obesity*.

8. *The treatment of Obesity is the most powerful therapy we have in medicine today, because it achieves so much.*

CHAPTER 4

WHAT CAUSES OBESITY?

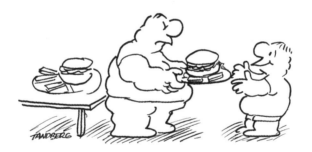

OBESITY BEING HANDED DOWN
FROM FATHER TO SON

WHAT CAUSES OBESITY?

"Heredity: the thing a child gets from the other side of the family"
MARCELLENE COX

Just look around you, we are not only fatter than ever before, but getting even fatter. Whatever is on offer to treat the problem clearly is not working.

If the cause of a condition is known and appreciated, the battle is half way won, as the saying goes. But with obesity it's not that simple. One of the main reasons people regain weight after successfully losing weight is the dreaded "Ah, Ha Syndrome".

"Ah, Ha, I've lost all my weight, now I can celebrate!"

It's like a free meal ticket for an eating frenzy, doing exactly the same things that made you fat in the first place. Most of us are willing to starve ourselves to lose weight, but rarely do we stay focused.

When asked what causes Obesity, most people will give the following answers:

"Eating too much" or "not enough exercise".
When asked for further information, they'll typically offer the following:
"Eating the wrong foods"
"Too much fatty foods"
"Psychological problems"
"Eating disorders"
"Abused as a child"
"Depression"

In a rational way, "eating too much" and "not enough exercise" *are correct*, but there are plenty of people who over-eat, don't do any exercise, eat the wrong foods and have hang-ups, but aren't obese.

Some psychologists hold the view that the obese are depressed, or have other issues, therefore they over eat for comfort. Over eating causes too many calories to be consumed. Too many calories results in obesity. Let's treat the hang-ups and their obesity will be cured.

But what about the thin people who have their *own fair share of hang-ups*, over eat and stay thin. **Why?**

A whole industry has sprung up around this question.

THE PRIMARY CAUSE OF OBESITY

Various studies show the metabolic response after a meal differs for those who are lean and those who are fat. It is called diet-induced thermogenesis. In my view, these metabolic differences have more to do with physiology than psychology.

Are fat people born or made?

"The scale is tipped heavily on the side of heredity, rather than environment"
The New England Journal of Medicine

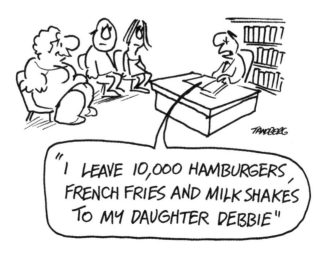

A patient once told me: "In my fantasy I'm slim, long legged and drop-dead gorgeous. In reality I am at war with my body. Having the perfect body isn't difficult, it's *impossible*."

Unfortunately; **your *genes* decide how you look in your *jeans*.**

The primary cause of obesity is genetic. When I started treating this disease I assumed, like most people, that it is a self-inflicted psychological condition. After treating thousands of obese patients I have come to the conclusion that this ominous disease is, first and foremost, a genetic condition and is therefore inherited.

It is sometimes called the "thrifty" or "famine" gene, but it involves a large number of genes. When it comes to something as crucial as survival, our bodies would never have relied on only one gene.

Why is the condition so difficult to treat? It is like the Medusa, cut off one head and the others take over. Obesity genes don't capitulate either, because our whole existence depends on it.

What is genetics?

It is basically a careless choice of parents. How do you determine the sex of a chromosome? You take its genes off.

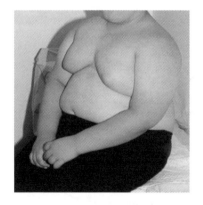

The seven-year-old boy pictured weighs 102 kg (225lb). He is understandably very upset, because he is called all sorts of names at school.

"Doctor I eat the same as the other kids. Why do I get so fat?"

Why on earth would he punish himself and eat to a degree that he weighs this much? Has he been abused? Does he have an eating disorder? Is he depressed? Is he just a glutton? Does his parents spoil him?

None are correct. *He would not have been able to if he did not have the genetic predisposition.*

In the main, obese people don't eat more than thin people - in spite of what some people might think. Various studies have shown that fat people often have similar intakes and activity levels to those of thin people. The thin stay thin and the fat stay fat.

Most of us, in a well-off society, gain at least a bit of weight as we age, especially around the midriff. How much depends on various factors like genetics and lifestyle. This fat gain is typically a survival mechanism. As we age, our reflexes and agility decrease, making it more difficult to hunt food, so we become more efficient in storing fat for survival.

What does this mean to you?

Knowing the problem is caused by genetics means *you don't have to feel guilty about it.* You were born that way. Guilt is still used by some as a tool to make fat patients feel culpable for their obesity, hoping that it will somehow give them the incentive to do something about it.

I believe this to be negative and dishonest psychology, and counter productive. You stood in the wrong queue and you were born in the wrong place and the wrong time. That is hardly your fault.

The odd couple - he is so skinny that when he is wearing a black suit, he looks like a rolled umbrella. She is so fat that she can't get the water *and* herself in the bath at the same time.

Efficiency

If we take two cars and put $50 of petrol in each empty tank, and one car travels twice the distance of the other before needing to fill up again, *which of the two cars is the most efficient?*

The car that travelled twice as far of course. *This is the difference between the obese and lean genetic types.* The obese are very *efficient* in using *and* storing calories. The skinny are *inefficient* in their handling of calories.

The primary cause for obesity is the genetics of an efficient metabolism, not gluttony.

SECONDARY CAUSES OF OBESITY

The secondary causes are mainly about **supply** and **demand**. We all have a huge demand to eat. The supply allows us to eat as much as we want. In times past the supply was erratic and even though our demand to eat was high, we could only eat what was available. Today we have a massive food supply and we don't have to spend much **effort** to find food.

Food is now on tap.

In addition, exploitative commercialism has taken over our food supply. Food outlets compete to make food tastier, creating an even larger demand to eat. We certainly don't have to catch the chicken, chop its head off, pluck its feathers, disembowel it, clean and cook it. And today's commercialism in delivering food straight to our mouths is compounded by a chemical industry never seen in the history of food.

If a person has a genetically *efficient metabolism* to start with, these modern circumstances will naturally trigger or aggravate their obesity. Your genes interact with the environment to produce the consequences of obesity.

TERTIARY CAUSES OF OBESITY

Some people don't have the genetics for obesity, but still become obese. Let me give you an example. Karen was always thin, but started developing menstrual problems and at the same time noticed a muscle weakness in her legs.

When she started to gain weight she cut back on her food, but this didn't help much, and by now she was feeling unwell and went to see her doctor. Dismissively he told her: "You eat too much. Take this appetite suppressant, eat less and come and see me in three months."

She objected: "You've known me since I was a baby. I've always been thin - my whole family is thin. There is something wrong with me. Aren't you going to examine me or do blood tests?"

He rejected her concerns. Karen tried his advice to no avail. In the end she joined Weight Watchers, watching her weight increase.

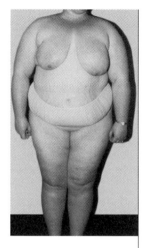

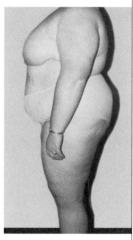

Karen

Karen consulted with me and after extensive investigations I determined that she suffered from Cushing's syndrome. She had a small tumour that was resulting in the overproduction of the hormone cortisol which, amongst other things, was increasing Karen's efficiency to store fat.

After the tumour was removed she practically melted away without going on a diet. The damage was done however, with skin damage and some psychological issues. To be fair to her doctor, she did not present as a textbook case.

There are other diseases too that can make the metabolism more efficient in storing fat.

Doctor induced obesity

Then there are the doctor induced or iatrogenic causes. Certain drugs like tricyclic anti-depressants can cause weight gain in people with a very low risk of genetic obesity.

Predictors of how much a person will gain excess fat are usually related to dose, length of treatment, female gender and younger age. If you are on any of the following medications it may aggravate or activate your obesity, but *you must at all times discuss this with your doctor first and not make decisions on your own.*

The following list contains the main "offenders":

Olanzapine	Imipramine
Clozapine	Paroxetine
Quetiapine	Venlafaxine (Efexor)
Respiridone	Valproate
Thioridazine	Lithium
Pericyazine	Gabapentin
Chlorpromazine	Topiramate
Olanzapine	Insulin
Clozapine	Ethanol (beer,
Tricyclic antidepressants	wine, etc)

Drugs that aggravate or activate obesity:

Alcohol (appetite stimulation, empty calories)

Tobacco promotes i-obesity (invisible obesity, discussed later in this chapter)

Marijuana (stimulates appetite)

Medications and drugs that assist in excess fat loss:

Caffeine

Ephedrine

Coffee

Tea

Phentermine (Duromine)

Diethylpropion (Tenuate Dospan)

Sibutramine (Reductil)

Summary of the causes of obesity

Primary cause:

1. Hereditary - an efficient metabolism to store fat

Secondary causes (DES):

2. **Demand** to eat
3. **Effort** to find the food - **Demand** and **Supply** driven
4. **Supply** availability
   - on tap
   - commercialism
   - processing, partitioning and adulteration

Tertiary causes:

5. Medical
   - Hormones
   - Doctor induced
   - Others

Fat or skinny depends largely on your genetic ability to store excess fat. Even doctor induced causes have little impact on some people, while some secondary and tertiary causes can unmask the primary cause.

Should it be called "obesity"?

What is a glutton? The person who took the piece of cake you wanted.

"Obesity" is a misnomer

It is derived from the Latin - obesitas or obesus. Translated directly, it means intensively over-eating and gluttony. But obesity is *not* just a simple matter of over eating and gluttony. What about overweight, plumpness, chubby, stout, portly, large or corpulent?

The term obesity *only* refers to a *possible cause* of the condition and does not *describe* what it really is, namely an over production of fat. The possible cause it refers to when translated from Latin is wrong anyway because, as we've discussed, lots of people over-eat constantly and stay thin. A more *descriptive* name would be more appropriate, especially if it addresses the cause as well, but this can be complex.

Adiposis means a production and accumulation of fat. You either have too much, enough or too little. Adiposis is a *descriptive* word, however it does not describe the cause of Obesity. Perhaps we need to invent a word.

In medicine the following words are commonly used to describe the quantity or size of something:

Hypo - too little
Normo - enough
Hyper - too much
Megaly - enlarged

Hyperadiposis is my usual choice. *Adiposity* is a state of being over-fat and also a contender.

The fat mass in the body can also be seen as an organ. It acts like an organ and makes its own hormones. This fat-organ can be over-sized, normal, or under-sized. When an organ is over-sized, for instance the heart, it is called cardiomegaly. If it is the liver, it is called hepatomegaly.

Adipo-hyper-trophy is also a contender, but it becomes a bit of a tongue-twister. After all, it is such an epidemic that we need to be able to pronounce it.

Hyper-adiposis, adipo-megaly, adiposity or adipo-hyper-trophy is an over production and accumulation of fat as in "obesity".

Hypo-adiposis is an under production of fat as in anorexia nervosa, famine and starvation. It would also apply in advanced forms of cancer.

Why a person is over (hyper) producing in fat (adiposis) is not relevant right now. It is caused by a multitude of factors with a genetic basis. All the causes cannot be incorporated in the name. The name refers only to the main and obvious *effect* of the disease, the overproduction of fat.

To call it "over eating or gluttony" is confusing the issue and is simply wrong. Obesity is not only non-descriptive, but an inadequate attempt to pinpoint the cause.

Perhaps an acronym can be used for Obesity, as with other diseases such as AIDS - Acquired Immune Deficiency Syndrome, or SARS, which can be even more descriptive and include some of its causes and effects as well. Since I am still thinking of a satisfactory name or acronym for obesity, I will use the one I find the most appropriate at present, namely **GOFES**.

GOFES stands for Genetic Over-Fat Environmental Syndrome.

It clearly indicates genetics interacting with a negative environment, leading to excess fat. It's easy to pronounce and the "o" reminds us of "obesity".

GOFES incorporates the causes plus a description of what it is - a syndrome. A syndrome is a group of signs and symptoms that together are characteristic or indicative of a specific disease.

GOFES is a condition of body-composition-change where the fat percentage has become too high, and in turn causes various unhealthy states.

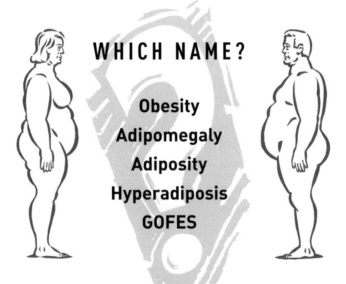

WHICH NAME?

Obesity

Adipomegaly

Adiposity

Hyperadiposis

GOFES

GOFES can be divided into two subgroups on the basis of obviousness and visibility:

- *Transparent-GOFES* (t-GOFES) - simply diagnosed by looking at a person

- *Invisible-GOFES* (i-GOFES) - you might look normal and be within normal weight parameters, but your fat percentage is too high. It can only be diagnosed by further investigation. *This is a seriously overlooked group.*

t-GOFES and i-GOFES can be further classified:

A. Increase of the fat mass in the body, distributing itself in genetically predisposed areas like:

1. Excess body fat mass all over

2. Android or apple shaped
   - excess surface abdominal fat
   - excess internal abdominal fat

3. Gynecoid or the so-called Venus pear shaped figure.

B. Decrease in muscle mass (sarcopaenia) with a resultant fat percentage increase.

C. A combination of both the above.

---

t G O F E S   a n d   i G O F E S

A. GENETIC DISTRIBUTION	*B. MUSCLE LOSS*	*C. COMBINATION*

1. All over
2. Android
3. Viceral abdominal
4. Gynecoid

---

i-GOFES is usually a transition between the genetically *efficient* fat storing group and the genetically *inefficient* cluster. While the weight to height ratio is normal, body composition is abnormal, with most of the fat percentage caused by muscle wastage. Whatever the case, they carry too much fat.

Preoccupation with t-GOFES is to the detriment of the i-GOFES who can *also* develop serious health problems. "If you don't look fat you ain't fat" is not the way to assess the GOFES epidemic.

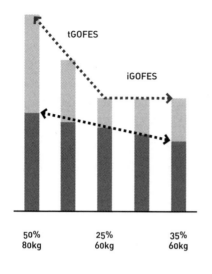

50%
80kg

25%
60kg

35%
60kg

This schematic presents the i-GOFES and the t-GOFES. The middle example is a 60kg (132lb) female with normal 25 per cent fat. The dark grey represents Lean Body Mass and the light grey fat.

She can develop GOFES either by;

- By increasing her fat percentage as depicted to the left. She gradually gains weight and her Lean Body Mass (LBM) increases as her body adapts to carrying the excess weight. She gradually increases her body fat to 50 per cent, weighing 80kg (172lb) - a 166 per cent fat burden increase from her normal weight and fat percentage.

- As her muscle mass decreases she develops i-GOFES. Her weight increases only slightly. She has a normal Body Mass Index and height-sex-weight ratio, but at 35 per cent her fat percentage has increased by 40 per cent. i-GOFES is common in older people with muscles and organs shrinking by as much as 40 per cent while their weight remains constant. As the muscles and organs shrink, they're replaced by fat.

Because obesity is the generally accepted, but inaccurate name, I still use it from time to time. But I mostly refer to it as Hyperadiposis, Adiposity, Adipomegaly or *especially* GOFES. In the past, when I requested blood tests for patients, pathologists would ring for clarification of these terms. Generally they'd remark, "that makes sense". I haven't had a query from a pathologist in a long time.

Is GOFES a disease?

In short "Yes". Anything that makes you sick is a disease. It can be argued that excess fat is not a disease in itself, but it can cause diseases. If low fat percentage does not cause damage and a higher percentage does, then *too much fat* is the primary disease. The genetic tendency to put on excess fat is not a disease, only the consequences.

Excess fat places a massive (no pun intended) burden and wear and tear on the body and metabolism.

Weight Gain Triggers

For those with a genetic predisposition to weight gain, the following are typical GOFES triggers:

Adolescence	Divorce
Smoking cessation	Prolonged stress
Menopause	Grief and bereavement
Middle age	After weight loss diets
Pregnancy	Changing jobs
Marriage	Quitting sports
Separation	Holidays

Synopsis:

1. Obesity is a misnomer. Adiposity, Hyperadiposis and Adipomegaly are better. **GOFES**, for the present, is the ideal description of this disease.

2. Your genes are the primary cause of **GOFES**. How it will be expressed depends on the food supply of the environment you live in. These genes date back from the last ice age and in today's environment they are redundant. But we may still need them again at some point in the future.

3. There are two types of "obesity", **t-GOFES** and **i-GOFES**. Both need treatment to avoid serious consequences.

4. Various genetic fat distributions have different health risk factors. *All* **GOFES** types are bad, some are worse than others.

CHAPTER 5

THE POLAR BEAR AND THE HUMMING BIRD

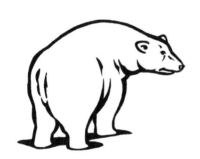
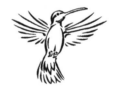

THE POLAR BEAR AND THE HUMMING BIRD

Please, come to the point!

"You have to be patient!"

It has always puzzled me why some of us seem to eat what we like and not put on significant amounts of fat, while others can't even look at food without gaining weight. I was searching nature for answers. Were there perhaps other examples of these variations in metabolism in the natural world? Was there something that I could use metaphorically to describe these human differences? What I found amazed me. The metabolic adaptations for food intake and fat storage in nature are extraordinary.

How this book got its name

Palm Springs, California, is nestled in a desert basin surrounded by the Sierra Mountains. The valley is warm, dry and pleasant, while the mountain peaks are covered in snow. It is a strange but remarkable sensation, lying next to the swimming pool in a warm desert, drinking one of the famous local date milkshakes, while watching people skiing on the snow capped mountains.

It was during a conference in Palm Springs, while enjoying an outside lunch, that I noticed a most interesting resident.

In the shrubs were tiny birds, not much larger than insects, darting from flower to flower. My curiosity got the better of me and I got up for a closer inspection. I even discovered one of their petite nests with a tiny egg in it.

Humming Birds have a very interesting metabolism, eating three times their body weight in a single day. Imagine if we needed to consume three times our body weight simply to survive!

They have a unique way of keeping warm or conserving their energy - a form of hibernation in which their metabolic rate drops to one-fifteenth that of normal sleep.

Found only in the Americas, Humming Birds are built for speed. Thirty per cent of a Humming Bird's weight consists of flight muscles, hence their high energy requirement. They have the fastest wing beats of any bird and their hearts beat as much as 1,200 times a minute. A Humming Bird's flight speed can average 30-50kph (20-30mph), and they can dive in flight up to 100 kph (60mph). In their non-stop pursuit of nectar, Humming Birds may visit over 1,000 flowers per day.

At the opposite end of the spectrum, crocodiles can survive without food for up to two years. In captivity, the big ones are usually fed just a chicken a month. Once a week can make them too sluggish.

Visiting Alaska and seeing pods of whales, I was told they migrate between Alaska and Hawaii to escape the winter freeze - an eight month return trip in which they don't eat at all.

They can complete this incredible journey because of their *efficient metabolism*.

Could this diversity of metabolism exist in the human race?

In the 1950s, a group of prisoners in the United States were encouraged to put on a certain amount of fat over a given time. They were selected from the leanest group of inmates, could eat as much as they liked and had access to all their favourite foods, snacks and desserts. To give them the motivation to stuff themselves, they were promised inducements. After a number of months of force-feeding, none of them qualified for these incentives, because they could not put on enough fat.

Sumo wrestlers, on the other hand, are selected from boys who have the natural ability to put on fat quickly.

Human comparisons

I doubt my patients would like to be compared to crocodiles, alligators or whales, even metaphorically. However, I eventually found another cuddlier animal for comparison - the Polar Bear.

Typically they don't eat for four months of the year, while pregnant females don't eat for eight months at a time.

Interestingly, scientists have found that when these animals dine exclusively on seal meat, their cholesterol levels drop lower than those of the fasting animals, because of the protective quality of the omega-3 fatty acids found in seal fat.

Life for these animals includes cycles of feasting and fasting, in much the way humans evolved.

Humans can be divided into a spectrum ranging from the Polar Bear to the Humming Bird in our ability to store fat. The majority of humans fall in the Polar Bear range.

The human metabolic spectrum

Some of us eat a lot and do not put on weight - human Humming Birds - while others eat the same and do put on weight - human Polar Bears.

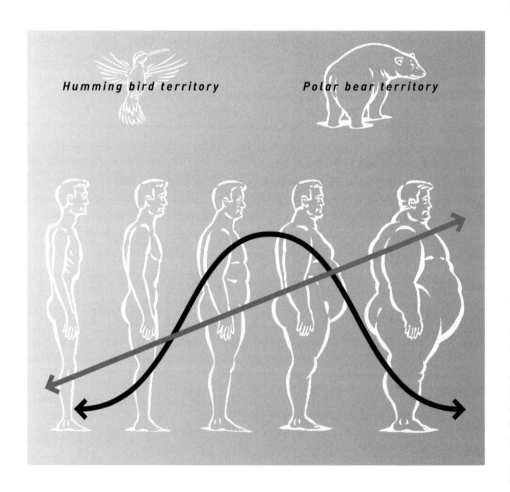

Humming bird territory   Polar bear territory

The dark grey line is the continuous spectrum between the *leanest* Humming Bird and the *fattest* Polar Bear. It depicts the spread of the genetic tendency. Some Polar Bears may control their **GOFES** and may look thin. But the illustration portrays only the genetic saturation potential. The average of the human population is the top of the grey bell shaped curve, right in Polar Bear territory. I estimate that about 70 per cent of the population falls in the Polar Bear range.

In some communities, like the Navaho Indians, the existence of these Polar Bear-like genes is even higher. Exposed to modern diet they are at high risk of becoming over-fat and diabetic at a relatively young age.

In my early days I was frantically looking for the "slower-sluggish metabolism' or so-called lazy metabolism, in fat people. I did thousands of metabolic investigations and tests and found they were nearly always normal. I have found some obese people to have low thyroid levels, but correcting this doesn't cause them to lose weight without additional encouragement. Metabolic studies comparing the lean with the obese don't show substantive differences in metabolic rates.

So, what is the difference?
Essentially it comes down to the respective *efficiencies* of the two metabolisms in the ability to store fat.

It is obvious when a Polar Bear can survive eight months without food, while a Humming Bird can barely survive without eating three times its own body weight in a day, that there are clear differences in their metabolic adaptations for different conditions.

Age and increasing fat percentage

Even Humming Birds seem to gain some fat as they get older. As we get older, degeneration sets in and we cut back on exercise. Our muscles waste and our hormone levels decrease. We also develop insulin resistance, stimulating our appetite and increasing our fat deposits. In short, our metabolism becomes more efficient as we get older. Under these circumstances it's easier to gain excess fat and, in fact, most of us do.

There is a good reason for this efficiency - it's called survival. Aging bodies find it harder to hunt food and therefore the body has to be more efficient in storing fat.

If the Polar Bear doesn't become over-fat, then this is not an illness and may even be advantageous. In many cases a Polar Bear with normal fat percentage is healthier than a Humming Bird with normal fat levels, but the Polar Bear's advantage is soon lost if it starts stacking on flab.

And the same applies to humans - "Polar Bear" genes aren't a disease, but if they cause you to develop **GOFES**, then you're facing a serious disease.

Is obesity a curable or incurable disease?

GOFES/Hyperadiposis/Adipomegaly/Adiposity (Old name: obesity) is a CHRONIC DISEASE WHICH IS NEVER CURED, but CAN ONLY BE CONTROLLED!

Acceptance of this can be difficult for some, but if you want to be successful with **GOFES** and your health, you better acknowledge it.

The 3rd characteristic of successful weight maintainers:
Acceptance of the fact that you are genetically different ("Polar Bear") and that this requires a permanent change of lifestyle.

Irritated doctor

A rather irate doctor phoned me: "How dare you tell my patient that she suffers from an incurable disease. Don't you have any hope for the poor woman?"

I tried to explain that if a disease was incurable the patient was certain to find out eventually. To control it, all the facts should be known and communicated. But he wouldn't have a bar of it.

Ironically, it eventuated that the patient he'd rung about was his wife, who lost 31kg (68lb).

Shortly thereafter I acquired another **GOFES** patient - it was the doctor. He was very apologetic about his previous behaviour. He admitted he was close to retirement and had lost patients to younger doctors opening in his territory.

I offered to train him in the treatment of **GOFES** and to send him some of my patients. It worked very well and he discovered new ideas in medicine and

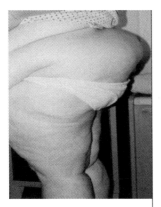

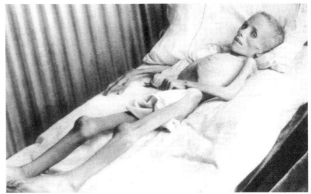

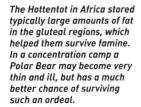

The Hottentot in Africa stored typically large amounts of fat in the gluteal regions, which helped them survive famine. In a concentration camp a Polar Bear may become very thin and ill, but has a much better chance of surviving such an ordeal.

even postponed his retirement. One of the first things he would tell his patients was: "Obesity is an incurable disease that can only be controlled. Look at me. I lost 36kg (80lb) - my weight is under control, but I'm not cured."

Why is it only some people suffer from GOFES?

To varying degrees, we all store fat.

In nature, lizards store fat in their tails and camels store fat in their humps. We humans are similarly adaptive.

The "Polar Bear" gene gives us a more efficient metabolism, increasing our potential to survive famine and holocaust, giving us an advantage over our "Humming Bird" compatriots. GOFES has helped us survive.

And providing Polar Bears don't become over-fat, they outlive Humming Birds. To have inherited the Polar Bear genes gives a person a distinct advantage in times of food crisis. *Polar Bears are survivors, but only if they don't develop GOFES in modern times.*

Synopsis:

1. The efficiency of your metabolism determines whether or not you have a propensity to get over-fat. This is inherited.

2. GOFES is an incurable disease that can only be controlled.

3. "Polar Bear" genes may be a drawback in modern times, but these genes have played a major factor in helping the human race to survive.

CHAPTER 6

WHY WE OVER EAT AND SHUN EXERCISE

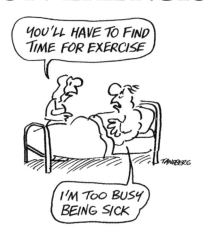

WHY WE OVER EAT AND SHUN EXERCISE

"Restlessness is discomfort and discomfort is the first necessity of progress. Show me a thoroughly satisfied man and I will show you a failure."

MARK TWAIN

Why *do* we eat at all?

"Getting enough to eat, and then getting rid of it, are two of the great problems in life."

ED HOWE

Obviously all living creatures are obliged to consume food to live. Not eating is incompatible with life. No matter how "sophisticated" we make eating and how much we culturise it, it is still a basic survival instinct. By having fancy dinners, BBQ's and the like, we are just toying with our basic instincts. *Something we tend to forget.*

We are what we eat. Human bodies are merely hairy bags made up of a chemical soup, consisting of proteins, minerals and various other substances. All the building blocks of our bodies are derived from what we have consumed at some stage. To maintain our bodies we use vast amounts of energy and nourishment.

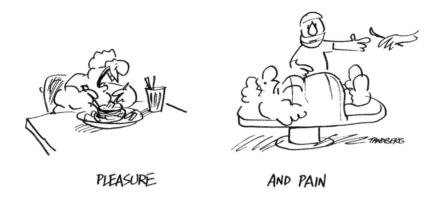

PLEASURE   AND PAIN

Eating as a survival instinct

Survival is controlled by the **Pain and Pleasure of Survival** (PPOS) phenomena. PPOS is all about the proverbial carrot and the stick approach. From a young age we soon learn to avoid the *Pain* and seek out the *Pleasure*. In this way we are steered towards survival.

To explain PPOS at work, let's use the following example: to be scantily dressed, without shelter, on a cold winter's night will be uncomfortable at first. The colder it gets, the worse the pain. Since death can result from hypothermia, our body will warn us that there is a threat to survival. This comes in the form of pain (stick), with the promise of pleasure and reward (carrot) if we do something about it - like getting warmer.

You rush inside, thawing out in a hot bath, and a relieving pleasure will be felt - your reward. If for some reason the tub water gets too hot, you will start feeling uncomfortable, increasing in intensity to pain. Again, you are warned to do something about it before serious damage is done.

Survival instincts are robust and can be ruthless. They ought to be - your life and very existence depends on it.

Pain and pleasure

To meet our energy needs, two basic criteria have to be met:
1. to *obtain* energy and nutrients
2. to *preserve* this energy.

To be able to do this the body has had to develop mechanisms to obtain and conserve energy:
1. *motivating* and giving the individual a powerful incentive to *obtain energy*

2. not only is the individual motivated to acquire the necessary energy, but to acquire an excess *amount* of it, using pleasure, satisfaction and comfort as a reward
3. *conserving* and defending this acquired energy by promoting inactivity
4. converting as much as possible of this excess energy to *stored energy* - primarily fat - ready for when it is needed.

The bottom line:

1. *we are genetically programmed to over eat, because under eating is incompatible with survival.* During ancient times as we found food, we ate like there was no tomorrow, because tomorrow food might have been scarce. We evolved on an erratic food supply.
2. we will, as soon as we get the opportunity, convert and store the excess energy. Most of us save some of our earnings for a rainy day- always mindful of unforseen eventualities. Some of us evolved to have **very** efficient metabolisms to do this. *When food is easy to come by, Polar Bears develop* **GOFES** *as a consequence of their efficient abilities to do so.*
3. we conserve and protect stored fat energy by not unnecessarily wasting it. Just as under eating is incompatible with survival, so is *exercise incompatible with survival.* Given the chance, we will avoid unnecessary physical activity.

Said one of my patients: "I'm suffering from an eating disorder - reverse anorexia nervosa."

THE PAIN OF DEPRIVATION

"You may proclaim, good sirs, your fine philosophy. But till you feed us, right and wrong can wait."
BERTOLT BRECHT

The specific survival mechanism that *makes us eat* is an offshoot from PPOS. I call it *Depalgia* - the Pain of Deprivation (POD). In ancient Greek "-alg" means pain. For example, neuralgia is a pain experienced in a nerve. *Depalgia is our survival pain.*

We have developed an interesting array of vocabulary to describe the various degrees, feelings and manifestations of the same thing. We perceive these various expressions differently, for instance hunger and appetite are perceived as poles apart, yet they are extensions of *exactly* the same phenomena at play, *Depalgia*.

POD as an "engine" that drives us to eat

The Pain of Deprivation is the blanket term for all the methods and systems at the metabolism's disposal that influence, direct and motivate our eating.

It is a system of intricate biochemical and neurological circuitry sending signals for us to eat and stop eating. While medical science has unravelled some of the factors that influence these signals, many remain elusive. The stop eating signals, for example, are generally only activated when we have over eaten. Suffice to say, POD (*Depalgia*) is the complete operating engine which is made up of many different parts.

POD in action

After a huge dinner you settle down to a night of television and a cup of sugar with a bit of coffee in it, followed by sandwiches with a nice thick layer of butter. And as you head off to bed you open the fridge door to see if everything is okay. Then you notice the rather large slice of cheesecake you didn't finish earlier.

"It may be off tomorrow, so I may as well eat it now," commencing to do just that at the fridge door. Why? Because it is there, and we are genetically programmed to overeat.

The so-called "hunger eating" and "non-hunger eating" don't really exist. The differentiation suggests "hunger eating" is "normal" and "non-hunger eating" is somehow "abnormal". But the only purpose of POD is to motivate feeding for survival.

POD at its worst is so strong it causes a grief-like reaction in some people, like the death of a loved one. Never underestimate its power and its life or death function in survival.

"Hunger is a mighty fine sauce"
SOUTHERN SAYING

THE PLEASURE OF EATING

"Hunger: one of the few cravings that cannot be appeased with another solution"

IRWIN VAN GROVE

Now where do the carrot, the pleasure, the sweetener and reward come in?

Depalgesia

Eating is the antidote for depalgia. Food intake is like a painkiller, a *depalgesic* for the Pain of Deprivation. An analgesic is a general painkiller. A depalgesic is a POD killer.

POE - the Pleasure Of Eating follows POD as an added bonus to further reinforce the eating cycle. We are rewarded with gratification - the pleasure of eating. No wonder many say they "eat for comfort". Unfortunately it is believed by many, including some intellectuals, that eating for comfort is deviant behaviour. In fact, it is very normal.

We demand food to control the pain, the reward leads to pleasure, which leads to overeating because we like gratification. We are genetically programmed to overeat.

Any eating behaviour we engage in is triggered by POD, otherwise we would not eat.

From A to B: it is all the *same* survival instinct with one thing in mind to make us eat.

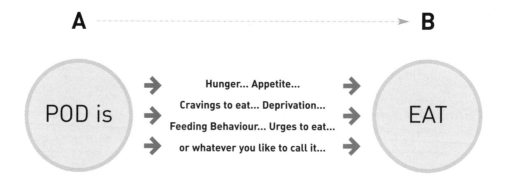

"Appetite: Something you always bring to another's table"
JEWISH PROVERB

Hunger is seen as the biological drive to find food and eat, while appetite is understood to represent a conditioned desire for food. I believe this to be wrong. It is all part of what we do when we are reared in an affluent society where excess is possible.

If a person takes in food without the agitation of POD, it is eating against the person's will, which is force-feeding. Like the foie gras ducks.

It is still the prevailing wisdom that we overeat because we are bored... need to reward ourselves... we're depressed... and the list goes on.

Trying to make all sorts of misleading categories out of the same phenomenon is not helpful or practical.

To control POD a little or a lot takes the same effort and requires very similar techniques.

POD gives us the incentive and motivation to eat. It creates a demand to eat for survival purposes. In short, anything that makes us eat originates from POD, no matter what we may call it.

POD may send out subtle signals like a vague feeling of "wanting to eat something", ranging up to very intense ravenous feelings of hunger and deprivation. Yet the survival goal is always the same: *to induce and seduce you to eat... and over eat.*

It is imperative for you to comprehend this phenomenon if you want to control GOFES in the presence of an abundant food supply.

Homeostasis is a word for describing the metabolism's way of creating conformity in the body. It has systems in place to keep the metabolism operating in a certain range - neither over nor under. For good health, homeostasis is essential.

For example, if your blood sugar is over a certain range the body will quickly release insulin to bring it to within normal limits. Your blood ph balance must be kept in a narrow range and if it strays into the alkaline range or the acidic range the body will quickly bring buffering systems into play. A distur-

HOMEOSTASIS

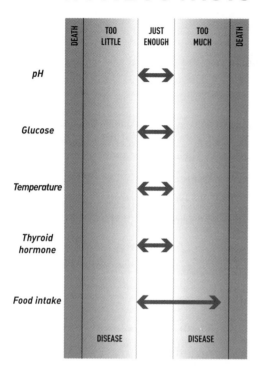

bance of these homeostatic mechanisms leads to a disease state, or pathology. In a worst case scenario this can lead to death.

But, when it came to POD the metabolism "deliberately forgot" about homeostasis in order to ensure survival. While some misinterpret this as a "disease state", they fail to take into account the basic survival needs. Overeating is the most normal thing to do. *Undereating* is abnormal, unless it is therapeutically engineered to lose excess fat.

According to homeostasis we should automatically adjust our food intake, up or down, depending on our needs at the time. *We do not*, for a very good reason - survival. If the supply is abundant we will eat copious amounts. Hopefully, the excess consumption can then be drawn on to supply reserve calories during inadequate intake - like money in the bank for a rainy day. If the supply is inadequate, we will involuntarily consume an *inadequate* amount.

We do not have the regulatory ability to know if we have had enough to eat. When a person says they have had enough to eat, interpret: "I have had too much to eat."

We are born over eaters. We never developed the ability to automatically know when to stop when we have eaten just enough for our needs. *We specifically do not have this capability. Do not try and waste your time looking for one.*

Unfortunately, human Polar Bear can consume as little as 20 tiny excess calories per day, and over 10 years can gain 20 to 30kg of excess fat as a result. This ability of Polar Bears is very useful in times of famine but not in times of abundance.

"I can't diet for medical reasons - it makes me HUNGRY"
ANONYMOUS

I was invited to a very good and well-known restaurant. The portion sizes were large. You actually got a huge plate with super-sized portions. It was excellent quality and a taste experience.

Opposite from me sat a couple I had never met. They were very jovial and pleasant. After a huge entrée, an even larger main course, the palate cleansers in between and a bottle of wine between the two of them, their joviality disappeared.

"Are you all right?" I enquired.

Patting his bloated stomach he responded: "If I have to eat anything else I will be sick. The food was too good."

Then came the dessert trolley. A good waiter doesn't ask: "Are you going to have a dessert?" No, instead they ask: "Which one are *you* going to have?"

POEx

As we've discussed, we **demand** a much higher intake of food than we require at any one time, and *exercise is incompatible with survival.*

This shunning of exercise is called the Pain of Exercise - POEx.

Feeling guilty you say: "I'm too lazy to exercise."

You know exercise is good for you, so why do you shun activity? Because you are programmed to act this way. Feeling guilt-ridden at your "lazy" tendencies is only based on the fact that you intellectually know the value of exercise. This is where choice comes into play. In times of old, survival involved exercise, but today you have choice. Don't lose sleep, it's absolutely normal to feel this way.

"Being normal is driving me crazy."

My advice: accept your inherent survival programming of shunning physical activity. Don't feel guilty about it, but do get proactive about it. Plan an exercise schedule and stick to it.

The physiology of survival is quite simple to understand in a superficial way. It is just common sense. Generally, it is wrong to view overeating as a so-called eating disorder.

THE SPECTRUM OF EATING BEHAVIOURS

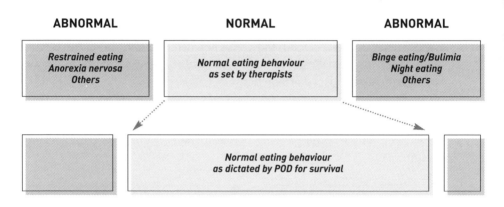

ABNORMAL

Restrained eating
Anorexia nervosa
Others

NORMAL

Normal eating behaviour
as set by therapists

ABNORMAL

Binge eating/Bulimia
Night eating
Others

Normal eating behaviour
as dictated by POD for survival

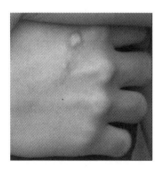

What is normal is much wider than commonly accepted and is more like the second level than the first. Too many obese are erroneously labelled as having eating disorders, when this group actually represents only a small fraction. So relax and deal with the real issues of POD/POE and survival.

I am not suggesting that abnormalities do not exist. The following patient of mine has a callous on the hand due to bingeing and purging by putting her finger in her throat. This is, of course beyond normal eating behaviour. However so-called experts too eagerly classify many eating behaviours as pathological.

Some medical literature also suggests psychological factors are in the main responsible for the large incidence of obesity. Are they suggesting the majority of us are crazy just because we are over-fat? Don't believe them. We are merely doing what we have been programmed to do.

Demand, effort and supply (DES)

As little as 150 years ago a rural labourer in Europe had to work two hours to be able to buy sufficient food to keep one person from starvation for one day. Allowing for winter months, a labourer with a family of five to seven had to work flat out just to stave off starvation.

In contemporary times a worker on the minimum wage earns enough to feed one person in less than 10 minutes.

While times have changed, we have always had a *huge demand* (**D**) to eat. This is triggered and fuelled by **POD**. In primitive times the *supply* (**S**) was often quite inadequate and unreliable. For much of history the *effort* (**E**) in obtaining this supply was enormous.

*For survival our bodies and metabolisms adapted on hard earned (**E**), expensive and low caloric dense food sources (**S**), accompanied by vigorous appetites (**D**).*

And the combination of low caloric dense foods, high activity levels and low body fat kept our arteries clean and our blood sugars and insulin levels low. Our bodies did not get rich food in excessive quantities, so we evolved on less caloric dense foods.

Think how much different modern-day life would be if our ancestors had been exposed to large quantities of high caloric dense foods and very low activity levels. They would have done the adapting for us!

We are creations of these circumstances. Being hungry (**POD**), accompanied by a limited food **supply** that kept us from overeating and the huge **effort** to source food, kept our ancestors metabolically fit and healthy.

We are like fish out of water as far as our metabolisms are concerned.

"There is no feast that does not come to an end"
CHINESE PROVERB

Given our programming to follow the path of least resistance, we will give in to our basic instincts of overeating and limiting physical activity, given the slightest opportunity. In prevailing affluent times where the food supply is very cheap and tainted, we are subjected to over-consumptive-malnutrition and sloth.

Given time we will probably evolve to adapt to our modern day diets and lack of physical activity and still be healthy. Will it ever happen? Probably not, since our present affluence is unsustainable in the long term. Then GOFES will disappear and the Polar Bears will live in an environment they were designed for.

To pander to pleasure and shun pain we *designed our environment to avoid the agony and seek the pleasure.*

In fact, as technology developed one of the first things we did was to over produce food to avoid the stressful effects of POD and starvation. Then we created labour-saving devices to avoid POEx. Not realising the power of our self-gratifying propensities, we have created a health epidemic of monstrous proportions. This epidemic may collapse health services in as little as a decade.

By the way, I am not advocating that we should go back to the bad old days where the struggle for survival was intense and the effects of POD and POEx were constantly endured and where the infant and maternal mortality rates were high and life-threatening infectious diseases struck us down in the thousands.

Instead of the environment determining our energy-in and energy-out equation, we designed our societal structures and technology for unlimited energy-in and zero energy-out. This has created a time bomb: the population explosion, the obesity epidemic and a host of previously unknown diseases. The environment that we created is not the same today as the ecosystems that created us in the first place.

We may be living in the space age, but our metabolisms are still caught up in the stone age. Humans have not had enough time to adapt to this excess of energy in-put and lack of energy out-put.

Human Humming Birds may not develop GOFES but effortless over eating still causes them to become diseased. But for human Polar Bears it's worse, since they have to carry the extra burden of surplus fat with its numerous metabolic and health consequences.

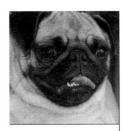

Pretzel ("PODzel")

My daughter's 14th birthday was a week before she was to have a serious spinal operation. She wanted a pet for her birthday and I was aware that she did not like "pretty" dogs. With this in mind I bought her a Pug. It was so ugly it was actually beautiful.

My daughter immediately fell in love with her and she was named Pretzel because her face resembled one.

I bought a book on Pugs at the same time.

In reading the book I came to the chapter on "How to feed your Pug". The author's tone changed radically.

"YOUR Pug is a ferocious eater. It is up to YOU NOT TO OVER FEED YOUR PUG. If you do it will get fat, sluggish and become diabetic and die young". And the author repeated, almost pleading, his warning *"do not over feed your Pug"*.

It immediately became quite clear what the author meant. Pretzel was a vicious eater. She had all sorts of manners and ways to beg for food. That's when the kids started calling her "PODzel", as I had explained the POD phenomena to them.

It became evident why owners easily spoil and over-feed them. We worked out a policy of only feeding her a measured amount each day. Pretzel's supply (**S**) is controlled and she stays the leanest Pug in the neigl   ɔd. If Pretzel was offered an unlimited supply of food she would have suffered the consequences. However, her owners *externally* impose control over her supply. In the past, our environment as humans was externally controlled and enforced. Pretzel has no choice and in the past we had no choice either.

To internally self-control POD, in the midst of plenty, can be a dreadfully difficult task. POD is the most basic instinct - it is ruthless and brutal in its task.

Governments and other bureaucratic social engineers will not do it for us and stop us overeating. Various agencies have spent billions and, in spite of their efforts, GOFES has soared. We're getting fatter by the minute.

Professor George Bray from Baton Rouge, Louisiana calls it the "fluoride option". Professor Bray is regarded as one of the foremost researchers in the field of GOFES. Dentists have known that the average person cannot be relied on to practice meticulous dental hygiene in order to prevent dental cavities. Fluoride in the water as mass medication has decreased cavities. Professor Bray thinks such a solution may be necessary to eventually control GOFES.

Demand, Supply and Effort (DES) control will form the foundation of any method to control GOFES.

When I was at high school my father noticed a lonely, hungry and somewhat sick looking wild pigeon in the garden looking for food. He took some seeds from the shed and fed the pigeon. The next day the pigeon was back. He got more seeds. Soon it brought some friends along and my father had to buy more seeds. In time the garden was full of hungry, begging pigeons. He bought even bigger bags of seeds. At one stage he had a large drum of seeds that had to be filled regularly.

One weekend my parents went away and I was given the task of putting the seeds out in the afternoon. I was early teenage and had a lot of other things on my mind, and I forgot. When I got home the trees were packed with hundreds of hungry pigeons all eagerly waiting for their handouts. They were very restless and hungry (POD) and it was almost dark. I put the seeds out as fast as I could. They almost got lost in the dark as they frantically struggled to find the seeds. It was a disturbing sight. The whole sorry scene left a lasting impression on me.

The wild pigeons became used to an effortless (**E**) over supply (**S**) of food. They built their nests nearby to be close to the food and structured their whole existence around it. When my parents came home I found my father had begun to doubt his actions and we worked out a plan to wean them off the over supply of food.

The process was not dissimilar to motivating unfit, overfed, TV-viewing couch potatoes to overcome their **POD** and **POEx** by eating less and getting some exercise. It was much easier rehabilitating the pigeons because they had no choice in the matter - adapt or die. Contemporary couch potatoes and butterballs *have a choice*, but they do not have the help of an external force to control their food supply. It has to come from within - internal control.

The following illustration summarises the effect of survival and eating. Take careful note of it.

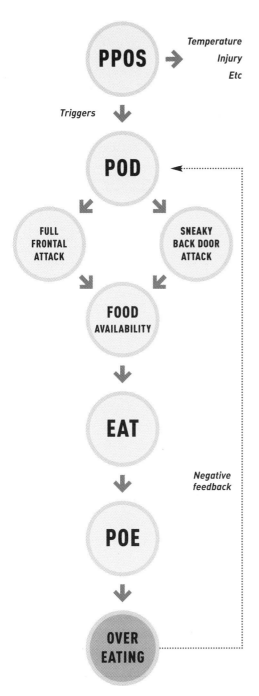

PPOS, the all over survival mechanism, triggers the various survival mechanisms. It also triggers **POD**, which is one of these mechanisms. The various triggers and cues of **POD** are:

- The sight of food
- The smell of food
- Talk and reminders of food
- Alcohol (very Depalgenic - triggering Depalgia)
- Insulin resistance (Insulin is one of the strongest **POD** stimulants)
- Circadian rhythms - if you are used to eating every night at six and one night you cannot, you will properly have a **POD** attack due to conditioning.

Once **POD** is triggered you will "suffer" its effects. We have developed many descriptions in our vocabulary to describe these, but primarily they fall into two categories.

1. The full frontal attack:

You are definitely aware of the fact that you want or need to eat. You may describe it as hunger, "I am starving" or "I am famished."

Your blood sugar may have dropped, your stomach gurgles and you feel weak. You may even feel you are going to "die" if you do not eat soon. A full frontal POD attack is transparent and easy to recognise. This type of attack is erroneously called "hunger eating". It is generally also easier to deal with than the following type of attack, which is shifty and causes the most problems with Depalgia (**POD**) control.

2. *The backdoor attack:*

These sensations of POD are more difficult to identify and are not usually as obvious to the sufferer. They are often described as "non-hunger eating". Still triggered by POD, you may experience what I'll describe as "POD Talk":

- "I am bored with my food" - meaning you want richer and more fattening food.

- You may experience feelings that you may perceive as temptations. It is just another way POD is trying to induce and seduce you to eat.

- You go to the fridge to get a glass of water - you see a piece of chocolate cake. POD kicks into action, spurring you to rationalise and formulate a plan: "There are no calories in this cake, because I got it as a present. Only if I baked it or bought it, does it have calories."

These back door attacks are at times incorrectly referred to as "non-hunger eating" as if it is not due to POD, but some sort of psychological problem.

Once POD (the stick) is triggered you will eat, unless the food is not available or you can successfully restrain the trigger. The limiting factor is the supply of food. If it is not there, you cannot eat it.

But what is in it for a living organism to respond to POD by proceeding to eat? Three things:

- pain relief - depalgesia
- reward (POE)
- nutrients and energy.

POE plays a significant role. When eating is pleasant we *want more*, leading to *overeating*. Remember, under eating is incompatible with survival. That is why it is made pleasurable to eat so that we can over eat. And because it is pleasant, we tell our friends, just like the pigeons and so it becomes a part of our culture.

It is not possible to constantly overeat and, through negative feedback mechanisms, POD is switched off when we declare, "I have had enough to eat", meaning in fact "I have had too much to eat".

This is a normal state of affairs. There is absolutely no reason to believe that you are acting in an abnormal way if you feel hungry (POD) and overeat (POE) or even binge.

The POD cycle can however be disturbed, leading to abnormality. Obvious examples are Anorexia Nervosa where for some pathological reason sufferers restrain themselves to the extent that their survival is in danger. Children with Prader Willi syndrome virtually cannot stop eating. After these children have consumed everything on the table they will literally eat the crumbs from the carpet.

Eating patterns and eating disorders

Just because a person is over-fat, suffering from GOFES, we cannot assume that they have an eating disorder. *By far the majority of GOFES sufferers do not have any abnormal eating patterns.* When a human Humming Bird is seen at a street café consuming a double thick milkshake with the works, we would not even look twice or make a comment. On the other hand if we see a human Polar Bear engaging in the same behaviour it attracts criticism.

There is no difference between these two behaviours. Both of them became aware of POD and gave in to it. *To give in to POD is normal and survival motivated.* Both indulge in the same behaviour, yet the Humming Bird stays thin and the Polar Bear gets fat.

Any normal aspect of human psychology and physiology can became abnormal leading to a pathological state. Eating behaviours can therefore become deviant. Generally however, many so-called eating disorders are not disorders at all. Categorising over eating as abnormal shows a lack of understanding of the relationship between evolved survival genetics and our recently created abnormal environment.

DES during various environmental situations

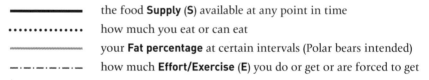

The illustration is not as difficult to understand as it looks, provided you take the following points into account. It depicts various scenarios of Hypo- and Hyper-adiposis depending on the DES situation.

The lines represent:

────────	the food **Supply (S)** available at any point in time
·············	how much you eat or can eat
～～～～～	your **Fat percentage** at certain intervals (Polar bears intended)
—·—·—·—·—	how much **Effort/Exercise (E)** you do or get or are forced to get

On the right of the illustration the up-arrow indicates our genetic demand and tendencies to over-eat. The down-arrow indicates our hereditary tendency to shirk exercise.

In between the two solid horizontal lines indicates the "just right" balance of food supply **(S)**, food intake and exercise **(E)** resulting in a normal fat percentage.

The vertical lines indicate different DES scenarios depending on the food supply.

96

- At top left the person is "under-fat" (Hypo-adiposis) and malnourished, because the food supply is too small, leading to under-eating and over-exercise to obtain this inadequate supply. Throughout history this situation existed during famine and other natural disasters.

- Between the next two vertical lines "just right", the food supply is adequate, but not excessive, and the amount of effort involved to get it is sufficient to obtain a normal fat percentage. *Therefore, the consumption of food is balanced with these factors of supply and effort* (Normo-adiposis). This situation existed in times of stability, where the food supply was relatively unadulterated.

- But then, about 50 years ago, things started changing as the food supply increased and became cheaper, and golf buggies and other POEx avoidance devices were introduced, with a corresponding drop off in physical activity.

If the supply is down so is our eating, if the supply is more abundant and cheaper so our eating is increased.

The ideal situation would be to be born a Polar Bear in primitive times and in modern times a Hummingbird. It's a pity that about 70 per cent of us are Polar Bears to varying degrees

- To put the matter therapeutically, returning to "just right", you have to manipulate your lifestyle so that your food supply (**S**) is controlled, so that you get some physical activity (**E**) and so that you control the demand (**D**) to eat. Then you can continue your journey in the "just right" zone without suffering from GOFES and its devastating health consequences. Provided of course, you *acquire the skills* to control and synchronise all these different factors (**DES**). That means you have to confront very normal basic instincts, realising that only our present environment is abnormal as far as our survival genetics are concerned. This is a very important concept and let me repeat it again:

Your survival instincts are normal, but your environment is abnormal.

You will not be able to control DES in the present socio-economic circumstances without a fight. If anybody tells you otherwise, they are insincere because they want to sell you something or are naive.

To control the food supply (**S**) is really the only way the problem can be solved. If governments and nature won't do it for us, we have to do it ourselves. Nobody will lose your excess fat and keep it off for you.

Some pharmacological agent may come along to change Polar Bear efficient metabolisms into inefficient Humming Birds metabolisms, but that will be like fluoride in the water. Will this agent be safe for mass consumption? Should you wait for such a theoretical eventuality that may never be ready in your lifetime?

The food supply is the key. Don't feel sorry for yourself, get on with the job, change your own food supply, lose excess fat and get healthy. You will never regret it.

Who will succeed?

Those who will succeed are the highly motivated, individuals who are interested in their health and are willing to take on the food supply and do the right thing. These people will have knowledge of the real issues involved. They will have to go against the trends. These Polar Bear individuals will be successful and this book is dedicated to them, as well as, to the Humming Birds interested in obtaining and maintaining Optimum Functional Health.

I sincerely hope there is a cure for every single GOFES victim on this planet, but at the moment it is a bit "Alice in Wonderland" stuff to expect such a cure.

If you don't fall into the self-motivated group, hopefully this book will motivate you to join.

Excess fat loss is the most powerful therapy we have in medicine today, because it achieves so much. You can have the best of both worlds - the benefits of an affluent society and the metabolic fitness of primeval times. It's up to you - this book will take you on this journey.

The 4th characteristic of successful weight maintainers: Understand that POD, POE and POEx are survival phenomena. They are natural and normal, but they demand control in an excess food supply.

Synopsis:

1. We are genetically designed to over eat, since under eating is incompatible with survival.

2. Exercise conflicts with survival and the need to conserve energy.

3. The unlimited food supply is the basic cause of the obesity problem. Unless the real issues of GOFES are recognised, the pandemic won't be controlled.

4. POD and POEx are not psychological pathologies. You should not feel guilty about feeling hungry - it is a basic survival instinct.

5. DES must form the basis of any program to control GOFES.

6. Polar Bears won't develop GOFES if they can't afford enough food, or if the effort to obtain adequate supplies is sufficiently demanding.

7. You need to be a pit-bull to fight a pit-bull.

CHAPTER 7

DEMYSTIFYING GOFES

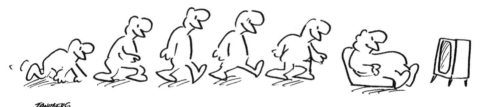

TANDBERG

DEMYSTIFYING GOFES

"Look... look the Emperor doesn't wear any clothes"
LEGEND

Now it's time to unlock the "puzzle" from the Introduction.

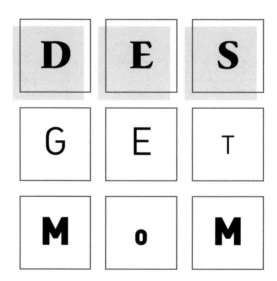

DES

D stands for Demand. With survival in mind, we have a very strongly developed demand to eat. The phenomenon responsible for fuelling this is the Pain of Deprivation (POD).

S stands for Supply. It refers to the quantity and quality of food that is available to eat.

E stands for Effort. This is the energy output necessary to obtain the food we need.

GET MOM

GET represents primitive or stone-age times and **MoM**, the modern or space-age times.

How DES (Demand, Effort and Supply) operates in these two separate time frames

GET - the demand to eat was great (**G**). The food supply was tiny (**T**) and erratic and the effort (**E**) involved to obtain it was enormous. This was the environmental-laboratory in which our metabolisms evolved.

Not overeating, mixed with a good dose of physical activity, kept us healthy. High degrees of metabolic fitness were maintained. Coronary artery disease, diabetes and other degenerative diseases of affluence were virtually unknown.

MoM - in modern times our demand to eat became even stronger because our senses are constantly stimulated. In more primitive times a cow may have represented a potential hamburger, but the effort to satisfy gratification was hardly worth it. Now demand is massive (**M**)

Today, not only is the food tastier than ever before, but it is instantly available in unsurpassed abundance. The supply is massive (**M**) and is now cheaper than ever before. And we can buy food 24 hours a day. The effort in acquiring this *massive-appetite-stimulating-supply* is zero (**0**) in practical terms. Such a **DES** environment has caused colossal abnormal changes in our metabolisms - changes for which our bodies were never designed.

Hence the health crisis of today - fatty livers, fatty organs, fatty marbleised muscles, diabetes, heart attacks and cancer. Humming Birds are suffering, even if they're not excessively fat, and the poor old Polar Bears are doubly sick due to the added burden of excess fat and its metabolic consequences.

Evolutionary processes have created an abnormal society and our bodies haven't been able to adapt to the change. Individuals aren't at fault and can't be held accountable if they indulge in completely natural instincts of over eating and avoiding physical activity. Some experts have branded our over-eating and shirking of exercise as abnormal. Hello!

The puzzle and its solution are so simple and so down-to-earth that the reality is not acceptable to many. A well-known commercial weight loss enterprise asked for my opinion on the "obesity epidemic" and my views on dealing with the problem. They market tested my comments and reached the conclusion that my views had no commercial value because they were too simplistic. Commercially, I can see where they were coming from. From a scientific point of view, these are the facts and if they are too simplistic to "market" then that just proves the point.

If something is too logical to "market" would you rather believe in the market or the simple facts? **It is important for you to understand these simple facts, since this understanding also forms part of the treatment.** Acceptance of these facts is a requirement for success.

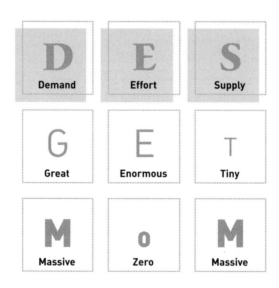

Scientists aren't always comfortable with simplicity. My sister-in-law, a very intelligent lady with a number of scientific degrees, told me bluntly: "this is too simple - almost child like." I am still trying to fathom what it is that motivates and compels people to think in mystical terms when it comes to GOFES. Is it perhaps due to the profound nature of POD, POEx and survival?

As an individual, you can only control your **GOFES** through a combination of **DES and metabolic changes**. Any successful weight loss regime has at its core Demand, Effort, Supply and Metabolism.

Demand to eat means you have to learn how to control **POD** even though we are genetically programmed to over eat.

Effort means controlling activity levels even though our bodies want to conserve energy.

These days, subsistence exercise is where you walk down the corridor, or to the bathroom, or to go shopping. It is not enough - we need to increase our subsistence exercise for good health and GOFES control. It is amazing how people circle like vultures around shopping centres for half an hour or more, just to juggle for the nearest car park to the front entrance. **POEx... POEx...**

One way to keep tabs on your subsistence exercise is to wear a pedometer. Aim for at least 5,000 steps a day. If you have done only 4,000 at the end of the day, go for a quick walk around the block or do 6,000 tomorrow.

Typically, our subsistence exercise is not enough for these modern times. We therefore need supplementary *deliberate exercise*. For example, gym work three times a week or some form of sport which is more demanding and vigorous than subsistence exercise.

The Environment (E) interacts with Genetics (G) in our DES model.

Genetics (G) determines the **POD**, **POEx** and our **Metabolism** (**M** - from Polar Bear to Humming Bird). The **Environment** (**E**) determines the prevailing circumstances, especially the availability and type of food, as well as labour saving devices. *Genetics and the Environment interact to create* **DES**.

If the metabolism is Polar Bear and the environment is modern day, then this will cause an individual to become **Over Fat (OF)** resulting in **GOFES**.

If unchecked, this will give rise to a number of nasty diseases and syndromes (**S**).

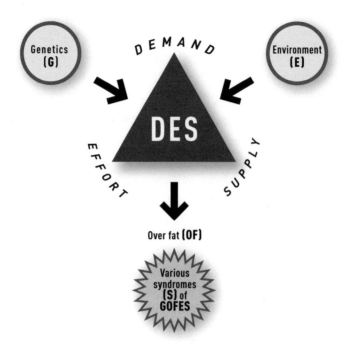

To treat GOFES we need to address **M** (metabolism) and **DES**. Orthodox medical practice has a tendency to research and treat the end results of a condition. *It may often be necessary to treat both the cause and effects at the same time, but the primary focus should be on* **DES/M** - *the primary causes.*

Whichever way you look at it, the modern **DES** of affluence and excess is bad for Polar Bears and Humming Birds alike.

Synopsis:

1. Why **GOFES** exists is not a mystery - it's a matter of simple survival. Various experts and special interest groups have mystified it. Jumping to conclusions is not half as good an exercise as digging for the facts.

2. The *propensity* to develop **GOFES** is not a disease, but the consequences are.

3. In treating **GOFES** the principal focus should be the control of the primary causes, **POD**, **POEx** and Polar Bear **Metabolism**.

4. It is negligent to treat the consequential effects, the diseases of **GOFES**, *without* addressing the primary causes of these illnesses.

CHAPTER 8

CONSTRUCTION OF A SENSIBLE GOFES TREATMENT PROGRAM

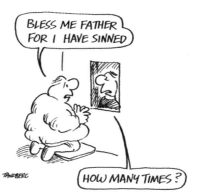

CONSTRUCTION OF A SENSIBLE GOFES TREATMENT PROGRAM

"Doctor, I've lost my teeth, hair, eyesight, hearing, and memory. You are NOT going to make me lose my waistline."

ANONYMOUS

Years ago a distraught young woman, Gloria, came to see me regarding her weight problem. A few years prior she was an up and coming actress. Gloria used to weigh on average 52kg (115lb) no matter how much she ate. She was very attractive and had plenty of boyfriends taking her out to all the best restaurants. She never gained any weight.

One day she was asked to do a photographic session for a magazine and she thought it would be very trendy to have the ultra slim look and lose two to three kilograms. Gloria achieved this easily on a diet she found in a magazine on women's issues. After the photo sessions she went back to her old eating habits, eating as she liked.

To her amazement she did not go back to 52kg (115lb) but went to 55kg (121lb). This necessitated dieting to get down to 52kg, but the moment she went off the diet her weight crept up to 57kg (125lb). I saw her almost two years later, in tears and without her job, at almost 80kg (176lb).

Gloria's history puzzled me a bit. If she was a genuine Humming Bird, as her past history suggested, she should not have gained this amount of weight. I medically investigated her thoroughly and could not find any medical cause for her weight increase. Was she a latent Polar Bear, unmasked by her "famine" (diet)?

Normally the body has an ideal weight, especially in true Humming Birds, but this set point is not necessarily stable in everyone. The Equilibrium Set Point (ESP) is non-existent in extreme Polar Bears, but very strong in extreme Humming Birds.

A person suffering from Haemochromatosis will store excessive iron, while a non-sufferer regulates their iron levels. The ESP or so-called thermostat is nothing but an equilibrium control mechanism. It works in Humming Birds as far as fat storage is concerned but not particularly well in Polar Bears. Haemochromatosis, like **GOFES**, is a survival mechanism from our primeval past. With the scarcity of nutrients, early man acquired the ability to store iron. So, in modern times with enough iron, some people will over store and get sick, just as Polar Bears over store fat and get sick.

In the following illustration, Gloria had a constant body weight of 52kg (115lb) which became her ESP. When she lost weight her body saw the prospect of famine and put in place a host of mechanisms to increase her chance of survival. Polar Bears are genetically very good at this.

Your body does not know the difference between a famine and a diet. Intellectually, you may know what you are doing, but your body follows instincts acquired over thousands of years. The ESP differs from most other equilibrium mechanisms in that it seems to have the ability to become aggravated during repeated famine. If you are a Polar Bear, it adapts to become more efficient in certain circumstances.

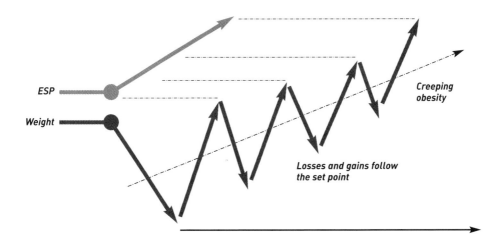

So, as Gloria started to decrease her weight, her ESP increased, protecting her against the next probable "famine". You are now ready for maintenance, but as so often happens, (the "Ah Ha syndrome" and the like) you start gaining weight almost immediately. The problem is, you do not go back up to your original weight, but adjust to your new ESP, which in Gloria's case had increased by two kilograms the first time she dieted, and a further two kilograms the second time.

The realisation that you re-gained the weight plus a bit more is a bit of a shocker.

Your response: "I better go on another diet."

Unfortunately it is now more difficult to lose weight than the first time, and what's more, your chances of getting down to your previous low weight are almost non-existent.

Instead of maintenance you almost immediately start gaining weight again. This time you notice it is easier than before to gain it and since your ESP has gone up further, you do not stop until you reach this new ESP. The process keeps on repeating itself with each subsequent loss and regain. In time you're in a spiralling cycle of increasing weight. I call it creeping-obesity. The western world has been dieting for the last 20 years and average weights have increased 15kg (33lb) as a result.

Polar Bears have a naturally high unstable ESP while Humming birds have a stable ESP. In between lies a group that appears to have a stable ESP, but this can be unmasked by repeated dieting or other trauma such as anaesthetic, mental illness or physical injury. Your ESP has a lot to do with brute survival and all manner of variations are possible.

This phenomenon, and the so-called drop in metabolic rate as you lose weight, have been used to scare GOFES sufferers to a state of panic. They are told to lose weight very slowly in order not to upset their metabolism and set point. It is also thought that with slow weight loss, our bodies can adjust to these new levels. However, in practice this is seldom the case.

There is no relationship between the speed of fat loss and a person's chances of regaining weight. The only exception is where the weight loss was unscientific and a lot of lean body mass was lost. In this case weight gain can be faster. Mostly, I find that slow fat loss ends up in frustration. Excess fat is dangerous, the faster you lose it the better. The old mantra "Don't lose too fast" is very vague. What is too fast anyway?

*"Don't worry about losing weight;
you will find it exactly where you lost it."*

ROBERT HALF

With this in mind, I have constructed all my treatment programs in two main phases and four stages.

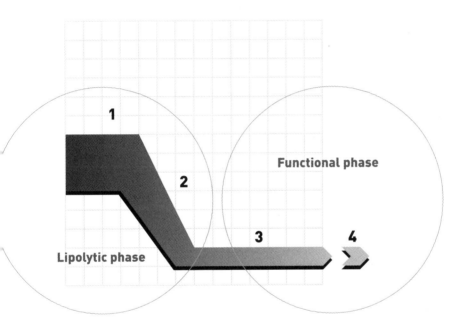

FUNCTIONAL LIPOLYTIC SYSTEM

The program as a whole is called the Functional Lipolytic System. Each of the two phases comprises two stages, and all are continuous.

PHASE ONE

The **Lipolytic (excess fat breakdown) Phase**, called by some patients the "Demolition Phase".

Stage One

Pre-preparation - a type of pre-school as you will. This stage is depicted as "fat looking" in the above illustration, symbolising the larger size of the patients before they start losing excess fat. This stage is also the preparation for the next stage, while giving patients the opportunity to decide whether or not to proceed to Stage Two.

Patients are also medically and psychologically assessed. The optimum time for this stage is about two weeks - longer in some cases. No dietary restrictions or modifications are placed on patients at this stage, other than an increased intake of water and a light walking program.

Stage Two

Excess fat losing stage - this involves strict therapeutic intervention and should be viewed as such by both patient and therapist. This stage takes as long as is necessary to lose all excess fat. Partial fat loss is not acceptable in that it is easier to maintain a normal fat percentage than to maintain a partial weight loss. A range of medical tests are recommended to patients during this stage.

Dieting involves going to great lengths to avoid going to great widths!

Stage 2 is a short-term goal. If you only have short-term goals you will only achieve short-term results. Research and experience tells us that the optimum time for follow-up is weekly.

PHASE TWO

The **Functional Phase** starts once the Lipolytic Phase is completed and is life long. Treating aging as with any other "disease", the aim is to lower your biological age to at least your chronological age, preferably less.

Stage Three

Once excess fat is lost you are neither stabilised nor cured. A fully structured *maintenance program* is now called for. It usually takes one to two years to learn all the skills to keep excess fat at bay. You will be asleep for a third of this time, so it's not as long as it seems! During this time you should remain on active treatment, although follow-up visits are further apart than the previous stage. This is actually the beginning of the treatment, since this is where patients develop their new lifestyles.

Stage Four

Here you stabilise the therapeutic benefits derived so far. After excess fat loss the body still sees itself as being "over fat". There is now much less fat, but all the hormones and blood vessels that used to feed and maintain the fat are still there. These factors are waiting, serving as infrastructure to fill your fat stores once again. This infrastructure needs to be toned down, otherwise permanent maintenance will be either impossible or an unpleasant struggle in an affluent society.

If you keep your weight and fat percentage stable for a year or two, this infrastructure will atrophy through lack of use - only then will you have stabilised. But remember, you will remain a Polar Bear for the rest of your life - never cured, although your genetics will now be synchronised with your environment.

During Stage 3 there is a huge gap between your ESP and your actual weight and you will be subjected to almost irresistible pressures to simply regain your lost excess fat. You have a few desserts and a bit extra on the side, and shock horror, a five kilogram gain in one week. Once stabilised however, the same behaviour will cause a much lesser gain. *This is the state you should aim for*. If you do not attain it, over time you will simply regain all the excess fat that you had lost - usually sooner than you might think.

Once you have stabilised you can accommodate the odd indiscretion. You must be stabilised before you go on your final maintenance journey. If not, your weight loss attempts will be short lived. The approach is always long term. Long-term goals - long term results.

"If you want to be young and thin,
Hang around with old fat people."
ANONYMOUS

What to treat?

Typically, the main emphasis and preoccupation today is to treat the secondary effects of **GOFES**. However, **GOFES** is the primary cause of over 40 secondary effects.

Take an example - GOFES induced hypertension. Statistics show that in only 36 per cent of cases will doctors even advise a patient to lose excess fat. And rarely will they tell you how to lose that weight.

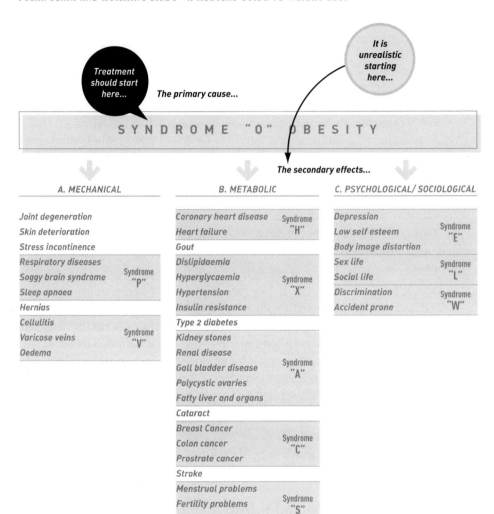

We can reduce the number of secondary side effects by clumping them together and calling them syndromes, but that's playing treatment-semantics.

As I've discussed earlier (Chapter 3), Syndrome X is a cluster that appears more often in a certain type of fat distribution and it is not to be ignored, but it is still caused by **GOFES**. Identifying that you are the victim of one of these syndromes means nothing if you don't treat the *primary metabolic syndrome*, **GOFES**.

The treatment of GOFES = The treatment of secondary diseases

The treatment of the secondary diseases on their own is not treating GOFES

Some of the secondary diseases may have been there so long that *a point of no return* has been reached. In these cases the secondary disease should be treated, but the primary **GOFES** should always be treated as a priority. For example, your hypertension will usually disappear if you lose your excess fat. It may have caused some kidney damage and no amount of weight loss will return your kidney function to normal, but you may be able to use less medication if you have lost your excess fat.

A fatty liver will usually disappear if a person loses excess fat. On the other hand, once a fatty liver has progressed to cirrhosis, a person has reached a point of no return and only a liver transplant can help you then. However, excess fat loss is still required.

A three-pronged approach

Three approaches are necessary, depending on your clinical situation.

1. **Prevention: GOFES** should *primarily* be treated to prevent any of the secondary diseases.

2. **Deal with the problem:** Once secondary diseases appear, treating **GOFES** on its own will often eliminate or at least improve the secondary effects. Some patients and doctors are horrified that I usually stop or reduce their medication while they are being treated for **GOFES**.

   People are conditioned to the need for prescription drugs. Reducing medication is not done lightly - your medical condition should be closely monitored as it may become necessary to reinstate some medication. If eliminating your medication is unsuccessful, the third option applies.

3. **Treat the problem *plus* the effects:** if a point of no return has been reached, then **GOFES** should *still* be treated, but a direct approach for these diseases should also be administered.

   The cure is in tackling the primary problem, which is *not* Syndrome X per se, or any of the other secondary diseases. The culprit - **GOFES** - should be dealt with. *A patient, once fully understanding this and being encouraged do so, will get* *much better results overall.* There will of course always be some people who cannot deal with **POD/POEx**, and their only hope is the bandaid treatment of the diseases caused by GOFES as they occur. This is not ideal, but we are all different and, unfortunately, this option is the easier option for the patient and therapist alike, and is more lucrative for the drug companies.

Synopsis:

1. In treating thousands of **GOFES** sufferers I have come to the conclusion that patients need to view their treatment program as a sequence of stages, each with a different approach, but with all forming a continuous spectrum.

2. The primary causes of **GOFES** need to be addressed. It is rather naive or perhaps negligent to only treat the consequent diseases without considering the core condition.

CHAPTER 9

DANGERS

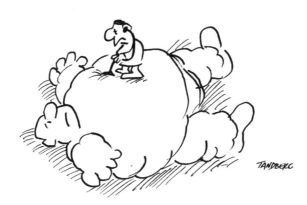

DANGERS

Living in the information age gives us unprecedented access to limitless stores of knowledge, but it has also engendered in us unrealistically high expectations.

It is your right to be informed of all the advantages of weight loss, but it is also important that you be informed of the potential disadvantages. Armed with all of the information you can adjust your expectations to a realistic range. The alternative is that when expectations are not met, the realisation can be depressing.

Are there any downsides to weight loss?

Not any that I know of. If however you are already in the normal fat percentage range, under this limit or about to go into a famine, it's better not to tamper with your fat percentage. No matter what is wrong with you, heart disease, cancer, liver or kidney failure, if you are a **GOFES** victim, *you will benefit* from losing excess fat. However, the method of losing it maybe different in these circumstances, since certain methods of treatment may not be appropriate for a particular individual.

Before attempting weight loss

A thorough medical examination is mandatory

Initially you should know if there are any *medical causes or contributing factors*, for your **GOFES**. Thyroid disease, Cushing's Syndrome and certain medications play a role in causing **GOFES**. Unfortunately, Obesity is often seen as simple gluttony and a lack of self-discipline, and serious disease states are missed because they are not considered.

Secondly, the secondary disease states that are *caused by* **GOFES**, should be identified and addressed. There are over forty potential diseases to look for,

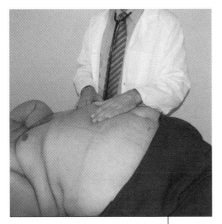

Many serious conditions can lurk underneath excess fat.

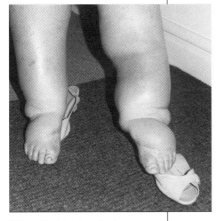

This patient has lymphedema - her mild GOFES was not the main problem.

including a host of cancers, diabetes, osteoarthritis, sleep apnoea and many more.

A medical examination should also look for any other medical conditions *not related to* **GOFES**, so they can be treated at the same time. Initiating a **GOFES** treatment program is the perfect time to fully assess a person's health.

And finally, a medical examination will determine an individual's suitability for a proposed treatment regime. For example, patients with heart or kidney failure will benefit if they lose their excess fat, however *the method that is employed* should be adapted to their state of health.

Knowledgeable medical supervision during treatment

Initial evaluation of **GOFES** sufferers should always be done by an experienced medical practitioner. Who else has the qualifications to identify and treat the medical conditions associated with and caused by **GOFES**?

The US Health Department is quite emphatic - it states that obesity should be investigated and treated by qualified medical professionals.

Nutrition and healthy weight loss

Certain mineral deficiencies during weight loss can be a health risk. In more severe cases electrolyte disturbances can be life threatening. It is impossible to go on a balance deficit diet and still get all the nutrients in optimum quantities for good health.

Anti-oxidants in optimum quantities are already deficient in our diets without the added stress of weight loss. The break down of fat creates an increase in free radicals and therefore an increased need for antioxidants. Some dieticians will argue that you can lose weight and gain *all your nutrients from a balanced diet*. Not in today's world!

To effectively lose weight, your calorie intake has to be lowered to achieve a negative caloric balance. This lowers your nutrient intake as well. The majority of patients will require a complete vitamin and mineral supplement. Magnesium, potassium, calcium and essential fatty acids - to name a few.

Lean Body Mass
Loss of Lean Body Mass can compromise the immune system and can even cause hair loss. Hence, the proper protein with all the essential amino acids in the correct ratios is essential during excess-fat loss. At a minimum this protein should be taken at least twice a day.

Carbohydrate loading
The concept of carbohydrate loading was initially developed in Scandinavia to improve the stamina of certain athletes. These athletes will "starve" themselves of carbohydrate and train very hard at the same time. A day or so before the athletic meeting they will suddenly stop or drastically curtail their training and "stuff" themselves with carbohydrate. This "squeezes" sugar into the muscles in the form of glycogen. Enhancing their energy, their strength is not improved but their stamina is.

The downside - the increased sugar levels also impacted their heart muscle and pancreas, causing damage to these organs.

Imagine: You have already lost 20kg (44lb), five more to go. You are fitter and leaner because you exercise regularly and have been eating a caloric deficit diet, meaning you are also eating less carbohydrate. Suddenly you get upsetting news - your stress threshold is lowered and **POD** gets the upper hand.

You give up your exercise regime and stuff yourself with chocolates and the like. What are you doing? You are carbohydrate loading - more or less like the athletes. You are harming your health.

You need to be weaned off your diet. This is one of the reasons I don't take on patients who want to lose weight quickly to fit into a bikini for their upcoming holidays. I know they'll "starve" themselves to lose weight and stuff themselves during their holiday - impairing their health through carbohydrate loading.

Beware fat city

Losing weight needs a carefully balanced program. If you don't follow all of the instructions you may look as if you have just been rescued from a prison camp. This will inevitably lead to criticism by others, sinking your spirits and giving you the perfect excuse to put on weight again. **POD** will then overwhelm your defences and you'll be back in fat city all over again.

Aggravation of your Polar Bear status

Losing excess fat may aggravate your GOFES problem. Your excess fat may reappear and you could ultimately weigh more than you did before going on your diet. It's vital that you have a pre-planned maintenance program ready to go once you have achieved your weight goal.

Alcohol

"Doctor, doctor, you've got to help me - I can't stop my hands from shaking!"
"Do you drink a lot?"
"Not really - I spill most of it!"

During Stage Two of your weight loss program - excess fat loss - you should not consume any alcohol.

Our "cellar dweller" culture makes it difficult to even dare mention you cannot have any alcohol during weight loss. Always remember, the driver is safer when the roads are dry, and vice versa. Drinkers are great believers in health. They are always drinking to other people's health.

Alcohol is mostly metabolised in the liver - so is fat. The two do not mix and you put undue stress on your liver by drinking while losing weight. Given the choice between combating an external poison - alcohol - and metabolising fat which your body believes it needs for survival, guess what? Your body will metabolise the foreign substance every time and burning off your excess fat will grind to a halt.

And if you're prone to **fatty liver**, that will be further aggravated.

Then there's **cancer of the pancreas** - usually more common among alcoholics than non-alcoholics. During fat loss, if you consume alcohol your chances of contracting cancer of the pancreas are increased to that of an alcoholic. And did I mention that cancer of the brain and oesophagus are also more common among regular drinkers?

"If you drink your brain will shrink". Yes, regular drinking over a 15 year period will shrivel your memory. During fat loss your nervous system becomes more sensitive to the effects of alcohol - there is no safe limit of alcohol during excess fat loss.

Don't drink and drive. You will spill it.
Beer kills brain cells, but only the weak ones.
Avoid hangovers - stay drunk.

A Swiss study has found that even small amounts of alcohol per day **stop the body burning fat for 24 hours**. Therefore, if you drink every day, you virtually stop burning fat altogether. Even in maintenance, when you resume alcohol intake, you should have at least three to four alcohol free days per week.

Did you hear about the new whisky diet? You don't lose any weight, but you couldn't care less.

Alcohol is **rich in calories**, but they're calories with very little nutrition if any. You certainly do not want to crowd out your nutritional calories while you slim down. During excess fat loss every calorie counts.

Unlike what most people think, alcohol is not a stimulant. It is a depressant. It depresses the frontal part of your brain so that it cannot inhibit the more primitive parts of your brain, making you less reserved.

One of the biggest **appetite stimulants** is alcohol. I once worked in the Adelaide hospital in Dublin, Ireland. My first night on duty I saw a young nurse carrying a tray full of Guinness. I assumed there was a staff party somewhere. I was quite surprised when she informed me it was for the patients. A long time ago Irish doctors discovered that giving patients a bit of alcohol stimulates their appetites.

Once your appetite is stimulated, and you cannot say "no", **POD** will overwhelm you and you simply will not say no. ***Booze is one of the top saboteurs of any fat loss program.***

Blood donation

Our blood is liquid living tissue, full of protein, cells, hormones and many other essential substances. It is part of your lean body mass. The fittest athletes take eight weeks to return to their pre-donation fitness level after giving blood. If you donate blood while you are losing excess fat it will be very good for someone who needs it, but it will be bad for you. During fat loss your reduced food intake will result in your body cannibalising your muscles and organs to replace donated blood.

Smoking

We should be kind to smokers because they do not have long to live.

One of the best things you can do for your health is to STOP SMOKING. It also interferes with your fat metabolism. The very best time to quit is at the *same time* that you are losing your excess fat.

For one to follow the other, affects both the mind and body. The discipline associated with losing excess fat can be tiring and to follow this with the discipline of quitting cigarettes can be very difficult. It's not unusual for these patients to end up being fatter than before while still smoking - the worst of both worlds.

Besides, you need to get fitter if you are serious about your GOFES predicament. How can you do this by being a smoker?

Once, without really thinking, I told a patient to stop smoking "NOW". This was at the start of the excess fat loss stage. To my surprise both projects were a great success. Since then I have had numerous patients who successfully did both at the *same time*. To kill two birds with one stone is much, much easier than killing two birds with two or more stones. *Stop smoking while you are losing weight!*

Cancer cures smoking

Not only does smoking mess up your fat metabolism, but also patients who smoke during weight loss suffer more skin tightening side problems than non-smokers.

It is claimed that smoking takes years off your life. So smoke and stay younger!

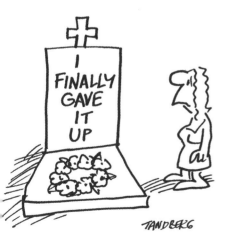

TANDBERG

121

Diseases must be treated concurrently

Few physicians seem aware of the latest discoveries strongly *linking* **GOFES**, hypertension, insulin resistance and heart disease, and the explosive knowledge *that you cannot treat any one of these diseases successfully without treating all of them - together.*

A physician for example, who gives over-fat patients hypertensive blood pressure drugs and sends them home is being negligent and leaving the patient at high risk of heart attack and even certain cancers. Obesity is a complex disease state. To treat in isolation any of the disease states that it causes is illogical.

The politics of weight loss

"It is much easier to be critical than to be correct."
BENJAMIN DISRAELI

When I became interested in the field of **GOFES**, related conditions and Functional Medicine, I naively thought that I would automatically have the support of all my colleagues and other interested people. What I did not realise was that I had stepped into a political minefield.

The overt and covert condemnation of my approach was astounding, and yet the majority of my critics had not even studied the subject or worked in the field.

On the other hand, I had support from many and had quite a number of doctors and their families as patients. These days I don't think twice about "uninformed" comment.

Your pursuit of weight loss won't be without its critics either. And typically the comments will come as you most need support.

"You should stop now - see, you look gaunt! You'll become anorectic!"

"There are too many carbohydrates in your diet."

"There are not enough carbohydrates in your diet."

In short, everybody is an "expert" when it comes to weight loss.

What is it that motivates people to put others off from losing weight?

Perhaps it's ignorance, envy or jealousy, or perhaps you're reminding your critics that they should be doing something about their own health and so they criticise you instead!

We all get used to family and friends with a certain body image. This is how we relate to one another. Your losing weight may come as a shock to them. Instinctively they do not know if you are the same person. Your body has changed... perhaps your mind has too? They become uncomfortable and at a subconscious level they may feel betrayed. Some will choose to attack as a form of defence, while you were expecting appreciation and acknowledgement for your efforts.

The politics of weight loss can negatively impact on your progress if you do not expect it. Understand the underlying basis for it and prepare a mental defence. Most patients will encounter it sooner or later.

Saboteurs in your life will try to push food on you. Controlling **GOFES** can be a lonely struggle. "Everybody" is an "obesity expert" and has an opinion. Some can be very overbearing. Don't be upset - take it for what it is.

"To avoid criticism do nothing, say nothing, be nothing."
ELBERT HUBART

Synopsis:

1. There are *no* downsides to excess fat loss.

2. Certain weight loss methods can be counter productive to your health.

3. You must not consume alcohol when you are losing weight. While losing excess fat is the perfect opportunity to quit smoking.

4. Be aware that you may suffer criticism during your efforts to control **GOFES** and regain your health. What we eat and the culture associated with eating are at the very heart of who we are - some people will be affronted by your "interference".

CHAPTER 10

THE DREADED SCALES

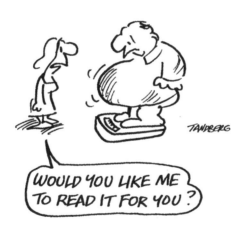

THE DREADED SCALES

"Nobody likes a liar - unless it's the bathroom scales"
A. BATT

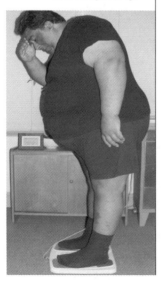

"Woh, I weigh 195 kg!"

Scales are a measure of weight. Weight is a measure of gravity. This is where it begins and ends for you in the treatment of **GOFES**.

A diet is not a "weigh" of life - it is much more than hopping on the scales.

The scales can show you've lost some weight, but what have you lost? Fat, water, Lean Body Mass, or a combination? All you should lose is *excess-fat*, but scales are a useless instrument for all but telling you how much you weigh. If you rely on scales for a psychological boost, you'll be sorely disappointed on more than the odd occasion during your **GOFES** control program.

The meaning of weight

What does this mean?

The 195kg (429lb) comprises clothing, Lean Body Mass, water and fat as in the table.

What percentage of each of these contributes to the 195kg?

The second column of the table indicates how much each of these components contribute as a percentage.

What makes up the weight	% of water?	% of water in this?
1. Clothing	x%	
2. Lean body mass Skin, Muscles, Organs, Bones, etc.	45 - 55%	80%
3. Water	25%	100%
4. Fat 1. Structural 2. Reserve 3. GOFES	20 - 30%	15%

How much water is there in each of the components? You can overlook the water in clothing, unless you are caught in a rainstorm. Fifty per cent of the weight of bone is water. Twenty per cent of the body's water is in the skin and most organs are made up of over 90 per cent water. On average we can say that Lean Body Mass is 80 per cent water.

Fat is quite dry in comparison to most other body tissues and is made up of only 15 per cent water. So, between 60 and 70 per cent of the body is water, depending on your age. Older people have much less water in their bodies than the young.

What you *do not* want to lose?

Ideally you want to lose your **GOFES** or excess-fat. If you lose anything else you will damage your health. There are two exceptions. It is really not a problem if you lose your old fat clothing. That should be a pleasure - other than the expense of replacing your wardrobe. And you will probably lose that small component of Lean Body Mass that was created and used to carry your excess heavy fat.

In the main, your purpose should be a body composition change and not weight loss per se. The aim is to lose your excess fat, while increasing your LBM, improving your *body composition.*

As we age the body is getting drier
A baby - 80 per cent water

A normal adult - 70 per cent water

An old person - 50 per cent

Fat versus water

Fat floats on water because water weighs four times as much as fat.

Greg

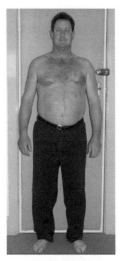

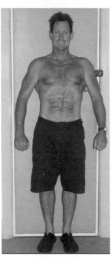

It follows that small variations in body fluid can dramatically affect your body weight and the reading on those bathroom scales. Unfortunately, doctors sometimes exploit this fact by giving patients diuretics or fluid tablets. A person may lose three kilograms - nearly seven pounds - overnight from taking one pill. You may be ecstatic, believing you have lost a lot of fat, but all you have lost is water. *It is bogus motivation.* These diuretics can also be dangerous if given for the wrong reasons.

Scales cannot tell you how much fat you have lost. Relying on scales to give you motivation and reward is the worst possible thing you can do. This motivation is misplaced and has nothing to do with changing your eating behaviour and dealing with **POD**. Indeed, if you rely on the scales to give you incentive, motivation and drive, you will at some stage become unstuck. It is imperative that you understand and accept the psychology of the scales.

Joyce, who lost 34kg (75lb) and kept it off for seven years, would not even look at the scales, in spite of the fact that I promote scales as a good maintenance tool.

"Joyce, what do you use then as an indirect way of determining your fat percentage?" I asked.

"I'll bring it in next time," she answered.

The next time I saw her, she took jeans out of a plastic bag and said: "these are my scales." She continued; "If I don't feel comfortable in them, I do something about it."

It worked for her and I guess different strokes for different folks.

Greg is a good example of a body composition change. He lost 27.3kg (60lb) in just nine weeks at the clinic. His fat percentage went from 35 per cent to 16 per cent. It is anticipated that he will decrease his fat percentage further in the next six months to a year, without much in the way of weight loss.

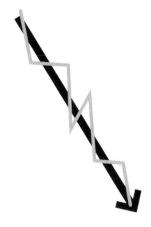

If scales aren't important then what is?

Body composition and fat percentage are really the only terms that you should be concerned about. Scales can't tell you how much fat you've lost and what your body composition is.

On a daily basis, you are not going to lose weight in a straight line as in the illustration, instead your weight loss will be fast one day, slower the next and some days you will even gain weight, to your annoyance. Scales can drive you to distraction.

If you "burn" one kilogram of fat for energy, it converts into two kilograms of water. So, while you've lost a kilogram of fat - which is good - you've actually gained a kilogram in weight - which is frustrating.

Are you going to be annoyed about the one kilogram weight gain that shows on the scales or the one kilogram fat loss that's not showing on the scales? Get perspective!

One kilogram of fat occupies more space than a kilogram of muscle.

1kg Fat

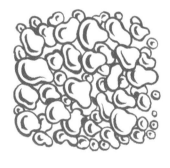

1kg Muscle

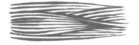

The reason is of course, fat is much lighter than muscle. You can lose a kilogram of fat plus gain three kilograms of muscle and still be thinner. Why? Simple arithmetic - you gained three kilograms of muscle and you lost one kilogram of fat, therefore you are two kilograms heavier. Why you are actually thinner, in spite of the weight gain, is that lesser space occupied by muscle versus fat. Losing fat makes you thin quickly. *Gaining* muscle makes you thinner if you *lose fat* at the same time. Back to those bathrooms scales - absolutely useless in determining what you actually lost.

When we work with fat percentage instead of weight, the result appears quite different as is portrayed in the next illustration. Weight loss occurs quite quickly at first and then slows down.

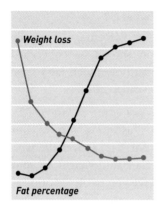

The fat percentage is just the opposite and speeds up. The logic: one per cent of an elephant's fat weighs much more than one per cent of a cat's fat, therefore the elephant has to lose a lot more weight to achieve a one per cent reduction in body fat.

While money loses value over time, kilograms actually *gain value* with excess fat loss. How is this possible?

We'll leave the money issue to the economists, but as kilograms are taken off a *progressively smaller* body, they become more and more valuable. As your body gets smaller, you need to lose less kilograms to lose a percentage point of fat. This is valuable information for those interested in controlling *GOFES*.

Fat loss is not related to weight loss

I use "fat points" as the primary measure of success in controlling **GOFES**. Though the kilogram relationship is constant, the value of "fat points" increase progressively as you lose weight. For example, once you have lost 10 kilograms, you may have lost 16 "fat points" while losing 20 kilograms could see you lose 35 "fat points".

This tracking method more accurately reflects what is actually happening to your body as you lose excess fat.

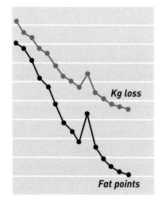

Remember, kilogram weight loss slows down the more you lose while the loss of "fat points" speeds up. By just concentrating on the kilograms you may become very despondent for no valid reason.

This method of measurement is derived from science. Losing "fat points" is very rewarding and motivating, but conversely if you gain weight you lose proportionally more points than kilograms as the following chart demonstrates.

More correctly, "fat points" should be called Lipolytic Dimension Points to emphasise the scientific nature of what is happening to you as you lose weight. Lipolytic referring to the breaking down of fat and Dimension referring to size. Once patients accept the rationale of these points they are more inclined to follow their regime and to lose excess-fat more quickly.

Fat loss versus weight loss

You've had a bit of a heavy weekend and **POD** got the upper hand. Monday morning you jump on the scales and to your surprise you weigh less. In your mind you don't feel so bad about the decadence of the weekend. The thought that you got away with it reinforces your negative cheating behaviour. Inevitably, a day or two later your weight goes up and you feel like it's the end of the world.

The scales are now determining your mood, particularly when you move on to weight maintenance. If you can use the scales as your motivator during excess-fat loss, in the maintenance cycle you'll miss the excitement of weight reduction. You then have to find something else to motivate you and once the scales start going up you're in more trouble than you bargained for.

You can approach excess fat loss in two ways:

- You can start with the scales and pin all your hopes on them.
- Or you can start with the instructions and concentrate on **POD/POEx** control and behaviour and the scales will take care of themselves. To gauge your progress you can look at the true picture, by checking your Lipolytic Dimension or "fat points" instead of kilograms lost.

Never weigh yourself more than once a week if you're in the therapeutic process of losing your excess fat. Even that may be too much. And if you can't follow this simple rule, how can you expect to follow the regime associated with getting rid of your GOFES?

The 5th characteristic of successful weight maintainers:
Forget the scales during the Excess Fat Loss stage - Stage 2 - concentrate on your prescribed instructions.

Normal fat percentage

Unless it is your aim to be within the normal fat percentage range, you will not really be in Optimum Functional Health. In other words, you have to lose enough excess fat to get into the normal fat percentage range for your gender.

"Doctor, I cannot weigh what I weighed 30 years ago. People will think I am silly."

How sad it is that we live in a society where it is expected that we get fatter as we grow older. If your fat percentage was normal 30 years ago, this is what you should strive for now, even if you don't quite get there.

Why is it so?

Lean people have healthier metabolisms. All the metabolic defects caused by GOFES *only* revert back to *normal* in the normal fat percentage range. If you only lose some fat you will only gain some of the benefits. Do you want it all or just a little? When it comes to Optimal Functional Health you should aim for HR/EC = ∞ as we discussed in Chapter 1.

Biological equilibrium is ONLY established in the normal fat percentage range. This is where you will be at your healthiest. Do you want to be less healthy and age faster?

Muscle to fat ratio is very important - ideally you should strive for more muscle and less fat. Muscles help burn fat. The more muscle you have, the easier it is to burn fat. Apart from being healthier, maintenance is just so much easier at normal body composition. Ironically, many of us care more about the health of our pets and cars than about our own health.

From a purely statistical perspective, maintenance is much easier if you fall within the NORMAL fat percentage range.

The top of the normal range can still be a bit plump for some people and the bottom of the range "too thin" for others. To a degree, you can choose what suits you best, however, it is always best to strive for the fat percentage you had as a young adult. Asians should aim for the lower end of the ranges.

You can weigh more than you were, provided...

Take note, we do not necessarily talk weight here. If you are female your fat percentage could have been 22 per cent at age 20, weighing 55kg. Now at the age of 48 you weigh 78kg, should you go back to 55kg? Not necessarily, but you should go back to about 22 per cent fat. You may have increased your muscle mass in the meantime and now 59kg will perhaps bring you to 22 per cent.

Some folks seem to be obsessed with a "fantasy weight" but that is all it is, a fantasy.

The 6th characteristic of successful weight maintainers:
Normal fat percentage range for your genetic body type.

Synopsis:

1. Scales are a useless excess fat loss instrument, but a good maintenance tool. The first step is to lock your scales away. You'll feel a lot better if you let your mirror do the talking.

2. Only weigh yourself on the days when everything goes wrong - the day is in any case spoiled.

3. Money loses value over time and kilograms gain value with successful excess fat loss.

4. Losing weight is not a behaviour. Understand the psychology of "weight loss".

5. The aim of GOFES treatment is to get you to lose excess fat until all excess fat has been eliminated, and then to keep it off. It's easier to do this than to balance the metabolic burden of having "some" excess fat.

6. Doctor says:
   "If you don't cheat when you eat;
   you won't wail on the scale".
   DR PETER LINDER

CHAPTER 11

DES CONTROL

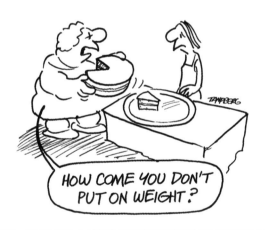

DES CONTROL

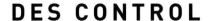

Most people would rather pray for forgiveness than fight temptation.

As Oscar Wilde said: "I can resist anything except temptation. The only way to get rid of temptation is to yield to it."

THE 23rd POUND

My appetite is my shepherd; I always want.
It maketh me to sit down and stuff myself.
It leadeth me to my refrigerator repeatedly.
It leadeth me in the path of Burger King for a Whopper.
It destroyeth my shape.
Yea, though I know I gaineth, I will not stop eating
For the food tasteth so good.
The ice cream and the cookies, they comfort me.
When the table is spread before me, it exciteth me
For I knoweth that I sooneth shall dig in.
As I filleth my plate continuously,
My clothes runneth smaller.
Surely bulges and pudgies shalt follow me all the days of my life
"And I shall be *pleasingly plump* forever."
ANONYMOUS

DES revisited

Demand Control (D) is in effect dealing with the Pain of Deprivation in the **DES** triangle.

How can you control your appetite for instance, toning down your inbuilt compulsion to eat?

Effort Control (E) will be mentioned only briefly here. How can you increase your physical activity for health and fat percentage control? Read on - when you get to Chapter 21 the issue of exercise is addressed in depth.

Supply Control (S) - managing your own food sources. In more drastic cases surgical intervention can be considered to shrink the stomach and physically restrict the intake.

Non-DES (Metabolic) - therapy techniques that do not fall strictly in the above categories. Some medications for instance stimulate fat burning and have nothing or little to do with Demand, Effort and Supply control.

*The various treatment techniques to manage **DES** don't always fall in just one category, but may overlap into another. Exercise, for example, falls into both Demand and Effort control. **To successfully manage GOFES a combination of <u>all</u> the DES and Non-DES categories need to be brought into play.***

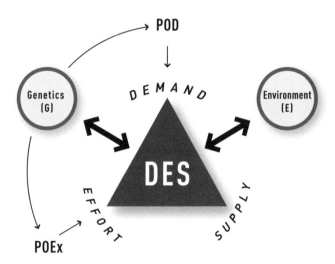

Demand management and control is aimed directly at **POD**. How can our body's insatiable *demand* to over-eat be controlled? Can **POD** indeed be managed?

Yes! Yes! Yes!

The surest and easiest way is to revert back to a scarce food Supply (**S**). This will *externally* enforce **POD** control for you. So, no matter how hungry you are, you have no choice. If it is not available to you in large quantities, you cannot over eat. Unfortunately, we do not live in a world of an *externally* controlled food supply and we have to learn how to *internally* control our own supply.

POD/POEx cannot be meek and weak and they are not - they are profoundly powerful, since they are essential to your very survival. For you to control these factors you too have to be ruthless - you cannot be meek and weak either. You will fail if you are. But given the right tools and a little practice, it's not that difficult.

However, complete control in an affluent society will require you to be obsessive. So remember, losing a battle or two is fine, as long as you win the war. You must learn to control **POD** if you want to lose your excess fat and keep it off.

A well off fat lady from an upmarket suburb was shopping in a chic shopping centre, when a beggar came up to her and said: "Madam, I have not eaten for four days." To which she replied: "I wish I had your willpower" and walked off.

This illustrates the **POD** phenomenon. The rich, over-fat lady can buy any food any time. Spurred on by **POD** she overeats and **GOFES** develops. She realises this and know she has to control her eating, *internally*, in the midst of plenty. For this she recognises she needs willpower. On the other hand the beggar does not have the money to buy food and in spite of the nagging pressures of **POD**, he cannot eat. His circumstances are *externally* controlled.

Unfortunately external enforcement is not an option for **POD** and Effort control - these are factors that you MUST manage yourself. Are you ready to accept this?

The following methods will assist you in controlling and managing **DES** and restraining **POD** - Mind over "platter."

Cognitive approach (Demand control)

This is about acquiring knowledge by use of reasoning, intuition, or perception and relating that knowledge to your thought processes.

It means you have to, *first of all*, have an *understanding* of *exactly* what the Pain of Deprivation is all about and the way it affects your body - understanding what actually drives us to eat and why. Forget about the "comfort eating", "non-hunger eating" stuff and anything else that doesn't take our genetic programming into account. It's better that you waste your fat energy rather than your mental energy!

You must have a true understanding, not just a fuzzy idea. Knowing what you are up against is paramount in controlling POD. If you are uncertain, review the chapter on POD now!

POD must be *confronted* or you will not be successful in controlling it. You must manage this yourself. Can you afford not to?

Various cognitive techniques can be used. A very frustrated patient of mine devised a very simple and effective technique. She was drawn like a magnet to the fridge to "treat" her **POD**. One mid-afternoon on another unscheduled excursion to the fridge, she got so distressed that she scribbled "**POD**" in lipstick on the "dreaded fridge" door.

Afterwards, on each subsequent impromptu foray to the fridge, she would see the lipstick POD - hesitate for a moment, and ask herself: "Am I here on legitimate business or is it POD driven?"

You can use all manner of different ways to adapt this technique to suit your own needs. It forced her to stop and think for a second. That's usually all you need to make the right decision.

POD - the mother of hunger, craving and appetite - lasts only three minutes at a time... just 180 seconds.

The first minute the cake will scream at you: **"EAT ME!"**

The second minute it will demand sternly: **"EAT ME!"**

and the third minute it will beg you meekly: "**EAT ME**...please...?"

When the sight of your favourite food triggers POD, it is designed to make you eat impulsively - right there and then. It is also intended to make you over eat - remember, under eating is incompatible with survival. Therefore, if you intellectually override the urge for three minutes it will leave you alone, especially if you then walk away from the food cue or trigger.

It works every time - just practice it.

Jossie, a 16 year old, developed GOFES after a complicated tonsillectomy at the age of six. I soon realised he wasn't a rocket scientist, but he knew what he wanted.

His main motivation for losing weight was that he wanted a "six pack" abdomen like a certain rock star he admired. About three weeks into the treatment we were at a stand still. I tried every trick in the book for another eight weeks to no avail and was ready to give up.

He was quite upset. "Doctor, why don't you just tell me what to eat? I wanna a six pack."

Then out of the blue a thought struck me.

"Jossie," I said, "from now on you can eat whatever you want, but before you stick anything in your mouth just ask yourself this question: is it ab or flab?"

I must have struck a chord, for his eyes lit up and for the next two weeks he and his mother phoned me a few times a day, wanting to know if particular foods were ab - for abdomen - or flab?"

Recently, when I saw him I estimated that he would have his "six pack" within the next six weeks.

Why did this mantra work so well for him?

First of all, it was simple. Secondly, it was linked to his goals of wanting a "six pack" abdomen. Additionally, it had an easy poetic ring and taught him in an indirect way about what was good to eat. There were no complicated instructions.

Why don't you create your own mantra? The sky is the limit.

POD - modus operandi

Understanding **POD's** modus operandi is essential.

The brain has various parts or levels, corresponding to the different parts of a computer by way of an analogy.

The *conscious brain* is the computer screen. What you are conscious of appears on the screen and is visible to you. However, on the hard drive there are large amounts of information that can be imported onto the screen if necessary. This is the *sub-conscious* brain. You can be made conscious of it if necessary. Thoughts, instincts, memories and images constantly go back and forth between the conscious and sub-conscious.

What distinguishes us from animals is that we have an *intellectual or reasoning brain*. In computer terms, this is the person controlling the computer.

Then there's the *spiritual brain*.

To eat is the strongest survival instinct that we have, designed to save the individual from extinction. The next strongest instinct is reproduction and is designed to save the species from extinction. These two instincts virtually compel all our actions and behaviours, directly and indirectly. If a species does not engage in both it will not survive.

Lets look at the following illustration:

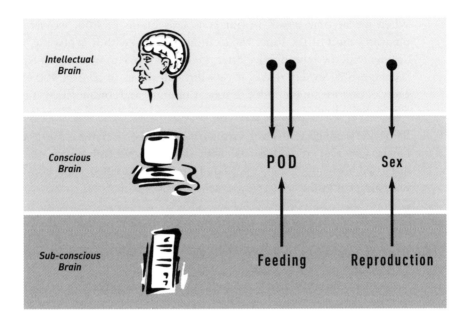

The main three brain areas are depicted in the above illustration.

At the bottom is the subconscious ("hard drive"). Next up is the conscious brain ("monitor"). Next is the intellectual brain ('the controlling person"). Higher up is the spiritual mind. Deeply imbedded in our subconscious brain are our two most important basic instincts - *feeding and reproduction*. We get reminded of them from time to time as they make their presence felt in the conscious brain. We then become aware and conscious of them as manifestations of **POD** and a **SEX DRIVE**.

As soon as animals such as dogs, become consciously aware of their reproductive urges, they tend to give expression to it, right there and then. Even in the most public of places. On the other hand, when we, as humans, get a sudden sexual desire in public, we do not engage in it there and then. It is illegal and not appropriate. Our *intellectual brains* kick into action reminding us of the consequences - we are civilised after all. We can think and reason on balance.

In this way it is quite easy for most humans to control their reproductive urges in public places, especially when sober.

While we can generally control our sexual urge, remember it's survival that is our primary mechanism and controlling our eating urges is another story.

When we become aware in our conscious brains of **POD**, we are caught unawares most of the time. The technique to deal with it is just the same as dealing with the reproductive drive, except you have to work much harder to accomplish it. Society makes it very difficult for us to control **POD**. Around every corner we are reminded of food. Culturally and commercially it is virtually forced into us.

Being the strongest survival instinct we possess, we have a battle on our hands. However, if you persist with the cognitive techniques that we've discussed you should, over a period of time, be astounded at the control you will gain over **POD**.

Keep practising. Just say "NO... NO" when you have to!

"The more I say NO the better I feel."
ANONYMOUS

Philosophy - Demand control

It is critical for you to alter your attitude and philosophy towards food deprivation. If you don't, you have no hope of managing it. When you feel deprived you should be grateful for it, in fact you should celebrate. *Unless* deprivation is associated with famine and or malnutrition, it is the best thing that can happen to boost your health.

Why is deprivation *bad* for you?

It is only ever bad for you if it is associated with malnutrition or famine. For any other reason it can only be *very good* for you.

- Hungry - wanting to eat, even if you don't need to eat
- Hunger - lack of food that can lead to sickness or death
- Starve - can weaken the body or cause death from a lack of food.

With a good quality therapeutic fat loss program, you may be hungry, but you will not be starving or suffer from hunger.

Why is deprivation *good* for you?

It is proof that you are alive! As long as you are alive and kicking you will experience the Pain of Deprivation. Accept it. Dead people don't feel hungry.

Deprivation is excellent for your metabolism. In fact, it is the single most important thing you can do for your metabolism. Nothing else improves it like deprivation. Only during times of hunger and deprivation can your metabolism do some housekeeping that is impossible when food is over-plentiful. We are not meant to constantly eat. Your body needs time to detoxify, burn some fat and give our insulin and sugar levels a change to re-synchronise. It is during this housekeeping phase that the body slows down the aging process.

For the first time in history we now have food on tap. The fridge is never further than 30 seconds away. We are in a constant state of assimilating and metabolising food of some sort.

The French and Japanese typically live longer than most races - traditionally they don't eat in between meals.

Attending a conference in Paris I met with a French doctor for breakfast. The conference wasn't due to start until early afternoon and so we went for a walk around Paris. By 11 o'clock I was quite hungry (**POD**) and wanted a cup of coffee. The aromas of freshly baked bread, pastry and coffee were extremely depalgenic (hunger stimulating). We ordered coffee and I was looking at the cakes. My colleague indicated he didn't want anything to eat.

"Aren't you hungry? I asked. "Yes I'm hungry, but what's the point? I'm going to have lunch in two hours!" was his reply.

The French are perhaps the leanest people in the industrial world. Unbeknown to the French doctor he was doing his metabolism a favour by keeping it hungry for longer. I spiked my insulin and denied myself the metabolic advantages of deprivation.

During earlier times if a person felt hungry (**POD**), he had to go and catch a chicken, slaughter it, pluck its feathers out - one by one, disembowel it, clean it, cut it up, marinate it in spices and then cook it. (Nowadays, all these processes are commercially taken care of.) This took lots of time and in the meantime the body was kept hungry. During these deprived time periods, metabolic processes kick into action that could not have taken place if the person was in not in a state of deprivation.

The body needs to be put in reverse gear on a regular basis. Taking in food and assimilating it requires a different set of activities and metabolic processes than cleansing and rest. During these fasting times our metabolisms get a real health boost.

With our constantly available fast food we kill off **POD** as soon as we become aware of any of its manifestations. The antidote for depalgia is to use the depalgesic, which is food. Eating is an appetite suppressant.

Patients who complain of feeling bloated are simply eating *too often*. The digestive processes need rest just like your muscles.

While we are not designed to "like" these feelings of deprivation, you should be grateful for them nonetheless. How can anyone lose weight without feeling hungry? It comes with the territory. It is proof to you that your weight loss efforts are working. In fact, during these times, your fat burning is *actually accelerated*. By the way, feelings of food deprivation are also good for people who are not trying to lose weight.

Behavioural modification (Demand and Supply control)

POD can also be controlled with behavioural modification techniques. How you eat, when you eat and certain behaviours associated with eating can be habits. How you implement these habits and behaviours go a long way in controlling **POD**.

We'll talk later about behavioural modification techniques. Suffice to know at this stage that certain eating behaviours can play right into the hands of **POD** and need to be modified if you want to control it.

BAT - Behavioural Aversion Therapy

If POD is very menacing, BAT can be a very useful technique. If you "imagine" that the piece of cheesecake you want to eat has mould on it, or the chef sneezed over it, the thought is usually enough to stop you wanting to eat it. Remember, you only have to keep temptation at bay for three minutes. With practise, this technique can be quite useful and strong.

The variations that you can apply are endless. You don't have to be overly dramatic. Just image the cheesecake to be full of additives like artificial vanilla - an old remedy for killing head lice! Or perhaps picture yourself being fat all over again - "once on the lips, forever on the hips".

I find that women in general do better with BAT than men. Maybe they have better imaginations. Nevertheless, the technique can be very useful for both sexes.

Fascinating psychology

There are instances of people who subconsciously suppress their survival instincts, even in the face of grave danger.

The following story illustrates this point. A five-year-old boy in America developed type-one diabetes and had to inject himself with insulin up to five times per day. He knew that if he didn't balance his insulin and blood sugars he would die.

As an adult he found himself on death row. For his last request he asked for his insulin and blood sugar test kit. He had completely divorced his diabetes from the rest of his life, even when facing execution.

I have sometimes noticed that people can become obsessive about maintaining their health and normal fat percentage, excluding other influences on their lives.

Exercise - Demand and Effort Control

Effort Control - exercise - has both indirect and direct **POD** controlling effects that fall under the category of Effort Control. More on this later, but regular physical activity has a wonderful affect on our ability to control POD. The operative word is "regular". I observe this every day with successful patients. Patients who exercise habitually do not necessarily lose weight faster, but they are much more successful in keeping the weight off. There appears to be a connection between regular exercise and controlling appetite (POD).

Nutrition - Demand control and Non-DES

Particular foods can be said to be more depalgenic - appetite stimulating - than others. So it makes more sense that you concentrate on the latter. Good chefs know instinctively what food and combinations stimulate appetite. They will be complimented for it.

High-energy, dense foods play havoc with insulin levels and you feel hungrier more often. High fibre and good sources of protein are much more filling and satisfying. A lack of some nutrients like protein, chromium and zinc can make it more difficult to control POD, pointing to the need for a nutritionally sound diet if you are to be successful.

Stress management - Demand control

We each have differing stress thresholds that vary from time-to-time depending on the circumstances. If your stress threshold is high you'll find it easier to control and override POD. If your stress threshold is lowered, POD can sneak up on you. Preventing your threshold from being lowered is a very important tool in controlling POD and we'll discuss stress management in Chapter 23.

Medication - Demand control and Non-DES

At one stage I was very much against using pharmacological depalgesics, more commonly known as appetite suppressants. However, over the years I have found them very useful and safe for a proportion of patients. Used properly they do work. They will not eliminate **POD**, but they do dull hunger and appetite, making it easier to control. A word of warning however: anything that completely blocks **POD** is incompatible with life.

The use of medication is controversial and it only serves to suppress appetite as long as you are taking the drug.

Used properly, pharmacological depalgesics are a safe long-term solution to the problem. They should always be prescribed by a physician experienced in their use and should only be taken in *conjunction* with other GOFES control approaches. For some patients I find them very useful during the maintenance stage.

Drastic measures - Supply and Demand Control

A point may be reached where a combination of all these techniques is repeatedly unsuccessful. This may call for direct Supply Control, where the supply of food is externally regulated.

A patient can be put in hospital or kept on a deserted island where the food supply is controlled - in the same way we control the weight of my daughter's pug "Pretzel". She gets a certain amount of food, which is controlled by us - and that's it. However, these methods are not very practical with humans, because they have to be reintroduced to society at some stage.

Supply Control may call for some form of surgery such as gastric bypass or gastric banding. In spite of the fact that the patient cannot consume more than a certain amount of food, they also report reduced appetite after such surgery. This is probably due to a hormone in the stomach lining called ghrelin. I find these treatments quite useful for a very small proportion of patients, but they are a last resort when all else has failed. There are risks and these should be discussed with the surgeon.

Acceptance - Non-DES

If all of the above fail repeatedly then accept your condition and join a "fat is beautiful" club until some revolutionary treatment comes along that can cure GOFES. Very occasionally I see patients who fall in this category. Some have gone on with their lives and appeared reasonably contented. Their Polar Bear status is just too extreme to control with any known methods.

Synopsis:

1. All categories of DES - Demand to eat, Effort and Supply control - need to be applied simultaneously to successfully manage GOFES.

2. Some approaches have effects across more than one category.

3. **DESM**

D Demand POD	E Effort POEx	S Supply	M Metabolic Non-DES
Cognitive	Cognitive	Cognitive	
Philosophy/Attitude	Philosophy/Attitude	Philosophy/Attitude	
Behavioural modification	Behavioural modification	Behavioural modification	
Exercise	Exercise		Exercise
Nutrition		Nutrition	Nutrition
Medications			Medications
Drastic measures	Drastic measures	Drastic measures	
			Acceptance

4. Appetite suppressants are an option for some patients, but only as an integral part of a formal treatment program.

5. **Ab or Flab?**

Refrain, restrain...
and use your brain
to combat the pain
of POD.

If you don't, you're a sod
and your arteries may clot
and your body will rot.
Stop being an if-not.

Use mantras as part of your strategy.

6. You must have a ruthless attitude in dealing with **POD**. It is a brute survival force and does not respond to a softly-softly approach. Why should it, after all its function is to keep you alive. It is human nature to think wisely and act foolishly. This is especially true when it comes to basic instincts like **POD**.

"There is no memory with less satisfaction in it, than the memory of some temptation we resisted."
JAMES B. CABELL

7. The following techniques facilitate **DES** control:

   a. Cognitive control
   b. Philosophy and attitude
   c. Behavioural modification
   d. Exercise
   e. Nutrition
   f. Stress management
   g. Medication
   h. Drastic measures
   i. Acceptance (if all else fails).

8. "Some live to eat - others eat to live" I believe we are all the same: we all eat to live and live to eat. We have to eat to survive (POD driven). We get pleasure in eating (pleasure of eating - POE driven). We are simply designed that way for survival. If you come to terms with it you have already made a big dent in controlling POD.

9. *What is the science behind POD?*
   It is the system covering *all* the mechanisms and methods available to the body to give us an *incentive to eat for survival*. Many building blocks of the physiology of the different parts of which POD is made up, *still remains elusive*. However, we know there are areas in the hypothalamus involved in addition to, neuropeptide Y, serotonin, amphetamine, opioid receptor blockers. leptin, ghrelin, CCK, OXM, GLP-1 *and many others also implicated*.

CHAPTER 12

MENTAL ATTITUDE

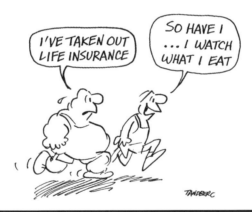

MENTAL ATTITUDE

"The greatest revolution of our generation is the discovery that human beings, by changing the inner attitudes of their minds, can change the outer aspects of their lives."
WILLIAM JAMES

Nobody can lose your weight for you. Your success depends entirely on you. Help is available and can be of great value, but in the end it is *you*. As we've discussed, in the past **external** factors helped early man to control **GOFES**. In today's environment you have to control it **internally**.

With today's copious supply of food, controlling our intake isn't easy. To be successful you need to change your mind-set. To use the cliché, we cannot change a lot of things in life, but we can change our attitude. The latter is essential to the long-term control of **DES** (Demand, Effort and Supply).

Speaking recently with a person from Crete, I mentioned to him that his people live longer and are perhaps the healthiest people on earth.

He chipped back: "That was before they became affluent."

It really says it all. **DES** has changed our internal ability to control our food intake.

Expectations

Our expectations should always be reasonably realistic. You might want stage two of the weight loss program to be over and done with as soon as possible, but it won't happen overnight.

You perform your own miracles. Be patient - results takes time.

Let's use a little common sense in promoting the premise "You can be anything you want to be."

"No matter how much he aches for it to happen, the 90kg six foot three inch, 16-year-old should probably forget his dream of becoming a jockey."
FRANK WALSH

Attitude

"If you find a path with no obstacles, it probably doesn't lead anywhere."
FRANK CLARK

If you are a nothing, it's because you do nothing and the latter can be hard work. If you are negative you will get negative results. If you are positive you will get positive results. It may be that you are negative in disposition. If so, you can improve your attitude tremendously by positive self-talk. It is an acquired skill. Once you get results, these results by themselves will motivate you.

Bob in the following photo (left) had already lost 47kg (104lb) when the photo on the left was taken.

Bob found it very hard to pass urine, since his abdomen was too heavy to hold away with the one hand, while using the other hand to direct the flow. It meant he was wetting his abdomen whenever he went to the toilet. He demonstrated to me once what he had to do to not wetting himself. He would

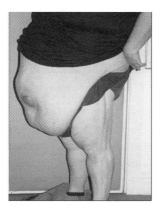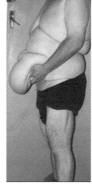

Bob

go to a wall at the back of the house, leaning with one hand forward against the wall so that his heavy abdominal area could pendulum away from the rest of his body. Then he would lift one leg backwards like a dog, grab his penis with the other hand and direct the flow below the kicked back leg.

He loved going to movies, but he could not due to his

disability. One day I saw him standing anxiously at the reception desk wanting to see me. It was a particularly busy day and I asked if he could wait until his appointment the following Friday.

When I called in the next patient he was still waiting. Then after the third patient I called him in. When I asked him what I could do for him he said: "Doctor please take a photo of this - I can go to the movies now without drenching myself."

With his weight loss his abdomen was now light enough to hold it with one hand so he could pass urine. It may sound like a bizarre incident, but unless a person has been in such a position it can sometimes be difficult to understand that something like this can make a person so excited. As they say, we shouldn't judge unless we've walked a mile in the other person's shoes. After this Bob was all fired up. It changed his attitude and there was no stopping him in his commitment to overcoming GOFES.

Make sure you work hard and smart to get the initial results, because from then on it will be a whole lot easier.

Be Ruthless

You cannot be meek and weak in dealing with the brute strength survival instincts of **POD** and **POEx**. You need to be a Pit Bull to fight a Pit Bull.

Moira

I like most people I meet - it is just my nature. In spite of this, every 10 years or so I come across someone I do not like. Moira was such a person. She was 21-years-old when I met her. She was spoilt rotten and, quite frankly, had an obnoxious personality. I even diagnosed her as a borderline personality disorder.

Moira was constantly trying to tell me how I should treat her. She was one of my most challenging patients and progress was very slow. After what was an eternity she eventually lost 15kg (33lb). Then a surprising thing happened, the next 18kg (40lb) went at record-breaking speed.

I put her on maintenance, quietly convinced that she would regain the weight in a few months. Reluctantly I gave her the "No-Belly Prize". To my surprise, six months later she was still keeping her excess fat perfectly at bay. A year later her weight was still under control and I presented her with the "Diploma of Maintenance" and told her it was not necessary to come and see me again unless she had problems.

Six months later she made an appointment and I was convinced she had regained all her lost excess fat.

She merely wanted me to weigh her and her weight was perfect. Every six months for the next three years she came to be re-weighed, each time with the same result.

The last time I saw her as a patient she had been on maintenance for four years and I told her: "I didn't like you in the beginning and I never thought you'd ever lose all your excess fat and keep it off. What's your secret?"

She looked at me nonchalantly and replied: "I thought you'd never ask". From her wallet she took a card with a variation of my logo drawn on it and the words...

Nothing tastes as good as thin feels.

"Doctor since losing this weight nothing can *ever* taste as good as I feel now. I was miserable when I was fat and I'm not surprised you didn't like me - nobody did. I play tennis now and I'm engaged. When my fiancé and I go out for a meal and I think I am starting to eat too much, I just look at this card. Nowadays I don't physically look at it so much, but I always carry it with me for good luck."

I just sat there and listened.

"I realise that when I was 21 I was just a spoilt brat. I was scared and insecure. All I knew was to be defensive and unpleasant. I can never go back to that again because nothing tastes as good as thin feels."

It became clear to me, in hindsight, why after 15kg of weight loss the rest just melted off her like a hot knife through butter. She saw results that inspired her to escape from her misery.

That was 15 years ago and Moira and I have always stayed in touch. She and her husband were house guests at one stage and were some of the most pleasant guests I've ever had. Moira has two lovely boys and always maintained her weight loss. Whenever she phones she greets me with the words: "Nothing tastes as good as thin feels".

With Moira's permission my clinic uses the adaptation she drew of my logo - an ecstatic looking person escaping the prison of **GOFES**. Slimming indeed sets you free.

The 7th characteristic of successful weight maintainers: Developed the right attitude.

Burn your fat bridges behind you. Set yourself targets - for instance when you drop below 100kg (220lb), make a pledge that you'll never ever top 100kg again.

I give my patients 100 per cent, but I expect 100 per cent in return.

Don't procrastinate! Do it tomorrow.

When is the best time to start?

Never. The time is never right. **POD** will make sure of that. There is always going to be your spouse's birthday, then afterwards a wedding.

POD is not designed to care for you in the midst of plenty - it's there for your survival in times of scarcity. Look at it objectively - take POD out of the equation - why wait until it's "Diet or Die?"

The best time to start is already gone. That was when you started developing **GOFES**. The second best time to start is always NOW. It may be your last chance.

Synopsis:

1. Start NOW in controlling your *GOFES*. If you wait until the iron is hot, you will be waiting for a long time. The iron always tends to become cold again. *The best time to start is when you don't feel quite ready to start.*

2. If you are negative you will get negative results. If you are positive you will get positive results. Feel confident in your ability to control **GOFES**.

3. "Nothing tastes as good as thin feels". Nothing feels as bad as excess blubbery flab feels.

4. Strong is he who forces his actions to control his thoughts. Weak is he who permits his thoughts to control his actions.

CHAPTER 13

GIMMICKS, MANIPULATIONS, MYTHS AND QUACKS

Never Before in Australia

As featured by the B.B.C. and highly acclaimed by the British

The Honest-to-Goodness Slimming Plan

Powerful New Slimming System that quite simply does all the work for you!

Now internationally respected behavioural researcher Christopher Roberts F.E.S.H. finally unmasks the hidden secrets that weight loss experts don't want you to know!

The Radically Simple Slimming System with an Amazing 90% Success Rate

GIMMICKS, MANIPULATIONS, MYTHS AND QUACKS

"They told me I was gullible... and I believed them."
ANONYMOUS

"Did you hear about the new diet miracle? Within two weeks you can lose $800."
ANONYMOUS

Treating **GOFES** is as much an art as a science. It does not however mean that the "art" should be misleading and fraudulent. Advice is a dangerous gift, be cautious about receiving and giving it.

"Doc, I can't stop singing 'The green, green grass of home'."
"That sounds like the Tom Jones syndrome."
"Is it common?"
"Well... It's not unusual..."

It would not be unusual for anybody to be conned by the mis- and dis-information* that is spread about **GOFES**, diets and lifestyle. It is a multi billion-dollar fraud industry. Why the fraud industry exists is open to conjecture, but perhaps one of the reasons is that the medical profession neglected this disease by placing it in the "too hard basket". The vacuum was then filled by those who identified obesity as a lucrative area to exploit.

*Misinformation is where a person is given erroneous information, but in good faith. Disinformation is deliberately fed information where the giver knows full well it is not the truth. *Both are dangerous.*

We are like sitting ducks when it comes to the aggressive marketing of these people who are literally "living off the fat of the land". What makes their task easier is that the target group is vulnerable and very susceptible to this type of promotion.

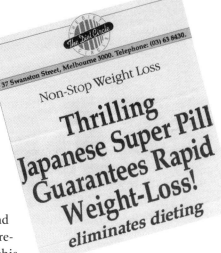

37 Swanston Street, Melbourne 3000. Telephone: (03) 63 8430.

Non-Stop Weight Loss

Thrilling Japanese Super Pill Guarantees Rapid Weight-Loss! eliminates dieting

Exploiting the Obese

- **What is the biggest fear of a person wanting to lose weight?**

Deprivation - **POD** and the restraint and discipline involved to control it. It is therefore hardly surprising that much of this advertising proclaims words to the effect: "Eat all you like and still lose weight" or "Eliminates dieting".

Claims that people can lose weight without deprivation are a prime example of disinformation.

- **Once the deprivation issue has been settled, what is the next thing a fat person likes to hear?**

"Guarantees rapid weight loss".

Instinctively you know you are not going to lose weight without deprivation of some sort, therefore sorting out your problem *rapidly* by not prolonging the agony is a very attractive option.

- **What else is dreaded by a prospective flab loser?**

"It's not a diet. No it's not *exercise*". The reluctance to face up to POEx - the Pain of Exercise - is exploited.

- **The psychology of being individualised**

The weight loss marketers try to give an air of individuality to their products, targeting our need to feel special. People are told they are a specific "body type" and need to eat only certain foods. The facts are that we all need basic nutrition with proteins, vitamins and the like and we can only lose weight if we are put in negative caloric balance, irrespective of body type.

Some people may have food sensitivities or allergies and they do have to avoid certain foods, but it is not their body type. The body type diets have been around for many years and have not done anything to reduce the

GOFES epidemic. Blood type is another gimmick to make people feel special. Blood is taken for very vague reasons and a diet is prescribed - it's pseudo-science.

The approaches vary in sophistication from gender, body types, blood types, personality types, to the spiritual and the bizarre.

Gimmicks

Most diets and gimmicks use dietary manipulations to make a person eat less. Some of these manipulations are good and others can be just plain dangerous. Eating certain food, at only certain times, is a way of eating less. One day you can only eat a certain group of food and the other day another, and so forth. To be charitable, this sort of manipulation may have value in the short term.

Association

A very common technique is to associate a famous celebrity's name with the diet or product. Retail aggressively - and it sells.

Choice of words

Dramatic adjectives are used. "Powerful", "Honest-to-Goodness", "Thousands of people have used Fat-Off daily". The naive and gullible are sucked in, and to a degree we're all a little naive and a little gullible.

Success rate

The success rates of these programs and products are advertised at 90 to 100 per cent. Who wants to pay for something unless it has a very high success rate? Fact: successful weight loss is measured over a five-year period and I've yet to see anything that has a success rate of 90 to 100 per cent over this time. Look around you - do you see a 90 per cent lean population?

Something based on science

Numerous metabolic pathways and studies are quoted - perhaps suggesting that a certain enzyme can be blocked using this and that product.

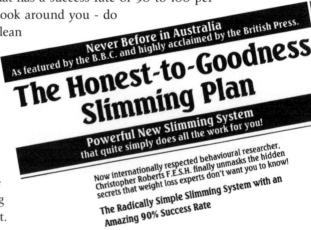

Never Before in Australia and highly acclaimed by the British Press.

As featured by the B.B.C.

The Honest-to-Goodness Slimming Plan

Powerful New Slimming System
that quite simply does all the work for you!

Now internationally respected behavioural researcher, Christopher Roberts F.E.S.H. finally unmasks the hidden secrets that weight loss experts don't want you to know!

The Radically Simple Slimming System with an Amazing 90% Success Rate

On the face of it, it makes scientific sense, but survival is profoundly strong and is not going to be conquered by blocking a pathway here and there.

It's easy to be blinded by science, but you only lose weight if you have eaten less. Talks of essential fatty acids and nutritional supplements make sense, but most of the rest is just hocus pocus.

Something new

Being human, we're attracted to the "latest", "newest" and the "revolutionary". If it can be promised: "Never before in this country", "Brand new research" or "The latest and greatest", a fat person will always be interested. A person losing weight and then regaining it does not like to repeat the same diet. *They want something new.* This is exploitation. Fact: if a treatment has worked successfully and safely in the past, it is best to go back to it. Scientific principles don't change.

Money back guarantee

Instinctively you know that the latest diet or product is not what it is cracked up to be. You may have been caught before, but human nature hopes it will work this time. It is like the definition of insanity - a person keeps on doing the same thing over and over, expecting different outcomes.

Wouldn't it be nice if you could at least get your money back in case it is ineffective? Hence the all-too-familiar marketing offer of a money back guarantee. What these commercial predators know is that less than two per cent of customers will ask for their money back, even if it is a total flop for 99 per cent of the purchasers. In some instances of course, these snake oil salespeople will simply disappear into thin air five minutes after launching and selling their product.

Block, Burn & Lose 1,000 Calories A Day - Guaranteed!

Jan Barron was overweight and desperate to lose weight. With just four months to go before her wedding she discovered the secret of the century... the BBL-1000! She shed 30kg (65lb) and five dress sizes in just nine weeks! Imagine losing that much weight, that quickly, without ever going hungry!

Here's why BBL1000 is so effective: This wonder-working tablet actually blocks sugar, carbohydrates and fat that would normally attach to your body. It helps your metabolism to burn faster and more efficiently. 100 per cent safe, with no unwanted side effects! Guaranteed results.

Key words in the above: guaranteed, secret, without going hungry, effective, 100 per cent safe...

Waiting in waiting rooms is not my strong point. On one occasion, to pass the time, I looked at all the magazines. At one point I noticed a full-page advertisement of a woman who lost 75kg (165lb) in a very short timeframe. Instinctively I knew it was impossible to lose this amount of fat so quickly. Allegedly, all she had done was to add a teaspoon of the advertised powder to a glass of fruit juice in the mornings and she was then able to "eat all she liked" for the rest of the day while "melting away".

As they say, if it sounds too good to be true, it probably is.

When it comes to **GOFES** it is too good to be true, but it must be true because it appeared in print. Whatever is in print, on TV or the radio must be true (yeah, right). There were even before and after photos to prove it. This was when I realised that she was one of my patients! What was more, I even took the photos!

When I got back to the clinic I looked in her file and noticed she had only lost 60kg (123 lb) and it took her much longer than claimed in the magazine.

A few months later we bumped into each other in the street and I remarked that I'd seen her in the advertisement. At this she turned bright red and said shyly: "Doctor, they gave me $15,000 for the photos."

This was in the early eighties - it was probably more like $50,000 in today's money. I don't have a problem with her being paid to advertise her weight loss, but I don't like the idea of other **GOFES**-suffering Polar Bears being mislead.

Miracles do happen

When Russell came to the clinic he weighed 212kg (466lb).

Ten months later he'd lost 100kg (220lb).

Russell lost a further 26kg (57lb), that is a total of 126kg (277lb). It took him 14 months in total and he has been keeping it off for over a year now.

With Russell's weight and fat loss graph we had to glue two pages together because it couldn't all be charted on a single page!

It is interesting to note that he was quite lean as a young man.

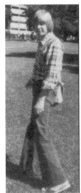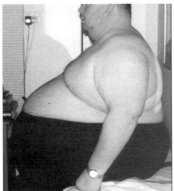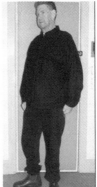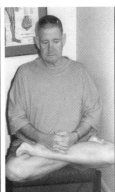

Russell

Russell was recently stopped at a routine police "booze-bus". When he had to show his driving licence he had some explaining to do. Luckily he had his before and after photos with him.

If you can't understand it it's probably nonsense

Numerous weight loss scams are perpetrated on a daily basis. Some of the unsophisticated ones are not as common these days, but there's "a new kid" on the block that blinds you with science. It refers to biochemical pathways that are "disordered" in a **GOFES** person, and uses scientific language that most people have never heard of. And, of course, they have products to solve the problem!

Good try, but in spite of all their efforts, unless POD is confronted and seen as something that can only be cured with a negative caloric balance, it won't work... no matter how many studies the would-be perpetrators quote.

"Have you wondered WHY people eat too much? Proper appetite control mechanisms are designed to prevent chronic ingestion of calories beyond your metabolic needs. Exciting new research has recently..." "What are the metabolic defects that cause excess fat mass?" Etc... etc...

I would personally like to know what "mechanisms" they know of that *"prevent chronic ingestion of calories beyond your metabolic needs".* Sorry, we are not designed that way. The "metabolic defects that cause excess fat" is another furphy. For Polar Bears, putting on excess fat is not a "metabolic defect". It is a normal survival mechanism. I do wish some of these commercial-driven things worked... they would be the answer to many problems.

Admittedly, some of these so-called "metabolic things" can play a role, albeit a small one. Even a person with an under active thyroid will only lose about 8kg (18lb) maximum if the problem is corrected. For the rest, only eating less will reduce your weight.

Fact: no matter what the biochemistry, we are genetically blueprinted to over eat and we do not have mechanisms to control how much we should eat for our individual metabolic needs - not even Humming Birds. We only know when we have eaten too much and never when we have had just enough.

"It is twice as hard to crush a half-truth as a whole lie."
AUSTIN O'MALLEY

Synopsis:

1. Don't be conned.

2. **POD, POEx, DES** and your Polar Bear status will always come into play and have to be dealt with for successful **GOFES** management and control. There is no other way. Anything else, at best, will only facilitate this.

3. *"Life is a system of half-truths and lies. Opportunistic, convenient evasion."*
LANGSTON HUGHES

CHAPTER 14

THE SCIENCE BEHIND LOSING EXCESS FAT

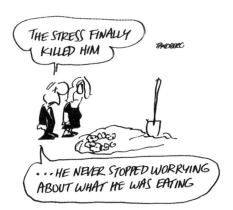

THE SCIENCE BEHIND LOSING EXCESS FAT

It is so simple and we all know it. When it is realised, we ask: "Is THAT it? We have been so conditioned that there is some secret involved that we are shocked by the simplicity of it all.

A physical law needs to apply in order to lose any excess fat at all. There is no other way. This law is: **The Law of Thermodynamics**.

It is mentioned only for the sake of completeness. You can forget about the name as such. How it operates in fat loss can be explained in the following way. The lady in the illustration stands on the scale with a worried look on her face. She has fallen victim to GOFES and its consequences. Her doctor has told her she has gallstones, diabetes, high cholesterol and osteoarthritis. She also has a lump in her breast, which has not yet been investigated. She feels bloated, uncomfortable and has low self-esteem. Additionally, she is on a cupboard full of prescription drugs. She is very worried about her condition and there is an urgency to do something about it.

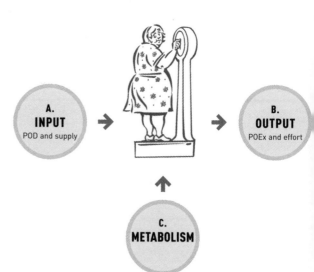

How can she get rid of this over-fat (**OF**) and improve the consequences of **GOFES**?

She must somehow be put in negative calorie balance in line with her individual Polar Bear metabolism - the number of calories coming in must be less than the number she is burning. The difference will be consumed from her stored energy, which is fat. Her body will consume her own excess-fat as part of her body's food requirement.

A. Input - *Supply and Demand Control*

Our example can control her input of food calories or fuel to the point where her input or supply is less than her output - or effort - of calories. But, the type of calories is also important - they must be nutritional calories.

Input < Output (less in than out)

Our example should go on a deficit-diet to put herself in negative caloric balance. This will of course bring her in conflict with **POD**.

"A successful diet requires an open mind and a closed mouth".

Silverware for dieting!

B. Output - *Effort Control*

Her output of energy can also be increased to exceed her input of calories.

Output > Input (more out than in)

In plain language - it means she must exercise, and lots of it if that is the only way she wants to attack the problem. This will bring her in conflict with **POEx** - the pain of exercise.

"Every time I feel like exercise, I lie down, until the feeling goes away."
WINSTON CHURCHILL

C. Metabolism - *Non-DES Control*

Our example's metabolism could also be transformed to be less efficient in its ability to store excess fat - metabolic manipulation. Just as a Humming Bird is genetically less effective than a Polar Bear in storing excess fat. Being able to change our metabolism to behave more like that of a Humming bird is of course, the answer to every GOFES victim's dreams. The outcome: no **POD** or **POEx**, just effortless fat loss on demand.

Very efficient *Less efficient*

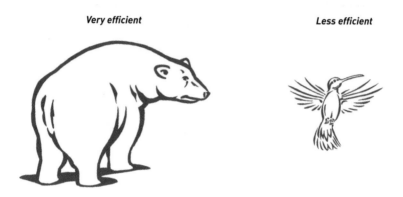

This will probably happen one day, but not in the foreseeable future. Survival is very complex and medication to achieve such change can be fraught with danger in the longer term. The intricate survival mechanisms that control what we are not going to be easily redirected without our bodies objecting. It is better to bite the bullet, deal with **POD** and **POEx** and become health conscious.

In summary

Supply (S) must be limited to decrease the input of calories. **Effort (E)** must be increased at the same time to expend calories. Additionally, methods need to be used to overcome **POD** and **POEx** and the metabolism needs to be manipulated to behave more *inefficiently*, like a Hummingbird.

For your own sake, please don't let anyone convince you that there's any other way.

Weight and Pregnancy

The misconceptions and disinformation about weight gain, or loss, in pregnancy is enough to drive any pregnant woman to distraction. "You have to eat for two" suggests you need to eat for two adults. It then becomes open slather to give **POD** free reign, harming not only the expectant mother but also the unborn child.

During pregnancy the body becomes a bit more efficient in storing fat for obvious reasons. Even Humming Birds become more efficient. During primitive times this was a desired adaptation. However these days, with our plentiful supply of food, it's easy for this to turn into overeating leading to excess fat and diabetes.

Midwives are usually horrified if mothers-to-be cut down on their food. Over-reducing your intake and eating rubbish can never be good, however you can cut down sensibly. You should gain between 7kg (16lb) and 12kg (26lb) during pregnancy - no more, no less - unless you are expecting twins or more!

In fact, if you are quite fat when you fall pregnant, you can cautiously lose weight for the first two trimesters, but not the last trimester. Study the graph. The light grey line is the minimum you should gain and the black line the maximum. The dark grey line is the average for western women. As you can see, during the first month of pregnancy you should not gain any weight at all - a fertilised egg does not weigh anything on the bathroom scales.

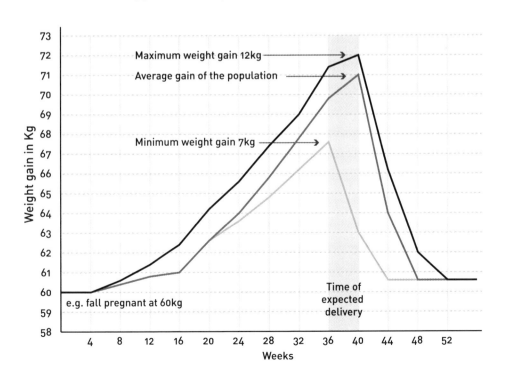

Even after three months you should gain a maximum of 1.5kg (3.5lb). Not much. Some women take off like rockets and gain in the order of 30kg (66lb) during pregnancy. Once you have delivered the baby, you should be back at your pre-pregnancy weight within six weeks. It is however, quite natural to have a permanent weight gain of 1/2 kg (1lb) after each pregnancy, but only for the first three children.

An interesting observation

I have noticed that women who gain too much weight during pregnancy are upgrading their Polar Bear status by doing so. Afterwards they end up with a worse **GOFES** problem than before.

Conversely, women who control their fat percentage during pregnancy downgrade their Polar Bear status, having less of a GOFES tendency afterwards. Think about it.

Synopsis:

1. The law of thermodynamics needs to apply if you want to lose weight. In other words, you need to be put in a state of negative caloric balance whereby your input is decreased by supply and **POD** control, your output increased by effort and **POEx** control and your metabolism made less efficient in storing fat in order to keep it off.

2. Don't be fooled by smooth talking uninformed "experts". There is basically only one way. Half measures do not work.

3. *"My doctor advised me to give up those intimate dinners for four, unless there were three other people eating with me."*
ANONYMOUS

CHAPTER 15

STAGE 2 MEAL PLANS FOR EXCESS FAT LOSS

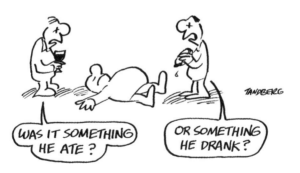

STAGE 2 MEAL PLANS FOR EXCESS FAT LOSS

"I may be fat, but you are ugly and I can lose weight."

Diet-induced weight loss may increase the risk of cardiovascular disease. To minimize this risk it is essential that nutrient ratios be maintained.

Two diets will be described - each is designed to maintain your nutrient ratios at optimum levels. Choose one or the other. You cannot mix them or go back and forth between them. I also employ other dietary regimes that require strict medical supervision, but for self-monitoring programs you should do very well on either the "Basic Lipolytic meal plan" or the "1/2 cup diet".

"It took a lot of will power, but I finally gave up dieting. People that say they are on a diet are just wishful shrinkers."

"Diets are for people who are thick and tired of it."

BASIC LIPOLYTIC MEAL PLAN

Lipolytic, meaning *lipo* for fat and *lytic* for the process of breaking down fat.

Construct a meal plan for yourself by using the following rules and guidelines. However, once you have done that, you have to stick to it and minimise changes to the diet to every two weeks until you have lost all your excess fat.

The instructions and considerations

In order to lose weight the diet must be a *balanced deficit diet. You have to be in negative caloric balance or you will not lose your excess fat.* Your own surplus fat will be strategically used as part of your diet. Make sure you understand, in no uncertain terms, that fat loss needs to be a strict therapeutic intervention - all or nothing, or you will be disappointed for a lack of results.

Even if you go to Siberia or Paris on business, you must still stick with the diet if in Stage 2 - the process of losing excess fat.

"Wait a minute - all or nothing?" This does not fit our general philosophical thinking, but *metabolic logic* and *mathematical logic* are quite different. Metabolic logic is based on brute survival. I often see patients who are frustrated with their lack of progress, despite considerable effort. On closer questioning it becomes clear that they have been a 100 per cent committed every day of the week except on Tuesday and Saturday. They're applying mathematical logic!

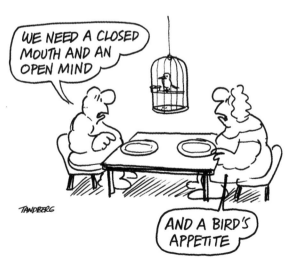

If a student gets 80 per cent for an exam it is regarded as very good indeed. The student is only penalised for the 20 per cent they did not know and is rewarded for the 80 per cent that is known. Unfortunately, when it comes to brute survival metabolic logic, it operates quite differently. While you may have scored 80 per cent in the exam, in a metabolic sense your final score is likely to be closer to 0 per cent. The 80 per cent performance does not count. Hard to accept? If you want good results in Stage 2 you need to be aware of this and to accept the inevitability.

Weight maintenance on the other hand is different - *it is not what you do 20 to 30 per cent of the time, it is what you do 70 to 80 per cent of the time*. I urge you to remember this.

Any construction of a caloric deficit nutritious diet must contain, as much as possible, all the nutritional lessons that will be described in a later chapter.

There are four components to the construction and implementation of the two recommended diets.

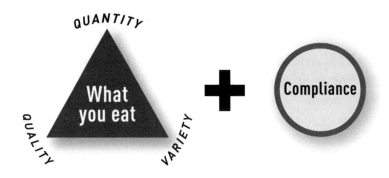

1. **Quantity**: "I am on three different diets. - it's the only way I can get enough to eat." The best thing for a person on a diet is to eat less. Size does matter! Portions are easily misrepresented. Quantity in this sense is calories. A small amount of food may represent a large quantity because it is caloric compact. However, do not eat less than the recommended quantities, unless you are under *direct* medical supervision. You may choose to limit your vegetables, but do not have less than 250g (9 onces) per day.

   Stick with the quantities - this is not the "over-eaters' diet" or the "all-you-can-eat diet". You cannot lose excess fat by talking about it. You must keep your mouth shut.

   Remember: you have to eat less in order for your excess fat to be consumed as energy. To maintain your body mass or deposit excess fat, you will need to eat more than the specified quantities. These quantities will vary according to how you control **DES** and to what extent you are a Polar Bear. You will soon learn how much food you require while successfully achieving weight loss, and the quantity at which you can continue to keep the weight off.

2. **Variety:** the smaller the variety that you allow yourself, the more successful your weight loss will be. A single-item-diet variety will always work. If bread or ice cream are your favourites you can go on a "bread diet" or an "ice cream" diet. You can eat as much as you like, but you can't have anything else. You will lose a lot of weight - guaranteed.

Whether you will stick with the single-item-diet for longer than a week is debatable and from a nutritional point of view it is ludicrous. However, to allow yourself an endless variety will make your excess fat loss attempts next to impossible.

The trouble with a diet is that you don't eat what you like and you don't like what you eat.

Decide exactly what variety you are going to have while losing weight and stick to it until you are finished.

This is the only really successful way. The smaller the variety from each group you choose, the more successful you will be. *You must limit your choices but it is variety that will ensure a nutritional balance.* The lower your blood pressure the better, but there is a cut off point - a dead person has no blood pressure.

Construct your diet plan from items that are easily available in your local area and things that you like, but to be fair, also include some items that are nutritionally good yet not necessarily to your liking.

"If you want to be lean whatever you like to eat don't, and whatever you don't like, eat."
MARK TWAIN

Variety:

Proteins:	choose not less than 5 and not more than 7
Vegetables:	not less that 6, but not more than 9
Fruit:	not less than 5 and not more than 7
Breads and cereals:	not less than 3 and not more than 4

Write it down - this is your Lipolytic excess-fat-loss diet - stick to it! It will work in spite of **POD** and the so-called experts who'll be trying to convince you to try their solution. And, if you wish, every two weeks you can construct a new diet by changing your choices, but then must *stick to your choices consistently for the full fortnight.*

"Doc, can I p-l-e-a-s-e have a bit of wine and cake for my birthday??"

I can understand your dilemma, but your enquiry is a **POD** driven question, based on profound survival instincts. By chopping and changing you will not achieve your goals. You must be very clear on this if you are at all serious about losing your excess fat.

If something is not listed on your list, it is not allowed.

"If you ask for permission the answer will be: It's forbidden."
YIDDISH PROVERB

The variety you choose needs to make nutritional sense, but remember, **one of the "secrets" of weight loss is that you do not only have to limit your quantities,** *but also your variety.*

Many experts do not understand this, and they give bulky lists of things you haven't even heard of and long lists of things you cannot have. **POD** loves to confuse people with too many choices.

3. **Quality:** During fat loss your nutrition should even be better than ever before. Your need for certain nutrients will be increased. To allow yourself even the tiniest amount of junk food is crowding out good calories. You cannot eat ice cream, pizzas and desserts during an excess fat loss program, and you must not drink any form of alcohol. If you pick up a piece of food to put in your mouth it must look as though it has been alive at some stage, coming from a plant or an animal. Every calorie counts. Only quality-calories are of any value during fat loss.

A healthy diet requires nutritional food for you to stay healthy.

4. **Compliance:** Sticking with your diet is entirely up to you - nobody can follow the instructions for you. The most difficult thing about a diet is watching other people eat. **POD/POEx** will do its best to sabotage you!

Wouldn't it be nice if a two week holiday lasted as long as two weeks on a diet?

- Use your instincts in making a decision on the following criteria on how many main meals and the quantities you are going to consume in a day:
  Gender: Male choose towards the larger quantities allowed. Female less.
  Age: Younger - more, older - less
  Activity: Sedentary - less, active - larger
  Polar Bear status: Less Polar Bear - larger portions,
  For faster weight loss choose minimum quantities and minimum variety, but individualise it more if you so wish. Stick with it!

- A main meal consists of a portion of protein plus a portion of vegetables, mixed or single.

- Your fruit, rice and bread can be eaten with the main meals or as snacks in between. It can even be had as a third meal if you have chosen to be on only two main meals per day.

- Decide when you are going to have these main meals - breakfast, lunch or dinner. They must be at least four hours apart. Keep the nocturnal and food peaks into account as discussed in a later chapter.

- Do not eat before 6am and not later than 9pm. 7pm is even better but not always practical with busy lifestyles. Liquids any time.

- **NO ALCOHOL** is allowed. No desserts and the like are allowed either. Wait for maintenance!

- *Sin Days do not apply during Stage 2.*

- Eat only fresh food - no canned food.

- A totally vegetarian diet is not recommended during weight loss. If you are a vegetarian, especially vegan, you will have to think carefully about your intake. In general, vegetarians do not lose weight as quickly.

- Compile a list - whatever *is not on that list, you simply cannot have*. This needs to be clearly understood. *Remember, you are on a therapeutic diet*. It's good if you feel your weight loss diet is restrictive, even though you have designed your own fat loss meal plan. **POD** *means you cannot lose weight without feeling hungry, deprived and practising restraint.* You have to accept this as the price you pay. Remember, the rewards are enormous and it is worth it - the most powerful treatment we have in medicine today is excess fat loss, because it achieves so much.

- You will need nutritional supplements. Magnesium, chromium and selenium to mention a few are very important and will be discussed later. Large doses of single nutrients can cause problems. In a supplement program it is very important to have comprehensive, balanced supplements.

- From the variety listed, you can make many traditional recipes including Chinese, French, Greek, Italian, Mexican, Japanese, Jewish, Turkish, Scandinavian and Thai. Stay traditional, but be aware of *quantity, variety, quality and compliance*. Stay with your instructions - remember you are on a remedial diet to rid yourself of your excess flab.

- Even if you are not religious, construct your meal plan according to your religious upbringing. You may find this very useful.

- On the second day of your diet fast from noon to noon, consuming only listed liquids. This will help with the onset of fat burning. If you choose to change your food varieties every two weeks, you should fast for a similar 24 hour period on each occasion to initiate the change, but do not fast more frequently.

- During the *first week* you must choose the smallest quantity and variety that is listed. Thereafter you can choose to move to an increased listed quantity and variety. Once you make this change, you must stick to it.

- Keep your cooking recipes simple. This is not a cookbook, but one of my next books will focus on recipes. Arrange your food neatly and attractively on the plate at all times.

  Divide your food into the following categories:

1. **Protein**
2. **Vegetables**
3. **Fruit**
4. **Grains**
5. **Condiments**
6. **Liquids**

"I've been on a diet for two weeks and all I've lost is two weeks."

POD INDUCED TALK

1. Protein

Quantity: 90g (3 onces), 95g (3.5 onces) or 100g (3.75 onces) (pick an amount and then stick to it) of chicken, fish, seafood or beef at any one main meal - not less not more. A good average is 95g (3.5 onces). If you are female or inactive opt for 90g (3 onces). If you are male and active opt for the higher amount. **Always weigh the portions - don't guess**, but don't worry about weighing the eggs. Do not mix proteins across any one main meal.

Variety: *choose a minimum of five to a maximum of seven.*

Choose from:

1. Fish fillets
2. *or* Prawns
3. *or* Squid
4. *or* Scallops
5. *or* Meat/beef/veal (lean cuts)
6. *or* Venison
7. *or* Chicken
8. *or* Turkey
9. *or* Pork (lean)
10. *or* Eggs plus whites of two to six eggs (egg whites are fat free)
11. *or* Egg Whites - five to eight
12. *or* Protein powder, such as good quality whey - this can be a very useful choice once a day
13. *or* Cheese - cottage or ricotta
14. *or* Tofu - bean curd, although this is not a complete protein.

Do not deep-fry anything if you want to lose weight. Grill, cook, bake and broil only. Make sure you get lean cuts. Be careful of soy and its products - it is vastly over promoted. Significantly, soy products are eaten only in small quantities in Asia. Soy contains toxins that need to be neutralised through fermentation.

2. Vegetables

Eat your COLOURS. Coloured vegetables are packed with Phytonutrients. **Quantity:** 220 (7.75 onces) to 250g (9 onces) a day. If you choose to have two main meals a day, have 110 (4 onces) to 125g (4.5 onces) each meal - choose a definite amount. You can have your choices mixed or single.

Variety: choose a minimum of six to a maximum of 10.

Choose from:

1. Asparagus
2. Broccoli (the best vegetable)
3. Beetroot (lots of phytonutrients, but high in GI)
4. Brussels Sprouts
5. Cabbage
6. Capsicums (any colour)
7. Cauliflower
8. Carrots
9. Garlic
10. Green beans - French style
11. Mushrooms (various types)
12. Onions
13. Salad Leaves
14. Spinach
15. Sweet Potato
16. Tomato
17. Zucchini.

3. Fruit

Quantity: be careful - while losing weight do not eat less than two or more than four portions a day. Irrespective of size, one item is one portion - for example, two small apples do not equal a large apple. You only need to weigh berries and grapes.

Variety: *choose a minimum of five to a maximum of seven.*

Choose from:

1. Apple
2. *or* Apricot
3. *or* Any citrus fruit - orange, mandarin, grapefruit etc - citrus is the best fruit
4. *or* Banana (only one per day)
5. *or* Grapes (half a standard cup only)
6. *or* Mango
7. *or* Pears
8. *or* Peach
9. *or* Plums
10. *or* Berries - strawberries, blackberries (quarter of a standard cup)
11. *or* Kiwi Fruit

4. Bread, cereals, legumes, rice and nuts

Here you have to employ a dietary manipulation with bread and rice (rice cakes). Only have bread in crisp form. Warm bread, freshly out of the oven, is very appetite stimulating. Without changing the nutritional value you can dramatically decrease **POD** by crisp drying the bread and rice - as you would with Melba toast which is placed in the oven at low heat until it is crisp or rusk-like.

Only have wholemeal bread and rice. This is especially important during excess fat loss to maintain the natural fibre in food.

Quantity and Variety: *choose a minimum of three to a maximum of four.* Have three or four portions a day - not three or four of each.

1. Wholemeal bread, wheat or rye - half a slice crisped (like Melba toast)
2. Matzos
3. Brown Rice - a measured half cup of cooked rice, once a day only
4. Rice cakes manufactured from brown rice.
5. Lentils - a measured quarter of a cup cooked, once a day only - Indian Dahl can be good for you.

5. Condiments

You can choose from a wide variety of the following. Be careful how it is marketed. It may contain sugars, cheap oils and other unknown substances. No butter allowed yet. You can have as many or as few of the different condiments as you like.

- Herbs and Spices - *any type* - they must not have been premixed with sugar and other substances, as is often the case with Thyme, Oregano, Rosemary, Coriander, Turmeric and Parsley, for example
- Chillies
- Tabasco sauce
- Pepper
- Ginger
- Extra Virgin Olive Oil 5ml (one teaspoon) a day
- Flaxseed oil 10ml (2 teaspoons) a day - keep refrigerated
- Sea Salt to taste - do not be concerned about salt when losing weight - ignore the prevailing "wisdom" about salt and use as much as you like
- Fresh lemon or lime
- Vinegar: white, balsamic (5 to 10ml)

- Natural Vanilla - this can have POD suppressing effects
- Pumpkin seeds - one teaspoon per day
- Almonds - raw, whole - eight only, counted not guessed!
- Fibre mix - psyllium, wheat bran, etc - the importance of fibre will be discussed in a later chapter.

6. Liquids

No juices - eat the whole fruit or vegetable. Don't drink your calories - eat your calories! No milk yet. NO ALCOHOLIC BEVERAGES - they cause weight gain - this is not the beer drinkers' diet!

- Water - it's important that you drink plenty of water for the health of your body. Depending on your size, physical activity and the weather, you should be drinking 10 to 15 glasses a day or more. Drink a glass of ice water after every meal - it can speed up calorie burning by 20-30 per cent.
- Soda Water - as much as you like, especially for your "mock gin and tonics" at parties. Ice, soda water and lemon looks like a gin and tonic!
- Tea - green or black - unlimited. NO MILK OR SUGAR.
- Chamomile tea - up to four cups a day.
- Coffee - black only. NO MILK OR SUGAR. No cappuccinos.
- Diet cordials, diet sodas, Diet Coke. Diet Coke plus lemon looks like a bluff "Coke and vodka" at parties. Unless you appear to drink like everyone else at parties, people will single you out for comment. Pretend - go through the motions with your pretend drinks and sham eating to keep others off your case. Go for an Oscar.

The listed foods are not part of a fad diet, they're just food. No gimmicks. We have thousands of years of experience with food, but only about 30 to 40 years of experience with protein supplements and the like. You have a little bit of choice within the confines of the diet, but quantities need to be strictly controlled because you are a Polar Bear who lives in a modern **DES** environment. You do want to lose weight, don't you now?

After 14 days - two weeks - 336 hours - take advantage of the opportunity to juggle the variety and break the monotony, but then you have to stick with those changes for the next fortnight. Too much tampering with your diet and you won't get the results you want. Stick to the rules.

*Remember - no matter what you do, **POD** will enter the equation and try its utmost to force you to make changes and eat more.* Can you blame it? It is just trying to protect you. Intellectually, you understand what you are doing, but your metabolism does not know the difference between a diet and a famine. If you override POD you will never regret the rewards of losing your excess fat.

P.S. This isn't a diet for life - it only applies while you are losing weight. As soon as you qualify for maintenance, different rules apply. With this diet you should lose between 15 and 25kg (33 and 55lbs) in 12 weeks or about 80 days. Some people will lose more, but this is a good average.

How fast you lose weight depends on:
1. Age - young adults lose weight faster
2. Gender - men lose weight faster
3. Polar Bear status
4. Initial size
5. How many fat loss attempts you have had in the past
6. Compliance with the instructions.

Important Summary
- Choose the variety you want to have within the guidelines
- Use the lower quantities of the listed foods for the first week
- Take the 24 hour, noon to noon fast on the second day of each fortnight - do not fast more frequently
- *Do not weigh yourself every day* - weekly at the most
- In the second week you can increase the quantities to the higher allowed level - if you wish
- After two weeks, you can change your food selection, but don't forget to fast on the second day
- Do not exercise heavily while you are losing excess fat - once you have been on maintenance for two weeks you can go for gold
- Before you attempt this deficit diet, consult your doctor - you may need medical monitoring. Get your renal and liver function checked and any other tests that you require.

The following is merely a sample menu constructed within the rules of this diet. It is very simple, effective and offers sound nutrition. The following is simplicity itself.

(1) PROTEIN

(Look out for total fat content)
Quantity: Fowl, Meat, Fish, 95g per meal.
Don't guess weight.
Variety: 7

• **Lean Beef/Veal**
or **Turkey**
or **Chicken**
or **Fish**
or **Prawns**
or **Egg** (+ whites = fat free protein)
or **Protein Powder** (the correct type)

(2) VEGETABLES (Complex Carbohydrates)

Lots of Phytonutrients./Anti-oxidants.
Eat your COLOURS.
You can have it single or mixed
Quantity: Max 250g/day. (125g per main meal)
Variety: 8

• **Broccoli**
• **Sweet potato**
• **Cabbage**
• **Carrots**
• **Cauliflower**
• **Spinach**
• **Mushrooms**
• **Garlic**

(3) FRUIT (Simple Carbohydrates)

Quantity: 2 to 4 portions per day.
Not less than 2.
Variety: 7

• **Apple**
or **Apricot**
or **Any Citrus**; orange, grapefruit, mandarin, etc.
or **Kiwi fruit**
or **Mango**
or **Peach**
or **Berries, Cherries, Strawberries** (1/4 cup only)

(4) GRAINS, BREADS, CEREALS

Easy to overdose in this category – excess will be
stored as excess fat.
Quantity: 3 portions per day. Not 3 of each.
Variety: 4

• **Whole meal bread (crisp dry)**
or **Matzos**
or **Brown Rice** (1/2 cup per day only)
or **Almonds** (5 to 10 per day – count)

(5) CONDIMENTS

Quantity and variety: as mentioned in the rules
Example:
• Sea salt • Pepper • Lemon • Curry Powder
• Herbs & Spices • Vinegar (White) • Mustard
• Sugar substitute • Flax seed oil
• Extra virgin Olive oil • Soy sauce
• Tabasco sauce • Oregano • Coriander
• Thyme • Cinnamon • Paprika
• Baking Soda (Aluminium free)
• Ginger • Miso (for Miso soup)
• Rosemary (Good Anti-oxidant)
• Pure Vanilla bean or extract (decrease POD)
• Turmeric (Anti-oxidant & anti-cancer)
• Vinegar: red, White Wine & Balsamic, etc etc

(6) LIQUIDS

Don't drink your calories – **eat** your calories.
Consult the rules

• **WATER**
• **Mineral water**
• **Soda water**
• **Tea:** Japan Green tea, ordinary tea, etc.
(Unlimited)
• **Black Coffee** (Up to 5 cups)
• **Diet drinks** (three glasses per day only)

An *example* of a main meal

Grilled chicken breast (100g/3.5 onces) plus spinach and sweet potato (combined weight 125g/4.5 onces), plus half a cup of brown rice and any variety of condiments together with one teaspoon of Olive oil.

Apple (one) for dessert.

Remember, sweets are the destiny that shapes our ends.

Green Tea - unlimited.

This diet will work if you stick to it. Modifying the quantities, particularly reducing your food intake, should only be done under experienced medical supervision. Keep the recipes simple, and make them as traditional as you can within the confines of the ingredients listed in this diet.

What to Expect

During the first few days you will have a *full on frontal attack of* **POD** and the feelings of deprivation may unnerve you a bit, but within a few days it will settle down, provided you have stuck with the diet. You may even experience headaches and dizziness. There is no harm in these and they too will disappear in a few days. If any symptom persists, consult your doctor.

After five days on your reducing diet plan you may not even feel the Full Frontal Attacks (FFAs) of **POD** anymore. Nevertheless, you always have to be aware of the SBDA's (Sneaky Back Door Attacks) of **POD**.

If you are on blood pressure medication your blood pressure may fall as your fat percentage reduces. Do not adjust your medication without your doctor's advice. Do not be concerned if your bowel movements are less frequent or smaller - you are eating less, therefore your output is less. You are not constipated. Your food intake is such that you may only have a bowel motion every three days. Do not use laxatives for something that is not really there to come out - you will damage your bowel. Add fibre and, if problems persist, see your doctor.

Downside

The only "downside" with the diet is that meal preparation may take longer, even if the recipes are kept simple.

In order to achieve optimum functional health you have to make a plan and nourish your body effectively. It is time and effort well spent.

Preparing an omelette with broccoli shavings, herbs and spices takes only minutes. A banana or mango "smoothie" with protein powder takes seconds. Put a handful of ice cubes in a blender. Crush it. Add as much or as little water to make it as thick or as thin as you like. Add the banana or mango with 10 to 20ml (4 teaspoons) of flaxseed oil. Add the protein powder. If you want extra fibre add a spoon of fibre mix. Blend and you have had a meal. It's that quick.

Suggestion: make double the recipe, put half in the fridge and the next meal is already prepared.

Sticking point or plateau
Consider some of the following options if you hit a difficult patch.

Red steak day: 200g (7 onces) of lean steak grilled with half a grilled tomato for lunch - clear liquids for the rest of the day.

Apple day: six apples from noon to noon with the allowed liquids.

THE 1/2 CUP DIET

Remember: This is an alternative to the Lipolytic Diet. Choose one or the other, don't mix them or go back and forth between them.

The cup is 1/2 full even though **POD** will try to convince you it is empty.

If it is not listed it is not allowed. Nothing except allowed liquids is authorized between meals.

The general rules that apply to the Lipolytic Diet apply to The 1/2 Cup Diet, and exactly the same condiments list and rules apply.

Breakfast
- Wholemeal toast one slice, with 1/2 teaspoon butter (if you wish)

    The following:
- 2 eggs
  or protein powder
  or 1/2 cup of cooked cereal, such as oats
- Milk if you wish - 1/2 cup
- Juice - 1/2 cup of tomato, carrot and/or other vegetable juice - mixed if you like.

Lunch and Dinner

- 100g (3.5 onces) of lean meat (any)
  or chicken
  or turkey
  or fish
  or protein powder (good quality)

- 1/2 cup of **cooked** rice (preferably brown)
  or plain noodles 1/21/2 cup
  or potato, especially sweet potato, 1/2 cup
  or pasta 1/2 cup (preferably wholemeal)

  If you choose these, preferably only for lunch

  or 1/2 cup of the following, mixed or single - always fresh:
    Carrots
    Green beans (French style)
    Beetroot
    Broccoli
    Spinach
    Tomato

- One of the following - always fresh:
    Apple
    or Peach
    or citrus - any
    or small banana - only one a day
    or tropical fruit, like mango. Bigger fruit like papaya, 1/2 cup

Liquids

- Plenty of water - at least twenty 1/2 cups per day
- Unlimited tea or coffee with no milk or sugar
- Diet drinks - a maximum of two a day
- **No alcohol** - not even 0.1 per cent of 1/2 a cup.

Stick to it until you have lost all your excess fat. **POD** will give you some resistance and excuses not to comply - of course. But remember, nothing t*astes as good as thin feels.*

It's something most of us do religiously: We eat what we want and pray we don't gain weight. A diet is the modern-day meal in which a family counts its calories instead of its blessings.

Dieter's Grace

> NOW I sit me down to eat
> I pray the Lord I do not cheat
> Should I reach for cake and bread
> Please guide my hands to the allowed instead.
> Amen.

Formula for Success

Stop doing the things you know you *should not do*.
Start doing the things you know you *should do*.

CHAPTER 16

EATING HABITS AND BEHAVIOUR

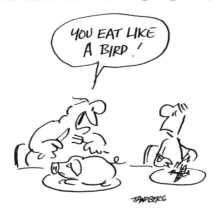

EATING HABITS AND BEHAVIOUR

"You are not just what you eat, but how you eat it."

The combination of what and how we eat encourages good health and helps control **POD**.

How we eat is about our behaviour associated with the simple act of eating. If you do not develop a system and protocol on *how* to eat and stick with it, **POD** and the oversupply of food will be out of control.

Control the eating environment and **POD** is a hundred times easier to control. This was easier in times past, particularly with the more sophisticated - sitting around the table at set meal times, saying grace and talking had various physical, mental and sociological benefits. Unfortunately the TV dinner has taken over. *There is no longer a defined moment when the meal has started or finished.* The attention is not on what is eaten, but on the television. Eating has become an automatic act.

Friends of mine gradually observed how their family had become dysfunctional with TV dinners, mobile phones and late night eating. Apart from their daughter starting to develop **GOFES** and the two sons often going to their bedrooms to eat and watch TV, the parents also felt stress in their relationship.

One Friday evening, after Ruth had prepared a nice meal, sitting alone with husband Sam, she said, "Our family has to return to our cultural eating habits". Sam immediately understood what she meant and a family meeting was called.

After their tough talking meeting with the kids it was decided to create a degree of decorum in the household. Dinnertime would be together, no TV or mobile phones. In fact, the telephone answering machine was to be switched on during mealtime with the message: "Our family is having dinner. Please leave a message and we will contact you later."

The outcome - they had a bit of trouble for a while bringing the kids into line and Ruth became interested in cooking again, particularly foods associated with their family culture.

I dropped in to see Sam at his business one day - his daughter Linda was there. She had lost 8kg (18lb) and what amazed me even more was that her attitude had changed.

Sam came out, noticing me but not acknowledging me at first, went over to Linda and gave her a kiss and a hug and then looked at me and said: "I've found my family again, and you know what? I feel much healthier and not so sluggish."

Food and how it is enjoyed can indeed be a powerful tool.

THE STOP START SYNDROME (SSS)

Eat, drink and be merry, for tomorrow we diet. I think I will plan to be spontaneous next Monday.

This can be a very destructive syndrome.

A typical example: you make a major decision in your life, for instance to improve your health and manage your **GOFES**. But instead of implementing it now, you set a date - next Monday, or your birthday, or you make it a New Year resolution.

"He who promises runs in debt."
TALMUD

Since you're going to be perfect from Monday, you can be as *bad as you like until then, and go on a rampage in the meantime!*

This becomes a destructive and vicious cycle, playing havoc with your chances of success. People become deluded into thinking they will *start, yet again*, and be *successful again*.

You cannot start all over again.

Unfortunately, the only thing we learn from from history... is that we do not learn from history.

Food Recording and PME

Recording what you consume can be a very potent tool in managing your eating. It helps focus your attention. You will think twice about putting it in your mouth if you have to write it down. Food recording also gives valuable feedback by highlighting problem areas and serving as a personal research tool.

If you notice that for the past few days you snack at around 4.00pm, there is a very good chance that you will do that again *today* at 4.00pm. What are you going to do about it? The value of food recording is that you can now start interacting with your food and activity diary. You could, for instance make sure that you are not around food at 4.00pm.

To make food recording even more powerful, use Premeditated Eating or PME. You sit down for a few minutes and visualise the next day, hour by hour. What you expect to do, where you will be and so on. Then you write out your food diary for the next day. You plan exactly what you will have, where and when. The next day it's just a matter of following your plan. If you eat something that was unplanned, cross out the premeditated food and write on top of it what you had instead. The plan is, of course, to have followed it perfectly by end of the day. This a very powerful management tool for **GOFES** and it can be surprisingly successful.

A business executive patient of the clinic found it so useful that he even wrote a software program to manage his eating program from his laptop. He claimed his work efficiency went up by 40 per cent. Not only did he have to plan his food intake in advance with PME, but it also helped to think through his other activities for the following day. PME can however be a difficult routine - we will fill in tax forms, census forms, surveys and the like, but when it comes to what we put in our mouths, paperwork seems to be taboo. The uptake on this powerful tool is therefore unfortunately low.

Those who are successful derive huge benefits from PME.

One patient, Louise, had a successful stint on **PME** but then ceased using the technique. When I enquired why she explained that visualising everything about the next day had led her to believe she was clairvoyant.

"I visualised an old school friend pushing a supermarket trolley in the mall where I planned to do some grocery shopping about eleven o'clock the next day. My friend looked really sick and weak. Guess what? The next day there she was and she told me she has breast cancer. I am scared now and I don't think I can handle this PME anymore."

Whether it was real or just an excuse, I leave it to the reader's judgement. Whatever the case, PME can significantly influence your ability to control **POD**, **GOFES** and your life in general. Just give it a go. Once practiced, the meditation session takes less than five minutes. To find these five minutes can be really hard, but not being able to find the time is depriving you of a very valuable device.

Premeditation intervenes in the stimulus and response chain and interrupts its compulsive nature. Do **PME** from time to time. You will thank yourself for it.

"Life can only be understood backwards, but it must be lived forwards."
MARK TWAIN

8th characteristic of successful weight maintainers: *Have a standard eating environment and do not eat on the run.*

Synopsis:

1. Eat more formally.

2. Cultural eating habits have developed for very specific reasons. Stick to them. TV dinners are not good for **GOFES** control. They are the result of commercial and other pressures and are at odds with your culture and your good health.

EATING HABITS MODIFICATION

Probably the best way to control the your supply of food is to **"Fat-proof your house"**. We can only eat what is there.

"Better shun the bait, than struggle the snare."
JOHN DRYDEN

"Every moment of resistance to temptation is a triumph."
ANONYMOUS

Modification of Eating Habits and Behaviour

HOW you eat is your **Eating Style**. This is just as important as **WHAT** you eat.

It is essential that you rehabilitate some of your eating style habits and behaviour in order to get rid of your excess fat and then to maintain ideal fat percentage. By the time you have lost all your excess fat, these **new healthy** habits should have become automatic and part of your every day life.

Remember: If you do not modify your old "fat habits" you will simply regain all the fat lost and maybe more.

Study the following often, until memorised and until *these habits* become automatic. Repetition is the mother of skill. You have probably heard some of the following, but **unless** you condition yourself to **APPLY** these rules, they will have no value.

1. The Purchase of Food

(a) Always make up your mind **beforehand** about what you **need**. Make a shopping list and **keep** to it! If you had not thought about a particular food beforehand, you probably do not need it. You also save money and time this way. **Need not Greed.**

(b) Make a list of all the shops where you intend to purchase. Stick to this list. Exotic shops should be avoided in Stage 2 therapy, as well as, certain bakeries with the aroma of freshly baked bread. Take only a limited amount of cash with you.

(c) Shop straight after a meal, or at least when you are not hungry. **Never** shop on an empty stomach - avoid temptation.

(d) Avoid buying food which may be difficult to resist later.

(e) Try to buy food which has to be prepared (raw meat, etc.) instead of instant and canned food which leads to impulsive eating. Make it difficult for yourself to eat straight away. Our distant forefathers had to hunt first before they could eat.

(f) Resist the free snacks (cheeses, crackers, ice cream, etc.) offered at supermarkets from time to time to promote sales. Resist "low calorie" cookies and "diet" snacks. These are traps.

2. Food Preparation and Cooking Habits

(a) Decide **before** a meal **exactly** what and **how much** you are going to eat - premeditated eating. Then keep to your plan! All foods should be eaten at meal times only, and not in-between or while preparing your meal.

(b) If possible, during Stage 2, let somebody else prepare your food to avoid nibbling and temptation. Stay out of the kitchen! Enter it only when absolutely necessary. **Limit your exposure to food.**

(c) Prepare your food separately in Stage 2 and use separate utensils. Fat deposits on utensils retard weight loss. This is not necessary during maintenance.

(d) Change the **preparation** and **appearance** of the food often. Beware of monotony. However, don't expose yourself to a large variety of foods in one day - you will eat more. People on gourmet foods usually eat 1,000 calories per day more. Keep things **simple**.

(e) Serve food from the kitchen, especially during Stage 2. Don't keep serving dishes on the table.

(f) Cut up food in smaller pieces than usual, or even into as many small pieces as you can.

(g) Do not taste while cooking. You will be surprised how many calories you can consume by tasting during cooking. While cooking, chew some sugar-free gum.

(h) **Pre-plan your menus.** If you are pressed for time, chances are you will opt for something that is quick and high in calories. Unplanned meals lead to indecision that can drive you into an eating frenzy at the nearest fast food shop.

(i) Cook only what you **need** for a particular meal. If you cook more, you will be tempted to eat it. **Need not Greed.**

(j) Prepare your food when your control is the highest. You can prepare, for example, your evening meal straight after you have had lunch.

3. Standardise your Eating Environment and Eating Triggers

(a) No other activity should be allowed when eating, e.g. reading, watching television, driving your car. Eating should be the **sole** activity.

(b) If you are eating at home, always eat in the **same** room in the **same** place.

(c) Always sit down while eating. No food should enter your mouth while you are standing.

(d) Use smaller plates and utensils and spread your food to make small portions appear larger. Arrange food artfully on your best china and glassware. Eat with finesse, style and control.

4. Serving of Food

(a) Only serve your food once, just the amount allowed in your meal plan.

(b) Avoid family style service. Everyone should serve themselves.

(c) Highly seasoned foods or high calorie condiments should not be served at meals, especially in Stage 2 therapy.

Modify your Actual eating Behaviour

Eat very slowly! Fat people usually eat fast. It is important to chew the food thoroughly. Put your utensils down after you have put the food into your mouth and don't pick them up until your mouth is empty. Chew each mouthful as long as possible so that you eat more slowly. For food to be absorbed it takes about 20 to 25 minutes. During this time you can eat a lot before you start to feel full. Therefore, the slower you eat the less you will consume. Be the **last** to **start** and the last to finish your meal. One guideline applies to fat and thin people alike: If you're thin, don't eat fast. If you're fat, don't eat - FAST.

(a) Wait at least three minutes between dishes.

(b) Never eat when you are agitated. Eat calmly. Relax. Avoid animated discussions during your meal.

(c) If you have problems, don't try and solve them with food. **Food solves nothing except malnutrition.** It is better to discuss your problems and try to find a solution.

(d) Know the difference between hunger and appetite. Hunger is a natural instinct to know that it is time to re-fuel your body. Eat only when you are hungry. Appetite is an artificially stimulated or created "hunger". Due to our culture and affluent society, the instinct of hunger is largely lost and it becomes difficult to distinguish between the two. If you eat only because you are truly hungry, you are unlikely to become fat.

(e) Concentrate on the taste and smell of the food. Eating should be a **pure** experience - enjoy your food. A **gourmet** is an epicure who enjoys food - a real connoisseur is highly selective and will often not each much. A **gourmand** is a glutton who eats everything in large quantities and often does not enjoy the food. Don't abuse food - be grateful for it.

(f) Let your spouse and children get their own desserts, chocolates, etc. Don't volunteer to have anything to do with food you should not have. Minimise temptation.

(g) Use utensils for eating all food, even traditional finger food, especially during Stage 2.

(h) It is well worth your while acquiring the habit of eating with chopsticks.

(i) Leave something for the dog. Don't clean your plate. Instead leave a bit of each food. A clean plate is a waiting plate. A plate with unfinished left over food at the **end** of a meal signals you are full and satisfied.

(j) The number ONE nutritional mistake is that we eat **too much!** - over consumptive malnutrition. Develop the EAT LESS HABIT. Eat less and less to live longer and longer.

(k) End each meal with a particular food - nothing more afterward. An apple is a good choice, slicing it thinly and eating it slowly. An apple then serves to remind you the meal is over.

(l) Those who indulge bulge.

When the Meal is Over

(a) Get up *immediately*. Don't linger unless all foods have been cleared away.

(b) Don't clear the table. Get up and out of the kitchen. The transition from ending the meal and clearing it away can be hard for a person who is accustomed to nibble as they wish. If possible, assign the job to someone else until new non-snacking habits take root. Leave the room for an hour to do something enjoyable (not eating!), then return to clear the table without nibbling.

(c) Dispose of leftovers straight away, directly into a garbage bin, otherwise you may feel tempted to eat it later. If you do not throw the leftovers away, at least make it less visible, for instance covering it with foil.

(d) Brush your teeth with toothpaste immediately after **all** meals. Use a sugarless mouthwash and floss your teeth at least once a day. Remember - take your toothbrush to the office if you have lunch there. This also signals that the meal is over and cleans the food taste from your mouth.

(e) If you are still hungry - take a walk! Phone a friend. Do something else.

(f) Perform mild exercise after each meal, for instance, walking. This is good for you, contrary to popular belief.

General

(a) Get organised! **POD** is sneaky. Do **not** keep tempting food in the house, especially during Stage 2. You may have an irresistible craving to devour tempting foods if you **know** they are **available. Your exposure to food must be minimised!** It is easier for fat people to avoid food rather than be **confronted** with tempting food. *Fat proof your home and office.*

(b) Avoid boredom. Keep occupied. Instead of thinking about food all the time - **do** something else! Whatever you do, keep occupied in a challenging way so that you do not become bored.

(c) Never skip breakfast - especially during maintenance. Generally, for most people, omitting breakfast has not shown to be of any value for long-term obesity control.

(d) If you want a snack such as an apple or orange, cut it in neat slices or segment it, then arrange it attractively on a plate. Don't just eat it. Eat and **enjoy** it slowly. Try sprinkling your fruit with fresh lemon juice.

(e) **Don't eat rubbish!** If you eat garbage, you become garbage. Apart from encouraging obesity, eating canned and fast foods regularly is a sure way of poisoning yourself, setting in train diabetes, heart disease and cancer.

(f) The first rule of nutrition: if it tastes good spit it out, because it's bad for you. Tongue in cheek, but with more than a grain of truth in it!

(g) Attempt to relax **before** and **during** meal times.

(h) If you feel a binge coming on:
- put something sour in your mouth, a slice of lemon or lime
- and/or a strong mint (sugar free)

- and/or brush your teeth with strong toothpaste. Or gargle with a strong, sugar free mouthwash.

(i) Behavioural Aversion Therapy (BAT).

(j) Don't fool yourself, you are not going to eat "just one", you will have another and another and another. If you never start, you won't have to finish. **Once on the lips, soon on the hips.** One is too much and a thousand is too little.

(k) Just thinking about food serves as a trigger to eating. **Deliberately** turn your thoughts away to some other subject.

(l) When you get an urge to eat, polish your fingernails - they will take time to dry. Or get your hands dirty with garden work etc. Do anything to delay eating. POD can be impatient and tends to back off if you ignore it.

(m) If you get an urge to eat something that you know you should not have at that moment, remind yourself, that you have only two choices: fat and unhealthy or lean and healthy. Make your mind up about what you want!

(n) Act thin.

(o) You can practice control. Once a week take your favourite food, for example chocolate, bring it to your mouth and say out loud: "I can stop myself from eating this."

(p) Eat + Eat = Fat. You are what you eat (and cheat).

(q) Remember: develop the "eat less" habit. We live on only a third of what we eat and the medical profession lives on the other two thirds!

(r) Don't over eat and abuse food: you will dig your own grave with your teeth. Fill your stomach only one-third with food, one-third with liquid and leave the other third empty - "that slightly empty feeling".

(s) Delaying, Substituting and Avoiding are three major strategies for interrupting eating behaviour:
   - Delaying... pause for a second for a chance to rethink the eating situation - go by a roundabout way to the kitchen or food. Store tempting foods in hard-to-reach places
   - Substituting... break the eating behaviour with pleasant activities such as music, hobbies, bathing, sleeping. Better still, break the eating behaviour with necessary activities such as opening mail, paying bills, washing the car
   - Avoiding... make food less visible or accessible. Avoid having tempting food in the house. Avoid saboteurs - people in your life who push food on you - by finding non-eating ways to spend time with the saboteur.

"There are a lot of things we cannot change in life, but we can change our attitude."

ANONYMOUS

Mental Attitude Modification

1. Fat Loss: "It's taking forever to lose excess fat. I guess this means I will be fat forever." A counter-argument: "I am losing slowly but surely, and this time I will learn how to keep it off."

2. Capabilities: "I've never been able to lose much fat before. Why should it work this time?" A counter-argument: "Maybe this will be the first time, and don't forget, this time I have some powerful procedures going for me."

3. Excuses: "Everyone in my family has had an obesity problem. It must be in my genes." A counter-argument: "That may make it harder, but not impossible. If I stick with the program, I will succeed."

4. Goals: "I will never eat chocolate cake again, and that will help me lose fat fast." A counter-argument: "These are unrealistic expectations and when I don't live up to them I will only get discouraged. I should pay more attention to the eating behaviours I have been learning."

5. Food thoughts: "I can just taste how good that ice cream will be." A useful response: "Stop that! I should think of something to do that will take me away from thoughts of eating."

6. "I'll never be able to eat tempting foods again". A counter-argument: "During maintenance, if I eliminate all fattening foods from my diet I'll most probably feel deprived and end up bingeing, so I'll have my 'Sin days', but I do realise that I will have to make permanent changes to keep my excess fat off."

If you are positive you will get positive results. Be negative and you'll get negative results.

Special Occasions

You must have a PLAN and stick to it.

Before you go out for a meal remind yourself that:

1. People do not invite you so that you can show them how much you can eat, but for your company.

2. You suffer from obesity, therefore your eating behaviour should be DIFFER-ENT to non-obese persons.

3. You are on a medical treatment plan and you are expected to stay on it. Don't cheat - help us to help you.

4. The best "organs" to celebrate with are your brain and heart and not your stomach and liver.

5. Observe those who eat little, are thin, and have interests other than food. Join them.

A big meal out or a function can usually be divided into five parts:

- Part One: The socialising before the meal where nibbles and drinks are served. Socialise with people who aren't so interested in food. The big eaters usually stand close to the nibbles. Only have a mock drink, like soda or mineral water with ice and a slice of lemon. Don't have any of the nibbles. If asked, say that you don't want to spoil your appetite for the main course.

- Part Two: At the main table, either don't have an entrée: "I don't want to spoil my appetite for the main course"... or order an entrée as a main course. Order first so that your choices are not influenced by other people. Remember, you don't have to have an entrée.

- Part Three: The main course. Avoid "I have paid for it, therefore I'll eat it". Eat very slowly and do not talk about diets. Keep on talking and always have a glass of water or a mock gin and tonic ready. It may be rude to refuse the main course in certain circumstances, but you don't have to eat everything. Shift the food from one side of the plate to the other so that it appears you are also in the act of gourmandising. Go through the motions. You must learn to bluff your way through. It is your health and figure and you have to be ruthless about it. Don't be meek and weak. You are invited for your company - not to demonstrate your eating capacity.

- Part Four: Dessert. "I am so full from the main course I couldn't possibly have anything else."

- Part Five: The cheese, biscuits, coffee, liqueurs, port, chocolates. Only have black coffee.

By being alert and following these rules you will save an enormous amount of calories. What's more, you'll feel good about yourself and in control and you'll be closer to your goal.

Negative Criticism

The Politics of Weight Loss

Most patients will encounter it sooner or later. This may interfere with your progress.

Saboteurs are people in your life that push food on you. Controlling obesity can be a lonely struggle. Generally the public views obesity as something to do with gluttony and lack of self-discipline. Usually not much support is forthcoming - in fact you may be negatively criticised for your efforts. Most of this negative criticism is based on jealousy, ignorance and envy. "Everybody" is an "obesity expert" and has an opinion. Some can be very overbearing. Don't be upset - take it for what it is.

Physical Activity

Inactivity leads to FAT! Need I say more? Physical activity also influences your eating habits and behaviour. It is essential to achieve moderate fitness in order to maintain Optimum Health. Couch potatoism promotes excess fat and disease.

Diets Are Better Than Sex

- Dieting won't make you pregnant
- You don't have to undress to do it
- You can do it any time, anywhere
- You can do it in front of anyone
- The quicker the diet the better
- You can doze off in the middle if you want
- You can always save a bit for later
- You can do it with your best friend's partner
- Afterwards, you don't have to lose sleep wondering if the earth moved for the cheesecake too.

ANONYMOUS

9th characteristic of successful weight maintainers:
Fat proof your house and work place. Do not keep tempting
foods laying around - keep it out of reach.

"POD TALK" AND EXCUSES

Physical POD - Direct POD feelings/sensations

Easy to recognise and identify.

Full frontal attacks.

1. "I am starving"
2. "I am hungry"
3. "If it wasn't for my huge appetite..."
4. "I have sweet cravings"
5. "I cannot control the urge to eat"
6. "I love my food"

Mental POD - Indirect POD rationalisations

Sneaky back door attacks.

Subtle and underhanded back door **POD** attacks, often catching you unawares in order to initiate any one of the following eating behaviours.

Calories That Don't Count

We have it on experience that the following foods are "calorie free" - tongue in cheek, but making the point.

1. **OTHER PEOPLE'S FOOD** - A chocolate mousse that you did not order has no calories. Therefore, have your companion order dessert while you taste half of it.

2. **INGREDIENTS IN COOKING** - Chocolate chips are fattening, about 50 calories a tablespoon. So are chocolate chip cookies! However! Chocolate chips eaten while making chocolate chip cookies have no calories whatsoever. Therefore, make chocolate chip cookies often but don't eat them.

3. **FOOD ON FOOT** - All food eaten while standing has no calories. Exactly why is not clear, but the current theory relates to gravity. The calories apparently bypass the stomach flowing directly down the legs, and through the soles of the feet into the floor like electricity. Walking seems to accelerate this process so that a custard tart or hot dog eaten at a carnival actually has a calorie deficit.

4. **CHILDREN'S FOOD** - Anything produced, purchased or intended for minors is calorie-free when eaten by adults. This category covers a wide range of foods.

5. **UNEVEN EDGES** - Pies and cakes should be CUT neatly, into even wedges or slices. If not, the responsibility falls on the person putting them away to "straighten up the edges" by slicing away the offending irregularities, which have no calories when eaten.

6. **TV FOOD** - Anything eaten in front of the TV has no calories. This may have something to do with radiation leakage, which negates not only the calories in the food but all recollection of having eaten it. Entire no-calorie dinners are now manufactured and frozen for this purpose.

7. **FOOD THAT DOESN'T TASTE GOOD** - this food doesn't count. This is an enormous category covering a diverse range, including airline food, cafeteria meals and dinner at your sister-in-law's. Also, dinners manufactured to be eaten in front of the TV.

8. **ANYTHING SMALLER THAN ONE INCH** - this contains no calories to speak of. For example: chocolate kisses, maraschino cherries, cubes of cheese.

9. **LEFT-HANDED FOOD** - If you have a drink in your right hand, anything eaten with the other hand has no calories. Several principles are at work here. First of all, you're probably standing up at a cocktail party. Then there's the electrostatic field: a wet glass in one hand forms a negative charge to reverse the polarity of the calories attracted to the other hand. I'm not exactly sure how it works, but it's reversible if you're left-handed!

10. **CHARITABLE FOODS** - Charity cookies, cake stalls, ice cream socials and church strawberry festivals all have a religious dispensation from calories.

11. **CAKES WITH WRITING ON THEM** - Primarily fat, starch and sugar, all cakes are horrendously fattening. However, the calories can be eliminated simply by

inscribing "Happy birthday, Charlie" or "Good Luck, Aileen" in coloured icing. And remember, not only is it unnecessary to decline, it's impolite.

12. **FOOD ON TOOTHPICKS** - Sausages, cocktail franks, cheese and the like are all fattening unless impaled on toothpicks. The insertion of a sharp object allows the calories to leak out the bottom.

13. **LEFTOVERS** - An extra pork chop, the crust of bread, half a Mars bar, anything intended for the garbage has no calories regardless of what happens to it in the kitchen.

14. **FOOD EATEN QUICKLY** - If you are rushed through a meal, the entire meal doesn't count. Conversely, if you have ordered something fattening and now regret it, you can minimize its calories by gulping it down.

15. **CUSTOM MADE FOOD** - Anything somebody made "just for you" must be eaten regardless of the calories because to do otherwise would be uncaring and insensitive. Your kind intentions will not go unrewarded.

16. **CHOCOLATE - sweet dreams:**
    - Chocolate is derived from cocoa beans and sugarcane. Both are vegetables.
    - Sugar is derived from either sugar cane or sugar beet. Both are plants, therefore chocolate is a vegetable.
    - To go one step further, chocolate candy bars also contain milk, which is dairy... so candy bars are a health food.
    - Chocolate-covered raisins, cherries, orange slices and strawberries all count as fruit, so eat as many as you want.
    - Diet tip... eat a chocolate bar before each meal. It will take the edge off your appetite and you'll eat less.
    - If you eat equal amounts of dark chocolate and white chocolate, you will have a balanced diet.
    - Chocolate has many preservatives. Preservatives make you look younger.
    - **Remember**: **"STRESSED"** spelled backwards is **"DESSERTS"**

17. **DURING AND AFTER ARGUMENTS** - It is a well known fact that food consumed during such times is all used up for the argument, and therefore none of the calories count, so to speak.

18. **I AM BORED WITH MY DIET** - A typical POD generated comment designed to alleviate deprivation.

19. **I HAVE LOST THE PLOT** - Actually, you lost the POD.

20. **WHY CAN'T I HAVE CHOCOLATE IN MY DIET?** - POD initiated question, again merely trying to remind you that you are in a probable famine and that you'd better stock up for survival.

21. **IF NO ONE SEES YOU EAT - IT HAS NO CALORIES.**

22. **FOOD TAKEN FOR MEDICINAL PURPOSES DOESN'T COUNT** - Hot chocolate, brandy, banana splits and ice cream (when your throat is sore!).

CHAPTER 17

AFTER YOU HAVE LOST ALL YOUR EXCESS FAT

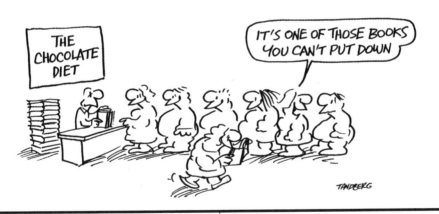

AFTER YOU HAVE LOST ALL YOUR EXCESS FAT

*"I am getting really good at dieting...
I only gained 8 kg on the last one."*
ANONYMOUS

Your only choice: Maintain and restrain or Regain and pain.

You can't hatch an egg before you've laid it. You can't do maintenance before you've lost your excess fat.

What benefits have you attained and earned by now?

Remember, weight loss is the most powerful therapy we have in medicine today, because it achieves so much.

Cosmetic benefits

Although the cosmetic advantages are only the cherry on top of all the other benefits, it is very important to your mental health and self-esteem. I have stopped counting how many patients have told me a variation of the following:

"Doc, when I was fat in the past, I would walk in shopping malls and see my fat reflection in the windows. I had a quick disgusting glance and looked away. I hated seeing myself.

"Now, since I lost the fat, when I see my reflection in the windows, I stop and admire myself. I go into shops and can now buy clothes off the rack."

A load off your organs

You cannot build the engine of your lawn mower into your car and expect it to perform properly. The load off your organs is awe-inspiring. Your body will thank you for it. Your joints, heart, other organs and metabolic systems feel as if they've won the lottery. If you have lost 20kg (44lb) it is equivalent to a bag of cement. Imagine a cement bag trimmed off your backside!

Risk factor reduction
Review "What Obesity can do to you" (chapter 3) and you will realise the risk reductions that you have achieved. You have really put into place life saving changes.

LIPID PROFILE:

	Before GOFES treatment	After GOFES treatment	Ideal range
Cholesterol	7.3	3.7	< 4.5
TG	4.4	0.9	< 1.1
HDL	0.7	1.3	> 1.3
LDL	5.1	2.4	< 2.0
Ratio	10.5	0.3	< 3.0

As an example, the above is the lipid profile of Jacob, before and after he lost his excess fat. He lost 26kg (57lb). It shows a dramatic turnaround and even if some may not be this dramatic, there is always improvement, especially during consolidation. The other metabolic improvements leading to metabolic fitness are too numerous to describe here.

Important point: while losing weight, don't bother taking your cholesterol levels. They are usually inaccurate during weight loss. Wait until you are on maintenance and then compare it with your previous **GOFES** levels.

Sociological and psychological
Many GOFES sufferers recount tales of failing at job interviews because they were overweight, but succeeding after losing their excess fat. While some will criticise you for losing your excess fat, you'll command respect from the majority.

Improved biological/functional age
GOFES is one of the leading causes of accelerated aging. Lose your excess fat, eat properly and exercise and you'll look and feel younger in a comparatively short period of time.

Optimum functional health

Just because you've lost all your excess fat, you may not have achieved optimum functional health just yet. You have laid the foundations and now you can build on them. It is in the first year on maintenance, when you consolidate your health to reach a state of metabolic fitness and optimum function.

Are there any downsides?

Decreased metabolic rate

This is a bit of a holy cow. When a person loses weight the body sees the process as a threat to its survival and tries its best to slow down your metabolism. This leads to a slowing of bowel action as your body attempts to gain the maximum nutrition from your reduced food intake. I prefer to see this as increased body efficiency - your Polar Bear metabolism will become even more efficient during "starvation".

Starvation involves losing strength and possibly dying from malnourishment. Losing excess-fat is about using a negative caloric balance to consume that excess-fat. Starvation results in the burning of your lean body mass. In fact, your nutritional intake during weight loss will very likely be higher than before. You should only be deficient in calories, and the deficiency will be derived from your surplus stores. *To do this properly is an expert field.*

So-called experts will use scare tactics in trying to dissuade you from this course of action, but excess fat is dangerous and you are a thousand times better off getting rid of it. The so-called "slower metabolism" actually improves very quickly once you move to maintenance.

When the metabolism is calculated per kilogram of body weight or muscle, fat people appear to have a slower metabolism. Fat people also burn less fat than naturally lean people, just as a car is more efficient if it burns less fuel. This is the genetics of a Polar Bear. Whether fat people lose weight or not, they burn less fuel and tend not to suffer from sluggish metabolism, indeed most fat people are energetic and alert.

Metabolism geared for a fat body

In maintaining a fat body the metabolism has various processes and hormones in place. Losing weight doesn't return the metabolism to that of a thinner body overnight. It takes time and you have to be patient. This is one of the reasons why **GOFES** is so intractable once established.

Redundant blood vessels

For every kilogram of fat, the body produces three kilometres of blood vessels to supply this surplus fat with oxygen and nutrients. Let's take an example.

A property developer finds a stretch of land and plans a residential development. As the land is fairly inaccessible due to a river and hills separating it from adjoining urban areas, he needs infrastructure before houses can be built. A highway, a bridge, streets, electricity, water and other services need to be established. The whole project may take three years.

Once the project has been completed a bushfire destroys all the houses. To rebuild the project would now take considerably less than three years to rebuild *because the basic infrastructure is already in place.*

Applying this analogy to fat loss, the infrastructure exists for the lost fat and is just lying in wait. Go away for a weekend, splurge a bit and you could gain a few kilograms in no time... you Polar Bear, you.

Building the body's infrastructure for all that fat takes time *and* loads of energy. It can take months to gain a kilogram from scratch. A malignant tumour also sends out signals to lay down blood vessels to help it grow (angiogenesis). In some ways, excess fat is like a malignant tumour and fat growth is certainly not benign in a modern-day **GOFES** patient.

For as long as that infrastructure exists, regaining weight will be easy. Keep your weight and fat percentage stable for a year or two and these vessels will clog up from disuse and atrophy. After you have reached such a state, stability will have been achieved. You will still be a Polar Bear and you will never be cured, but you will be stable, in spite of your genetics and your environment.

One of the major problems is that people don't keep up the maintenance long enough for that infrastructure to atrophy. Those blood vessels need to be made redundant so that your body has to go through a more time consuming process to rebuild them. Once these vessels have deteriorated you have a much better chance to keep the excess fat at bay. More on this subject later as we delve into what you can do to get rid of these superfluous blood vessels.

Increased Equilibrium Set Point - ESP

Your ESP is the point at which your body becomes increasingly efficient at depositing fat. After weight loss your ESP can increase and it may be necessary to lower it.

The ESP was discussed in chapter 8. The Set Point is the weight your metabolism wants your weight to be. To a degree it will defend this point, especially in Humming Birds as part of their genetics. If you are a Polar Bear the ESP you have would represent an unstable set point.

Our bodies do not know the difference between a diet and a famine even though we intellectually know what we are doing. Therefore, in order to prepare for the next famine as it were, the ESP is raised after each diet, especially in Polar Bears. This means that the person can become potentially fatter than before.

It takes time to lower the ESP to manageable levels. *It will only do so if you are persistent with your maintenance.* By way of illustration analyse the following diagram:

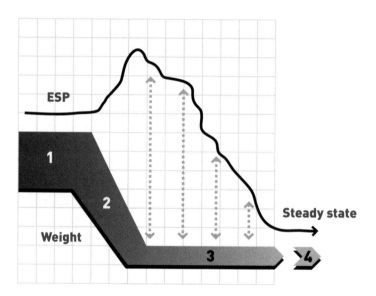

As you lose weight, if your ESP goes up you are subjected to almost irresistible pressures to simply regain everything you have lost. Your body is convinced you are in a state of famine and is only interested in brute survival.

If you persist with your weight loss, and provided you stay in the healthy fat percentage range, your body becomes "less alarmed". In an unpredictable way your ESP starts moving downward. The longer you maintain the more stable your body becomes and the easier it is to maintain your weight loss. Eventually you will reach a stage where maintenance becomes manageable. You have entered Stage 4. Your excess blood vessels have become dysfunctional and your hormones and other metabolic processes are now geared for a lower fat percentage. You are now stable.

To reach this point takes at least a year, but for many it could take two to three years. Be patient and persistent.

It is important that you remember that this is not a cure. Although it is now easier to maintain your healthy fat percentage, you are still a Polar Bear and there is nothing you can do about that. Your body still retains all the genetic tools at its disposal to develop GOFES again. The present DES situation, especially the supply state of affairs, is not in the Polar Bear's favour, BUT, by keeping the weight off you stand a chance to live longer than most Humming Birds.

I have noticed that most of the commercial concerns in the field of weight loss seem to give their clients a guarantee. As a medical doctor I believe this is unethical - all I can guarantee is that I will do my best to help you, but I can't guarantee the outcome.

Nevertheless, I'm prepared to give you the following written guarantee!

GUARANTEE

DEAR PATIENT,

I HEREBY CERTIFY THAT IF YOU DO NOT FOLLOW

THROUGH WITH THE MAINTENANCE PROGRAM

STAGE 3 YOU WILL PUT ON ALL THE EXCESS FAT

AND WEIGHT YOU HAVE LOST AND POSSIBLY MORE.

SIGNED: DR. HENDRIK

That's no guarantee!

How can it be? **GOFES** is an incurable disease and if you don't acquire the skill of keeping weight off, you'll never achieve success. Your "Set Point" or ESP is abnormally elevated after significant weight loss and unless you lower the bar during maintenance you'll be in a perpetual state of instability, which will inevitably lead to weight regain.

Be patient - the rewards are immense.

10th Characteristic of Successful Weight Maintainers:
Participation in the Maintenance Program (Stage 3) and follow up

The "Ah Ha Syndrome" revisited

"Ah Ha I have lost all my weight - I can celebrate!!" Following a therapeutic period of intense fat loss and the deprivation involved, it is just human nature that we want to have a bit of a holiday. As the scales go down, so does the incentive and the "Ah Ha Syndrome" becomes all the more powerful, spurred on by POD. Unfortunately, this is just when we need the most discipline.

One of my patients, a clinical psychologist, has an interesting theory why some people regain their excess fat. It's a lot like love.

There is a certain high in weight loss. People feel marvellous. It is exciting to see the excess fat melt away and to be able to buy new clothes and meet new people. But once they go onto maintenance, the excitement is lost as their weight stabilises. The high is lost. Some people feel so despondent that they need to regain weight as they seek once again to find the high associated with losing weight.

POD/POEx is now quite sneaky

This phenomenon no longer employs the full frontal attack, but it hasn't given up the battle and has plenty of other ways to compel you to eat. POD somehow knows you can now recognise the full frontal attack and can deal with it. It now switches to Sneaky Back Door Attacks (SBDA).

Just because you don't feel "hungry" doesn't mean POD is less active. If GOFES is to be controlled, then you need to control the Sneaky Back Door Attacks.

Recording

Once you formally hit maintenance - *and it is a formal process* - and you have earned your No-Belly Prize, then you are officially on Stage 3. One of the first things you have to do is weigh yourself daily. This is quite different from what I said before, but the circumstances are dissimilar.

For years I have tried to identify the mechanism that regulates our eating just enough for our needs. *I have come to the conclusion that we don't have such a mechanism.* We therefore need an "external speedometer" to gauge our caloric needs, otherwise we will constantly over eat as we are programmed to do.

"Dieting is the penalty for exceeding the feed limit."
ANONYMOUS

Calorie counting is one way of trying to do this, but it won't be long before you'll give up in desperation. What other methods could there be? Your bathroom scales could be the "speedometer" that keeps tabs on your fat percentage in an indirect but convenient way, but you must do it correctly.

Rules for weighing:

1. Weigh yourself first thing in the morning *only*, after you get up. Never any other time.

2. Without clothing. If you wear underwear, weigh yourself then every day with underwear. You need to *standardise* your weighing as much as possible.

3. Before you had any breakfast or anything to eat and drink. If after breakfast you realise you forgot to weigh, then skip it for the day. You have to have an empty stomach.

4. Before you weigh, go to the toilet.

5. Always use the same scales. Bathroom scales tend to be different.

6. Take your scales with you if you go away. It's easy to put them in the boot of the car. If you are serious about GOFES management and control, you need to

do this at least for the first year you are on maintenance. Some people tell me they weigh themselves at a chemist shop when they are away. I cannot see how a person is going to do that in the nude first thing in the morning. Besides, the shop's scales will be different from your scales anyway. If you are a type one diabetic would you take your insulin with you on holiday?

7. The way you stand makes a difference on most bathroom scales. Note for instance where you put your toes and always stand exactly in that position. If you bent forward a bit to see the dial better, then you always have to adopt this body position. If you get glasses in the meantime and it's no longer necessary to bend forward, you still have to adopt the original position.

8. All you really want from your scales is not to see exactly and correctly what you weigh, but whether you are gaining or losing weight - *that's all*.

This will give you quite a good idea about your metabolic weight.

How can this be used to determine your caloric intake?

Let's say that for arguments sake you weigh five kilograms on your first maintenance morning. I've deliberately chosen an unrealistic figure to convey the message that it is not really the actual figure that counts - it's about *gaining or losing* weight from that baseline figure.

While you'd like to maintain this baseline for the rest of your life, you'll soon realise you can't do it. Some days you will gain and on other days you will lose, but like anything in life, there are *limits*. These *metabolic limits* are within a two kilogram range. You can only strive for an average weight of five kilograms, varying up to six or down to four kg in our example.

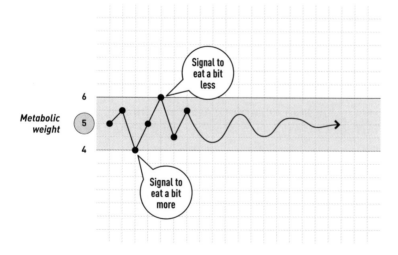

Looking at the illustration, the first day you weigh five kilograms, then you notice the next day you've gained half a kilogram. This is not a problem.

The following day you notice you have lost a kilogram. This is not a problem either, but it becomes the **signal** for you to eat a little bit extra for the next twelve hours. You know this, of course, first thing in the morning, before you've had anything to eat and drink. Armed with this information you can take some very important steps for the day, although POD will try and convince you otherwise.

Over the following two days you notice your weight is up to six kilograms. This still isn't a problem, it's just the **signal** for you to eat a little less over the next twelve hours. If you take evasive action your weight should come down a bit the next day.

The longer you maintain, the more stable you become and the easier maintenance becomes.

Why you have to keep your metabolic weight in a two kilogram range:

1. Our food intake is externally controlled and we do not have internal signalling mechanisms to tell us when we have had just the right amount. We only know when we've had too much. We need an *external signal* to allow us to monitor our food intake over a period of time - hence the scales. All that most Polar Bears need is 20 to 30 little calories extra per day, over and above their needs, and it can translate into 20 or 30 extra kilograms (44 to 66 lb) over a 10 year period. Those 20 or so extra calories just keep adding up.

2. The excess blood vessels need to be well and truly put to rest. This can only be achieved within a metabolic range of two kilograms, and you can't monitor such a narrow range without scales.

3. After a while your weight will start to follow a pattern that is specific to you. This becomes very important information in controlling your **GOFES** in the long term. Recognising these patterns and understanding them will help you keep **GOFES** at bay.

The next step is to jot down your daily weight on a graph.

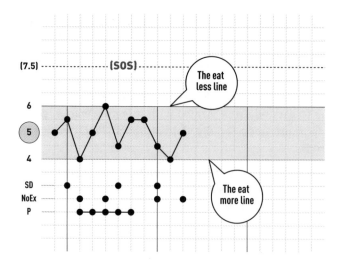

Your metabolic weight should always be circled in red. In this case it is five kilograms. The four kilogram 'green' line is the "eat more line" - green for "go". The six kilogram red line is the "eat less line" - red for STOP. Further up at the seven-and-a-half kilogram mark is a dotted line, called the emergency line or SOS line. You can call it what you like, as long as you know that drastic action needs to be taken if you happen to get there. Why is the emergency line not a solid line? It is because the dots symbolise the flashing lights of the ambulance that's coming to take you away.

Tip: Format your graph in pen, but always record your personal data in pencil. Keep it neat... it is your life.

SD - Sin Days

SD stands for Sin Days - "Party" or "Free" days if you prefer. This is the 9th Lesson of Nutrition. More on this in a later chapter.

POD can't be controlled all the time because we are not naturally inclined to restrain hunger and cravings.

Sooner or later a situation will arise where you become vulnerable and lose control. Without Sin Days, you'll become so deprived and frustrated with the incessant POD stimulation you'll end up in an eating frenzy that could take weeks of recovery.

Isn't it better to act before "giving in to **POD**"? If YOU deliberately "give in" to **POD** YOU are in control. You get it out of your system as it were. Over a period of time you will gain powerful information about your ability to deal with **POD** as it affects you. Although you can't win all the time, make sure you win the war. If **POD** wins the war you will be in Fat City again.

These "Sin Days" or "Free Days" or "Party Days" or whatever you want to call them, need to be:

1. **Well planned.** You can only have a Sin Day if you are not at your "eat less line" (the red line). Your Sin Days should be designed to prevent you going on a feeding rampage.

2. **On a regular basis.** One day per week, such as a Sunday, is ideal. We have a need for it, otherwise we feel too deprived.

3. **There are three distinct types of Sin Days.**

   - *Spontaneous Sin Days...* it just happened. You didn't plan it. Maybe you lost a bit of control. Make sure you record it on your graph - you need to keep tabs on it and see what patterns emerge.

   - *Planned Sin Days - Regular...* Sundays are good for Sin Days. It's easy to get back into a routine on a Monday, but if you choose Saturdays you may be tempted to merely continue and have another one on Sunday as well. However, you can make it any day of the week that works for you. "Sundae, Monday, who cares?"

   - *Planned Sin Days - Special Events...* such as birthdays or food festivals. If your birthday is in two weeks time, plan it as a Sin Day in advance. A day or two before your birthday, deliberately eat a bit less so that your weight goes down to the "eat more line" - the 'green' line. Then when you wake up for your birthday, you have to eat a bit more. This works well because you can eat within your two kilogram margin before you have to eat less again.

4. **Approach your Sin Days with caution.** Sin Days are not a right, but a privilege. They can serve as a springboard to catapult you into GOFES territory again. "One is too much and a thousand is too little". This saying from Alcoholic Anonymous is spot on here.

5. **Start cautiously.** Sin Days are not a licence to consume everything you want. There are certain foods you should permanently avoid. Why stick rubbish in your mouth?

NoEx - No exercise

The emphasis here is on "NO". Record these. Anything less than 20 minutes a day is a NoEx day. Plotting these will provide you with powerful information about your ability to control POEx - the pain of exercise phenomenon.

P stands for periods - menstruation - ladies only

When you have your period, record each day as a single dot, but then join them with a line. It is a single, continuous event. A number of women seem to have POD problems associated with their period and it becomes necessary to study individual behaviours and patterns objectively. Remember, quality information is powerful.

You might wish to use the graph to record other data that you think is pertinent in controlling your **GOFES** *or even other aspects of your life.* The data may reveal some interesting biorhythms. Asthma or diabetes sufferers may want to record this information on their weight graphs.

I have heard some interesting stories about what people record. A patient came in once and said: "Doctor, you've saved me a lot of money". I thought how could that be? I'm not a financial adviser.

She was on maintenance for four years and was still plotting her weight graphs, even though they are only required for the first year or two. I'd heard she was a frequent litigant.

"Doctor, I had to come up with a certain date for one of my cases. It had to be very specific. All I knew, it was about two-and-a-half years ago, but I couldn't work it out.

"Then a brain wave struck me. I'll look at my weight statistics. There it was - I found it. You saved me a lot of money."

The vertical lines from the "eat less line" indicate Sundays. It is merely a convenient way of breaking the graph into weeks.

In order to use this technique effectively you need to know certain concepts, rules and jargon.

The half kilogram rule

Only record 0.5 kilograms. If your scales indicate you weigh 57.2kg (125.8 lb), then round it up to 57.5kg (126 lb). Never round it down - don't give yourself the benefit of the doubt. Less than half a kilogram on bathroom scales is not of any use to you anyway.

The one kilogram rule

If you gain a kilogram *you have to get rid of it.* Even if you gain just one kilogram every six months, it may not sound much and nobody will really notice one or two kilos on you at first. In ten years time it will be at least 20kg -

equivalent to a bag of cement - and everybody will notice it, especially on your bottom and hips, and you'll have a beer keg instead of a "six pack".

The extra kilogram rule

When you have gained say two kilograms, *you have to lose three kilos*. If you have gained five kilos, you have to lose six. To correct the damage you cannot relax until you have lost this extra kilo. You have to aim to hit the 'green' line - the eat more line.

Visit or "test" the green line

Even if your daily weight is kept well within the "eat more" and "eat less" lines, you must deliberately, at least every week or two, eat less until you actually touch the 'green' line. *This is very important.* The constant tendency is always to go up. By aiming for the 'green' line you're more likely to control your weight.

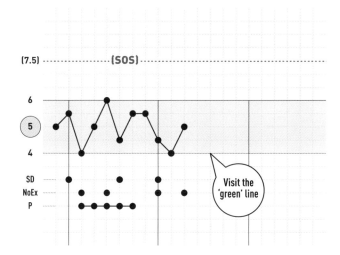

LRCP - lapse, relapse, collapse and prolapse (perhaps, perhaps!)

During maintenance your GOFES is in remission - but never cured. Maintenance will be a succession of lapses, relapses and remission. This will be your life story. It is normal. You just have to nip it in the butt - so to speak!

I worked out some time ago that I have probably lost 300kg (660 lb) or more in the last 25 years, but during this time I have never gone more than five kilograms over my metabolic weight. As soon as I gain a bit, especially when away from home, at the earliest opportunity I get rid of it.

L = lapse. It signifies any weight that is between the "eat less" and "SOS" lines. When you have a lapse, the one extra kilogram rule applies. Cut down until you have reached the 'green' line and then relax (but don't relapse!). A "shift" is also a lapse and needs to be addressed. You must learn to recognise these signs because they serve as early warning that trouble is on the way.

A "shift" means you are still in your metabolic range, between the "eat more" and "eat less" lines, but if you analyse the "shift" you'll see you have actually gained half a kilo which *you have to get rid of.* Apply the extra kilogram rule. Flush it out and do not stop until you have reached the 'green' line.

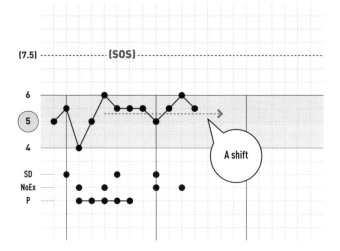

R = relapse. If you have hit the SOS line, you have relapsed. This calls for urgent remedial action, even if you are on holidays and have a meal booked with your favourite movie star. At the clinic our patients are required to phone us immediately and present themselves as soon as possible. Relapses can continue until you reach your starting weight. In this case you have **collapsed** and have to start all over again. What a mess!

Continuing gaining weight past the point of collapse, such that you are fatter than ever before, and you have **prolapsed**. Collapsing is bad enough, but prolapsing is the worst possible outcome of any attempt to control **GOFES**.

Everybody will lapse and relapse in maintenance. It is part of the treatment to anticipate and deal with it as it occurs.

A long time ago I told a patient with the rather unusual name of Bossby that he would lapse and relapse during maintenance.

He fired up and said: "Doc, maybe lapses, but I'll never have a relapse".

To my surprise - and there always a few in medical practice - he did not have any relapses for two-and-a-half years, but then came the inevitable relapse. We all do, unless you are an extreme Humming Bird with a stable set point.

What happens if you collapse or prolapse?

Please don't give up. A patient at the clinic was so embarrassed that she wrote me the following poem:

Doctor, Doctor do not pale,
For as a patient, I did fail,
but I am back again,
Fat and keen.
Please dear Doctor, make me lean.
Your patient,
Lorraine

Maintenance - Some Additional Points

Exercise

People who over value the role of exercise in **GOFES** control will be disappointed every time. Exercise just does not work on its own. Over exercising can take you from your comfort zone into the danger zone and accelerate the aging process. Exercise is very important, but above all, it is what you put in your mouth that will carry the day.

POD is more difficult to deal with than **POEx** and that is why we would rather exercise and suffer **POEx** than **POD**.

POD > POEx

Sleep habits

Disrupt your natural sleep rhythms, suffer sleep deprivation and you'll soon see POD and POEx take over your life. More on sleep routine later.

Inspiration and motivation

Concentrate on when you were over-fat and miserable, and not so much on what you can look like once you lose weight. This psychology works better in controlling **GOFES** - it's better to focus on the goals you have achieved and how much better you look and feel at this point in time with your weight loss to date, rather than the promise of the future.

Synopsis:

1. Maintain or regain. Your body needs attention or your physique will fall apart.

2. Record your habits and rhythms and obtain quality information on which to base your GOFES strategies.

3. You will never regret controlling **GOFES**. It will be the best investment that you have made in your life.

4. The treatment of **GOFES** is the most powerful therapy we have in medicine today, because it achieves so much - hopefully this is sounding familiar by now!

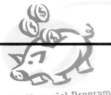

10. Financial Program

1. Nutrition Program

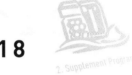

2. Supplement Program

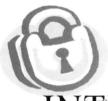

9. Protection and Security

CHAPTER 18

INTRODUCTION TO THE 10 PRINCIPLES OF GOOD HEALTH AND MAINTENANCE

8. Time

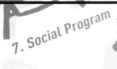

7. Social Program

6. Philosophy

5. Rest and Recreation

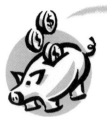

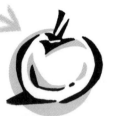

10. Financial Program   1. Nutrition Program

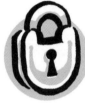

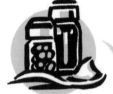

9. Protection and Security   2. Supplement Program

THE PRINCIPLES OF
GOOD HEALTH AS AN
INTER-CONNECTING
CHAIN AND GRID, ALL
WORKING IN SYNERGY
TO FORM A SYSTEM OF
HEALTH PROTOCOLS.

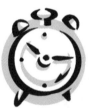

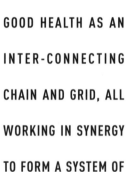

8. Time   3. Exercise Program

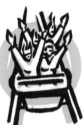

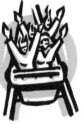

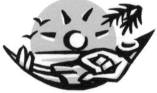

7. Social Program   4. Hygiene Program

6. Philosophy   5. Rest and Recreation

INTRODUCTION TO THE 10 PRINCIPLES OF GOOD HEALTH AND MAINTENANCE

"I don't like principles. Prejudice is more honest."
ANONYMOUS

Move into a brand new house with a newly landscaped garden and do nothing to maintain it, and within six months the garden will be a shadow of its former glory.

The body and mind have very specialised and regular maintenance needs and if left unattended for too long, the pain and cost in correcting the situation can be intense. Often the damage is irreparable.

That said, whatever you do for your health will always be of some benefit, but there are few second chances for health, lack of care and negligence.

Planning is bringing the future into the present, so that we can do something about it NOW.

It must be a pity to die of something that you could have prevented. Losing weight is the ultimate prevention tool.

In all my experience with **GOFES**, of the people who don't follow up with a formal maintenance program, I have only come across two who maintained significant weight loss for five years or longer.

What is the single most important characteristic of people who keep their weight off - who control their **GOFES** in the long term? Years of research leads me to believe it's because they're *health conscious*. Without health consciousness, in spite of other supporting characteristics, it is virtually impossible to keep fat percentage normal in today's society.

11th Characteristic of Successful Weight Maintainers:
They become health conscious and act on it.

For that reason, I have put health concepts together in a system of 10 principles. Following these principles will assist you to become health conscious. An Age Retarding Program will alert you to all the health issues.

For an Age Retarding Program to be successful every potentially harmful habit and action should be identified and eliminated.

Aging is an ailment and should be seen and treated as such, even though it is a natural process.

Chronological, Biological and at Risk Age

Chronological Age (CA) - your *birthday age*. If you were born 33 years ago you are 33 years old.

Biological Age (BA) - you can be biologically younger or older than your chronological age, depending on lifestyle and genetics. This is *the age that you function at*. It can also be called your **Functional Age (FA)**.

Risk age (RA) - determined by comparing an individual's chances of dying with others in the same Chronological Age **(CA)** group based on identified risk factors. *Risk Age* **(RA)** *is not related to Biological Age* **(BA)**.

Age-Retarding versus Age-Acceleration

Biological Age (BA) is on the y axis and Chronological Age (CA) is on the x axis.

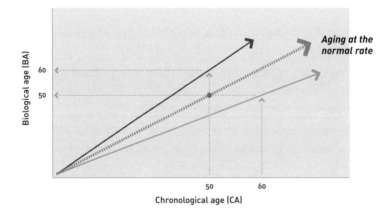

CA = BA

If a person is chronologically 50 years old and 50 biologically, then **this person is aging at the normal rate**. The body functions and metabolism are operating as would be expected for a normal person who is 50 years old.

CA > BA

If a person is 60 years chronologically, but biologically and functionally 50, then that person is 10 years "younger". In other words, they are 10 years younger than their Chronological Age. **This person is in age retardation.**

CA < BA

If a person is biologically 60, but but biologically and functionally 50, that person is obviously 10 years older than their actual age. **This person is in age acceleration.**

It stands to reason that one should aim for age retardation, as even the normal aging rate will bring on health problems way too soon. The 10 Health Principles are built around the concept of age deceleration, which not only promotes health, but also is the main chance you have to maintain your weight - your normal fat percentage - and control **GOFES**.

As this graph illustrates the older we get, the more likely we are to die from any number of causes. Increasing age increases the risk of accidents, heart disease, cancer and many other contributors to declining health.

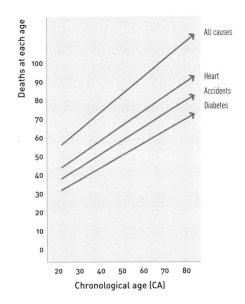

Age-specific death rates from various causes

227

Functional Age Monitoring - the Advantages

- **No matter what the outcome, it is motivating**

  If it indicates your aging rate is slower (**CA>BA**), then this is a great motivation to keep on doing the right things. If it indicates an accelerated aging process (**CA<BA**), then it motivates the person to do something about it and slow down the process.

- **Early warning system**

  Regular testing is important - ideally every three months, however once or twice a year will suffice. In a perfect world the tests will show that you are aging at a slower rate than normal. Even a slower rate than normal can be deceptive - in the event that your last two tests indicate acceleration, this could point to potential problems.

  An Age Delay Program should not be undertaken without the means to monitor it. You need proof that your efforts are working and to what degree. In addition, you need to make sure the program is not harmful - an unmonitored Age Delay Program could speed up the aging process.

  Occasionally you hear of people who are chronologically 60, but biologically 20. The majority of these claims are bogus. A 63 year old claimed to me that he was biologically 25. I offered to test it for him and to my surprise some of his biological makers were in the mid-thirties, but when I did a comprehensive test program I found his Functional Age to be 46 to 50. Still excellent, but far from the 25 he claimed. If you can achieve a Functional Age 10 years less than your Chronological Age, you are doing very well.

  The grey bell-shaped curve represents the Functional Age ranges of a person who is chronologically 60. From aging at the normal rate (**CA = BA**) to biologically 40 and in age retardation (**CA > BA**).

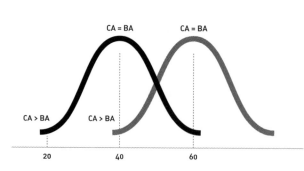

The black graph shows the biological age ranges of a person who is chronologically 40. When this person is biologically functioning at age 20, they're in age retardation (**CA > BA**).

The point is that a 60 year old may function at the level of a 40 year old, but will never compete with the lower biological ages that a chronologically 40 year old can achieve.

In spite of age retardation, we are still aging relentlessly. In 10 years time you will be 10 years older and the signs of aging will show.

Biological Age (**BA**) must be interpreted correctly. Even though you may be functioning at a younger age than your chronological age (**CA**) and you may look younger, there will always be aspects that will reveal your true age. Sad, but true.

It is therefore important to understand that the concept of Functional or Biological age is not a promise of immortality. Nevertheless, you may be surprised to know how rewarding it is to slow down the aging process. It is an important health concept - for example, **age retardation and monitoring can help to control GOFES.**

- **Other benefits of age rate monitoring**

It is important to point out there are limitations of Biological or Functional age testing and monitoring. You should be relatively healthy for it to be worthwhile. In the presence of another disease, other than aging, the accuracy declines. It can also be costly and so only the highly motivated will subject themselves to testing once or twice a year.

Functional Age assessment works very well with **GOFES** *since both are reversible,* and addressing these can reverse the progress of diseases directly associated with aging and GOFES. Monitoring of the Aging Rate (**AR**) is valuable for early detection of disease.

Sophie, suffering from **GOFES**, and a number of its associated diseases, as well as menopause, attended the clinic for the first time at age 54 (**CA**). She was put on an intensive treatment regime for **GOFES**, its accompanying diseases, and age retardation. Her Functional Age was 72 (CA54< BA72), which meant she was about 18 years older than she should have been. She was suffering from accelerated aging.

At age 56 (**CA**) her Functional age had come down to 47 (CA56>BA47). This was quite dramatic and although it is not usual, she was a very committed patient. Within two years her Biological Age Index (**BAI**) was now less than one, which meant she enjoyed a state of delayed aging.

- **A test is just as good as a retest**

This is not where the story ends because the most important of all these measures is the Aging Rate (**AR**). Sophie's was less than one, which of course is the desired outcome.

On Sophie's subsequent test series her **AR** was still less than one, *but had declined from minus 13.6 to minus 3.6.* As can be seen on the graph her **AR**, although still less than the normal aging rate *was accelerating.* This sometimes happens and is often a "correction" or "catch up" after such a dramatic initial drop in AR. Just to be sure, I repeated the test series three months later.

This time the **AR** was still less than normal aging but was in incremental acceleration. There were a number of possibilities. Maybe she was reverting back to her old **GOFES** life style, but this was not the case. Perhaps her treatment wasn't doing what it was supposed to do.

The other possibly was that she was developing disease somewhere in her body and was sending subtle warning signals in the form of accelerating aging. I contacted a physician friend whom I always refer to as a "medical detective" because of his special talents in diagnosis. He reported back to me and said he could find nothing wrong with Sophie. I told him that he should think outside the square and examine the situation with a magnifying glass.

After the second try he phoned me: "Are you psychic or what?" Sophie's cancer was early and curable. Not everybody is so lucky.

About 27 per cent of men who have a normal PSA (Prostatic Specific Antigen) are found to have prostate cancer. A result within the normal range, but with a slight increase in value, can still be predictive of prostate cancer. Therefore, a normal test should still be viewed with suspicion. Similarly, an accelerated Aging Rate (AR), even if it is less than one, may mean some pathological process is at work somewhere in the body. It is worth looking for, particularly if the patient is living a lifestyle that would normally be expected to retard aging.

You may not want to read the following because of its technical nature. If so, skip it and go on the next chapter.

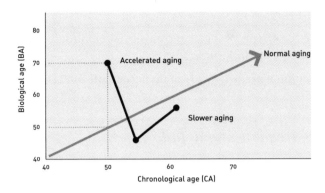

Sophie:

Chronological Age (CAn)	54	56	59
Biological Age (BAn)	72	47	54
Difference	18	9	5
Biological Age Index: (BAIn = BAn/CAn)	1.33	0.82	0.92
Aging rate: (ARn = ΔBAn/ΔCAn)		-13.68	-3.6
Incremental Aging rate:			10.08

A measurement of Relative Aging is the Biological Age Index (BAI):
BAI = BA/CA
<1 = Retarded aging (CA<BA)
1 = Normal aging (CA = BA)
>1 = Accelerated aging (CA>BA)

BAn = the most recent measurement
BA1 = the first measurement, BA2 = the second measurement, etc.

The Rate of Aging (AR) covers the whole test series. Thus from the first to last test series:

Aging rate **(AR) = ΔBA/ΔCA**
$$\Delta BA = BA2 - BA1$$
$$\Delta CA = CA2 - CA1$$

>1 = Accelerated aging BA>CA
1 = Normal aging CA = BA
0 to 1 = Retarded aging BA<CA
0 = Halted aging
<1 = BA reversal

Incremental Aging Rate (IAR):
Is AR, but only between the 2 most recent test values.

Synopsis

1. **GOFES** control is a health concept. We need to control and monitor it, as we would with any other aspect of our health.

2. Humming Birds also get immense benefits from living an **Anti-GOFES** lifestyle.

"If you fail to plan, you are planning to fail."
ANONYMOUS

CHAPTER 19

1. NUTRITION HEALTH PROGRAM

Financial Program

1. Nutrition Program

1. NUTRITION HEALTH PROGRAM

The first link in the health chain

The Nutrition Program **is the Supply** *in DES (Demand, Effort and Supply).*

Behind important philosophical questions like:
"What is life and consciousness?"

Are other important questions like:
"What is for breakfast, lunch and dinner and snacks in between?"

"Diet and religion are closely connected.
We eat what we want and pray not to get fat."
ANONYMOUS

No matter what we ponder in life, having food on the table overrides all else, after all it's about survival.

Our eating behaviours are governed by the Pain of Deprivation (POD) and supply. Our environment determines the quantity, quality and variety of our food. In days of old when food was more nutritious, natural and less plentiful, eating was hardly an intellectual pursuit. Today, our instincts are the same, but the quality and quantity of food has changed for the worse.

We have a propensity to eat anything, good or bad, especially if it looks good and is tasty. We have always been opportunistic eaters, but today opportunity abounds. Commercially, these factors are exploited to the hilt. Sure, we have acquired knowledge, but it's almost a case of paralysis from analysis.

WHY? Allow me to repeat it again. We are all genetically programmed to over eat. We will eat whatever the food supply will dish up to us. **POD** drives us to it - for survival. The food industry capitalises on it.

What's wrong with the following advice from the National Heart Foundation?

EAT LEAST	EAT MODERATELY	EAT LOTS
Butter, Coconut oil	Lean meat	Bread
Cooking margarine	Poultry	Unprocessed cereals
Meat fat, Poultry skin	Fish	Rice, Pasta
Cheese, Cream	Nuts	Fruit
Ice cream	Seeds	Vegetables
Cakes, Pastries	Eggs (2 per week)	Salads
Snack foods	Low fat dairy products	Grains
Take-aways		Baked Beans
Salt, Alcohol		

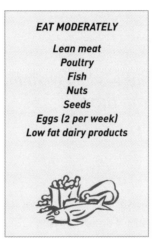 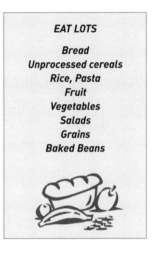

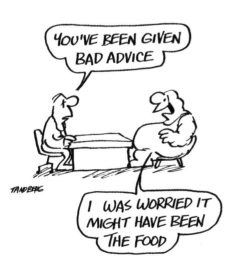

We should not be eating lots of anything - not even good food. The suggestion of "eating lots" is like music in our ears and panders to **POD**.

"Experts" are aware of the Pain of Deprivation and they know that talk of reducing quantities will scare people. The mere mention of reducing our supply of food stirs the survival instincts.

When it comes to GOFES, the primary issues are evaded rather than confronted. *Dodging and not enough confrontation are two of the main reasons why we never really make much progress in the treatment of* **GOFES**.

Two thousand years ago the Romans discovered that "eating lots" affected their health. Wealthier Romans noted that peasants were often much healthier. Gladiators refused to eat the refined breads and food, because it made their "limbs weak".

"Quid me nutrit me destruit" -
"What nourishes me also destroys me."
LATIN SAYING

"A man begins cutting his wisdom teeth the moment he bites off more than he can chew."
MARK TWAIN

Dose related response

Up to a point, food nourishes us, beyond that it becomes toxic. Most of us dig our graves with our teeth. Food in adequate quantities is healthy, but oversupply results in the slow release of poisons that have degenerative effects. This is why Polar Bears with **GOFES** fall victim to a broad range of health consequences.

Controlling the quantities we consume is something we have to do *ourselves*. No-one is going to do it for us. And the best place to start is by developing the "eat less habit".

Portion distortion

"Gluttony is the source of all our infirmities and the fountain of all our diseases. As a lamp is choked by a superabundance of oil, and a fire extinguished by excess of fuel, so is the natural health of the body destroyed by intemperate diet."
MARION L. BURTON

The French and Japanese traditionally consume considerably less calories than other industrialised nations, even though they are living amongst an abundant food supply. Culturally they have developed the *"eat less habit"*. Eating between meals is a rarity and portions are smaller.

McDonald's in the US versus McDonald's in Japan - not only are the Cokes and the Big Macs larger in the US, but the servings of French fries are three times the size. Super-sizing-portion-distortion!

"My doctor says I should stop drinking and eating expensive food - it will help me pay his account."
ANONYMOUS

Super sizing leads to over eating. Not only are we genetically programmed to over eat, but we're also driven by the view "I've paid for it, therefore I'll eat it". And it's not always *physical size*. With calorie-dense foods, sometimes a "small portion" may still be portion distortion. *Energy value* per volume is a more accurate measure than mere size.

I'm told that in the fifteenth century a Japanese Emperor toured a number of fishing villages and was disgusted by the crude way the peasants ate. On returning to his palace he decreed that his subjects should clean up their eating habits. Being a disciplined people they obeyed and developed strict eating rituals based on small portions, very neatly arranged. As a result they culturally developed the *eat less habit*.

We need to apply the discipline of CRAN: Caloric Restriction with Adequate Nutrition - *Under Nutrition, not Malnutrition*.

Presentation as a way to eat less

Presentation plays a big part in Japanese and French cuisine. Arranging the different morsels very neatly causes people to eat less. You may be sceptical of this, but try it yourself.

Separation of the different foods and dishes is another way to eat less. First the salad is served and you are expected to eat it on its own, then the meat by itself and so forth, not like a mixed grill or buffet. This slows down eating, making it easier to reach satiety before too much is consumed.

A patient who lost 115 kg (253 lb) liked to arrange his Stage 2 (excess-fat loss) food as attractively as he could. "You have to touch the bite size pieces twice," he told me. "Once while arranging it on the plate and then as you put it in your mouth." He thought about his food.

Speed of eating

You will eat much less if your eating takes longer than 20 minutes.

It takes about 20 minutes to feel full. If you eat very fast you can consume quite a lot before you reach fullness. This is even more relevant with junk food, because it is so calorie dense. Survival dictates that we eat fast - in primitive times we had to eat quickly before a predator took our food. We are still programmed that way. To change that programming we need to *start low, go slow.*

Inducing excessive eating

Advertisements that promote low carbohydrate or low fat foods induce you to believe these foods are healthy and good for you. "Because it's good for me, more is better"... it's NOT! Often with low fat foods the fat calories are removed and replaced by processed white sugar and syrup calories. Better to eat less of healthier quality food than more of engineered rubbish.

The first rule of nutrition is:
if it tastes good spit it out, because it is bad for you.

Little snacks,
Bigger slacks,
Little pickers,
Bigger knickers!

Eat less and less to live longer and longer.

The first lesson of nutrition is: we eat too much
  - super sizing portion distortion
  - develop the eat less habit

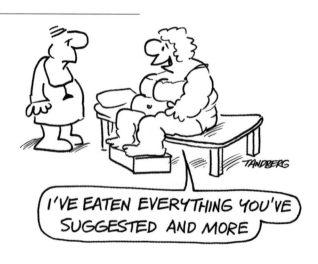

I'VE EATEN EVERYTHING YOU'VE SUGGESTED AND MORE

The explosion in nutritional knowledge

Nutrition today means confusion - bewilderment - perplexity - misunderstanding - mythology. What was the "in thing" last week is now the definite "out thing".

School of Nutrition		
As of today		
BUTTER	GOOD	•
MARGARINE	•	BAD
CHOLESTEROL	GOOD	•
FAT	•	BAD
FISH	GOOD	•
MEAT	•	BAD
WINE (WHITE)	•	BAD
WINE (RED)	GOOD	•
BEER	GOOD	•
TEA	GOOD	•
SALT	GOOD	•

Motto: Paralysis from analysis

We are living in a society that is over supplied with "experts".

With nutrition you only need a few basic facts about nutrition.

It is my mission to take the mystique out of nutrition.

It is important to note that even the dairy corporation is a commercial concern, in the business of selling milk and milk products, and not an independent scientific body.

Gurus, governments and experts have told us for the last 20 years to eat less fat. We followed their advice and ended up fatter and sicker than ever and diabetes soared to plague proportions.

Nutrition is a science that needs to be seen as a whole - more on this later. I would have left it at that, but unfortunately we are so far gone with nutrition that, in order to protect yourself, you need to acquire a bit more knowledge about the subject.

Remember, we don't have the natural ability to know when we have had enough to eat. We only know when we have over eaten. We are opportunistic eaters - nature supplied and we ate. Whatever is dished up we tend to consume - good or bad.

I hear your protest: "Hey, wait a minute. I'm aware of what I'm eating."

Maybe you are, but it doesn't hurt to be a better-informed, health conscious person.

Remember, we are genetically programmed to over eat and we don't have the natural ability to understand the quality of the food supply. If it looks and tastes good, we have a natural tendency to think it is good and nutritious. *Today, this is very far from the truth.*

Food instincts are acquired over many generations. We can't afford to throw out those instincts in favour of modern food. We did not evolve on margarine, 97 per cent fat free foods, white bread, ice cream, soft drinks and other adulterations of our food supply.

Simple time proven recipes are much better for us than what a food technologist can ever engineer.

The second lesson of nutrition is: KISS - Keep It Super Simple

Unfortunately, to keep it simple we need a basic knowledge of nutrition. We need to be able to make prudent decisions.

The purpose here is to give you the tools to get rid of your excess flab, keep it off, become and stay healthy and decelerate the aging process.

Nutritional basics

The third lesson of modern nutrition is: understand the evolution of our food supply and its metabolic consequences.

The evolution of our food supply can be divided into three distinct periods.

PERIOD ONE: PALAEOLITHIC/HUNTER GATHERER

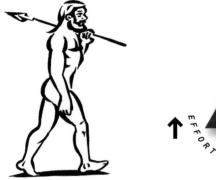
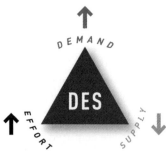

We evolved on the Palaeolithic or hunter gatherer diet. Our metabolisms are still stuck in the stone-age period even though we are living in the space-age.

DES (Demand, Effort and Supply) operated in the following way.

Demand to eat (POD): This was of course very strong and we had enormous appetites to give us strong inducements to hunt and gather in order to be able to eat and survive.

Effort: To find and hunt the food was at times a significant and challenging undertaking.

Food supply: Typically, this was scarce and erratic. We had a diet of wild meats, birds, eggs, fish, bush vegetables, tubers, tarty bush fruits and some-times nuts. When times were harsh we ate insects and rodents, and some even became cannibals. We were and still are opportunistic eaters.

It was in this environment that our present day metabolism was conceived.

PERIOD TWO: EARLY TO LATE AGRICULTURAL

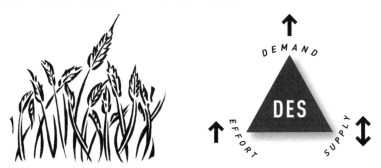

Agriculture developed when hunter gatherers noticed that some of the gathered plant food left on the ground would "grow" by itself. They deter-mined that putting some of this plant food on the ground and letting it grow, eliminated the need to travel huge distances in sourcing food. Over time the practices became more sophisticated and developed into modern agriculture.

Some even noticed that certain of the wild animals were not particularly frightened by their presence. They concluded that if they provided food and protection for these animals they might become a ready food supply.

Agriculture is arguably the most important development in human history. It offered a more secure food supply and gave us the freedom to move into the age of industry and subsequently technology.

During this time **demand to eat** remained a constant.

Effort was reduced. **Supply** became more plentiful and less expensive, *outstripping our metabolism's ability to keep pace with change.*

Grains and cereals were introduced some 10,000 years ago and while this led to wheat and gluten sensitivities, we persevered because of the advantages of an agricultural society over that of the hunter gatherer.

Domesticated animals took the place of wild foods, we discovered alcohol and became more calorie dense. The latter had some advantages at the time.

But about 120 years ago, especially in the last 50 years, we were catapulted into the third period. This happened so fast that we had no time to metabolically adapt. On a day-to-day level we did not even notice it, but on a metabolic level it was revolutionary and extreme. Old genes and new food.

PERIOD THREE: COMMERCIAL / DRUG / AGRICULTURAL

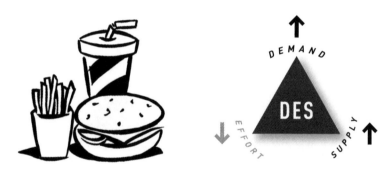

By now we were so urbanised and our technology so far developed that we could virtually play with our food supply at will. Our comfort zone had shrunk. Just a pity it was not done with our metabolisms in mind, they were still in the Stone Age. Our technological achievements and sophistication had outstripped our metabolisms.

Space-age-**DES** is much different than the **DES** we evolved on. For Polar Bears, **GOFES** and its consequences are the result.

POD is now more intense and stronger than periods one and two. Food is now ubiquitous. The sight and smell of food are some of the most potent triggers of **POD**. Food itself is much more appetising than ever before. Sixty years ago the only gourmet meal was the Sunday roast and a dessert. Nowadays, we have gourmet breakfasts, snacks, desserts and other delicacies on demand.

From all of this most of us developed insulin resistance, which *additionally* stimulates **POD**. Add alcohol to the equation and we are ferociously hungry all the time.

Effort is now zero. It takes negligible energy to open your wallet to pay for a ready made hot fried chicken and the accompanying French fries. Even the effort to eat it - the chewing - has diminished.

Supply of highly processed fast foods and alcohol is such that most of the population doesn't *get or want* enough vegetables and fruit. Our food supply includes refined sugars, saturated fats and large quantities of chemicals that never existed in the history of food.

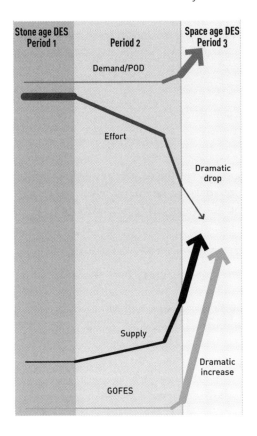

What do you get if you have a graph like this? You guessed it - **GOFES** - disease. So, what are you as an individual going to do about it?

In short:

Our modern food supply is different from our original in the following ways:

- It is abundant in unlimited quantities.
- Available 25 (sic) hours a day, eight (sic) days a week.
- Ready to eat without any effort or preparation. All processes have been commercially taken care of.
- Much more *palatable* than in the past, therefore more appetite stimulating than ever before.
- Advertised aggressively and promoted commercially, creating an artificial "need".
- Calorie dense. More calories per volume and weight.
- The result: excessive consumption of calories.

Our adulterated, tainted and hazardous food supply

Nature provided certain foods to eat. We evolved on it and our metabolisms are suited for this type of food. Some animals eat grass, others eat insects. Humans are designed to live off certain foodstuffs. I like to call them "Nature's Formulae" - formulated by nature to suit our unique metabolisms. Or perhaps our metabolisms were formulated to suit the food that was around - the food has changed, our metabolisms haven't.

In Period Three we have highly qualified food technologists interfering with nature's formulae. We have products that are peddled as "food" which, from a nutritional point of view, are often garbage and trash. Be reminded: if you eat garbage - you become garbage.

You need the full spectrum of nutrient dense foods.

The fourth lesson of nutrition is:
take nothing away from food and add nothing.

Generally we do not want to believe or accept the degree to which our food supply has been contaminated and altered. Pointing this out gives rise to derision from some so-called experts: "You are exaggerating. You don't know what you're talking about".

The issue of food is exceptionally emotional, often steeped in egos.

Even if we know our food is not appropriate, we are so busy we eat whatever is dished up as long as it is attractive and tasty. Remember, we are opportunistic eaters. In a moment of intense **POD** the majority will eat anything put in front of them. Therefore the food industry spends a lot on the appearance, taste and texture of food.

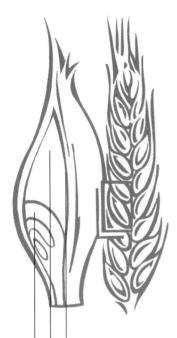

Endosperm
*Carbohydrates
and Protein*

Bran
*Fibre, B vitamins,
chromium and
other minerals*

Germ
*B, E and K
vitamins, iron and
other minerals*

Taking things away

Taking away natural substances from food is devitalising it - stripping it of nutrients and enzymes. In the illustration, the bran and wheat germ contain just the right amount of B vitamins and minerals to digest the endosperm in one grain of wheat. For good nutrition, nothing should be taken away, nothing should be added. By removing and adding things you end up with a completely different food having different effects on your metabolism and health.

Adding things

- There are numerous substances in our food supply. Some people classed as allergic to milk are not really allergic to milk, but to the antibiotic residue in milk. The cause - adding antibiotics to cow feed to prevent mastitis.

- Various hormones have found their way into our food supply over the last 50 years or so. At one stage hormones given to cattle caused cancer. These hormones are no longer allowed, having given way to other "safer" hormones.

  Hormones added to chicken feed in Puerto Rico were so excessive and passed on to humans to such a degree that even five-year-old girls developed breasts, pubic and underarm hair. While hormones don't usually find their way in our food supply to such a degree, the average girl now reaches puberty two years earlier than was the case 50 years ago. The long-term consequences have yet to be evaluated.

- Post World War I - brilliant colours were synthesised from coal tar and used as food additives to make food more attractive. Many of these additives were toxic and gradually banned, however we still use a number with questionable safety.

- Hot on the heels were artificial flavours. Given choice, we would not consciously add these to our diet as part of good nutrition:
  - Vanilla (Piperonal) was used to kill lice
  - Banana (Amyl Acetate) used as an oil paint solvent
  - Cherry (Aldehyde U7) used in plastic and rubber dyes.

The technology to deliver processed food items consists of such nutrient destroying processes as:
- Boiling and freezing of the food
- Bleaching and then dyeing
- Dehydrating and then reconstituting
- and involves thousands of chemical additives and dozens of processes unknown in the history of food.

When it comes to good nutrition - WHITE IS NOT RIGHT.

A man walks into a doctor's office. He has a cucumber up his nose, a carrot in his left ear and a banana in his right ear. "What's the matter with me?" he asks the doctor. The doctor replies: "You're not eating properly."

- Contamination of our food supply is common. Pesticides, industrial wastes and biological contamination are so common that it has become impossible to avoid these today. Ground water is so polluted by landfill that it is not safe to drink. Most of us have chemicals in our blood that have come from pizza boxes and various plastics.

Americans and Australians eat so much of these artificial additives, other chemicals and preservatives that the average person takes in about 2.5 to 5kg (5.5 to 11lb) a year of these substances - a baby's weight.

A patient of mine, who is the fifth generation of funeral parlour owners, told me that his dad and grandfather told him that if you got a call at four o'clock in the morning that a person had died, you better get up, get the coffin and the hearse and put the body in the fridge, because the moment we die we start decomposing. However, nowadays if you get such a call you just tell the relatives to put a blanket over the person and you'll pick the deceased up later in the day.

This is because we do not "go off" as quickly as we used to, because our bodies are saturated with preservatives from our food supply. I considered this to be a bit of a woolly story, but I phoned a forensic pathologist and he told me there was some truth in it. It seems as if we are mummifying ourselves while still alive.

"I personally stay away from health foods. I need all the preservatives I can get."
GEORGE BURNS

In some countries they add a plasticiser to highly refined cornstarch which when warmed is stringy like cheese. An artificial cheese flavour is added, together with a yellow dye. It ends up looking and tasting like "cheese". This is put on pizzas. This can be very confusing in making good food choices. You may be under the impression that you are consuming protein and calcium. It may look like cheese, taste like cheese, but "there ain't no cheese". If it walks like a duck, quacks like a duck and looks like a duck - it is a duck... that's an adage that doesn't necessarily apply to cheese!

Most of us love chocolate. The Incas and Aztecs first introduced it to the Conquistadors and from there it spread all over the world.

We are not the only creatures that love chocolate. Cockroaches love it too. A cockroach is a very interesting little animal and can withstand about hundred times the radiation we can. It will probably outlive us in an all out nuclear war. Apart from this, they are not really fussy where they live. Often they are found in the filthiest of places, collecting infested filth on the hairs of their bodies.

When chocolate beans are harvested and put in the sun to dry, cockroaches swarm out of the sewers to help themselves to the chocolate. They drop their filth and defecate. When the beans are ready, a half-hearted attempt is made to chase them away, but it is an impossible task.

Up to four per cent of the weight of chocolate may legally be cockroach parts!

Sugar is an important ingredient in chocolate and, depending on the type you buy, an ordinary little square can contain half to a full teaspoon of sugar. Various preservatives and other chemical products are added - and don't forget all that milk with the antibiotic in it. Most people who are allergic to chocolate are not really allergic to it per se, but to the cockroach protein that it contains.

In some places you can even order "deep fried Mars Bars". The latter is stored in the freezer and when a customer orders one, it is dipped in batter and put in boiling oil with all those fatty acids. Kids and adults alike are seen walking out of the shops with oily chocolate dripping oozing from the sides of their mouths.

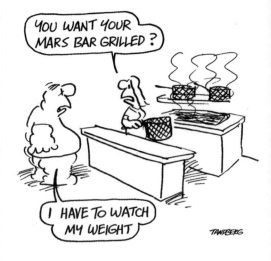

Deep fried pizzas have also made their appearance. A pizza is made up and then stored in the freezer. Six months later, or whenever some one wants a deep fried pizza, it is taken out of the freezer and immersed in the boiling oil. A patient told me they don't taste too bad! Maybe, but it's bad food.

Livestock are not "free range" any more, they are just like us, confined to small spaces without exercise, pumped full of hormones and bad food. This results in faster market-ready animals. Their metabolisms also evolved in the Stone Age. Today this produce is highly prized for its fatty liver and marbleised meat - but these are diseases! *We are already diseased, yet we are eating diseased animals.*

A commercial chicken is ready for the table some 35 days after hatching, while a free-range chicken takes 100-120 days to be ready. The commercial chicken makes good commercial sense, *BUT* what about our health? If you examine the commercial chicken you will notice that the meat is very white and the fat looks almost like the meat itself, at times almost indistinguishable from the meat. The free-range chicken on the other hand, has darker meat and the fat is yellow and quite separate from the meat.

Ask any surgeon - operating on an athlete is quite different to operating on the unfit fat "commercial patient". Little wonder it is suggested that the health system is economically unsustainable and facing collapse within 10 years.

It reminds me of the famous horse breeder who sells his thoroughbreds for hundreds of thousands of dollars. At one sale he escorted a potential buyer to the stables to have a look at his horses. Having missed breakfast, the horse owner bought himself a hotdog and a can of cola on the way to the stables.

A litre of cola contains a cup of sugar. Sugar is 99 per cent pure and as such is pharmacologically speaking a drug. It is also used as a preservative, since nothing will grow in it.

Japanese studies tell us the aluminium can containing the cola leaches aluminium into the drink through micro cracks in the covering plastic. Aluminium is regarded as toxic to the nervous system. The linkage with Alzheimer's disease is, however, controversial.

A few years ago it was reported in a medical journal that cola drinks are good spermicidals (killing male sperm). It was even suggested that if a woman was raped and could not get immediate medical help, she could douche her vagina with cola to avert a possible pregnancy. Recently an "expert" disputed that and said it was only weakly spermicidal. Whatever!

A kidney physician who did a conference tour and sabbatical around the world on kidney disease gave a few of us a talk at a restaurant about the latest factors in kidney damage. He mentioned how cola drinks can damage kidneys due to the high phosphate content.

I could not help noticing one of my fellow doctors drinking cola, trying to look nonchalant, putting it down and then pushing it slowly away.

Back to the racehorse breeder. The hotdog bun was made of white flour. White flour is not white but is bleached white. What is more, going from wholemeal to white flour sees the removal of 26 nutrients. Food marketers have taken to replacing three of these minerals with artificial nutrients and calling it "enriched flour". Enough said!

On this devitalised bleached bun was a layer of butter. Butter is much better than margarine, apart from containing a heap of saturated fat with a few pesticides and antibiotics. Admittedly it also contains some good stuff - milk and cream. What put me off butter was when I found out about a preservative used in butter in some countries. As medical students we dissected dead bodies, or cadavers, that had been kept for up to 18 months in this very same preservative.

In the dissecting hall the smell was conspicuous. This caused some students to change courses. If you work with a cadaver without gloves, the skin on your fingertips goes numb because this preservative acts like a fixative.

I almost forgot - the racehorse breeder. His frankfurter had a red colour. In days gone by the dye caused kidney cancer and has since been banned. Quite often these days, nitrates are used for the colour. This can cause stomach cancer in certain people, especially if they have a low Vitamin C intake.

You would not buy the meat used in the frankfurter if it was displayed in a butcher shop. It is mostly from old cattle - the reject bits. When it arrives at the processing plants the workers commonly call it "slush". Then, the processing commences. Various chemicals are added, and spice extracts, together with devitalised white flour. In the end it doesn't taste too bad.

Arriving at the stables the prospective client was admiring the thoroughbreds. While the breeder was chomping on hotdog and cola, the client looked at him and asked: "Do you mind if I ask you a personal question? Would you give what you're eating and drinking to your horses?"

"Of course not!!" the breeder exclaimed, "they're far too valuable!"

Is it not strange that we will eat food and give it to our children to eat, but we wouldn't dream of giving it to our pets because "it isn't good for them"?

Most Americans and Australians are on the Standard Australian Diet or the Standard American Diet - the **SAD** diet. If you take 2,000 calories of the **SAD** diet you are better off eating 2,000 calories of dog food. Pet food is often better formulated than human food.

The **SAD** diet is made up of 40 to 45 per cent saturated and other bad fats and 30 per cent sugar. That leaves about 30 per cent for nutrition.

The SAD diet

Our diet has become hopelessly polluted, unbalanced and poisonous for our Stone Age metabolisms.

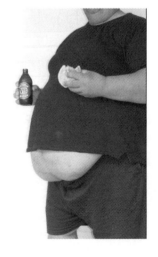

Many patients on the second stage of GOFES treatment ask me in a POD way: "Doc, when can I eat normally again?"

What we regard these days as "normal eating" is highly abnormal for our wellbeing. You have to make an attempt to avoid the garbage as much as you can, even though this is almost impossible at times. Just keep on eating normally and you will get a normal stroke, normal heart attack and other normal diseases.

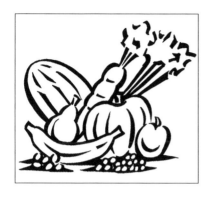

100 calories of nature's formulae and 100 calories of junk

The above two squares symbolise 100 calories each. The first comprises nature's formulae and the second junk. As you can see the volume and mass difference is quite substantial. You need to eat much more in volume and usually mass of the junk, than nature's formulae, to achieve the same feeling of fullness.

The junk is very calorie dense. This has various nutritional and metabolic consequences. The junk is absorbed much faster into the blood stream, raising insulin levels. The insulin response to foods will be discussed later, but it has important consequences for *GOFES*.

Eating disorder

A patient with a bingeing disorder was referred to me. I'm normally sceptical of so-called bingeing "disorders", but Bev's was definitely a disorder. Prior to consulting me she had seen psychiatrists, psychologists, naturopaths, faith healers, coaches and counsellors.

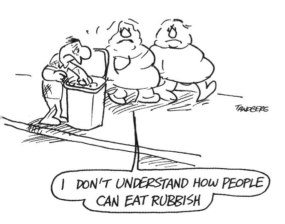

I DON'T UNDERSTAND HOW PEOPLE CAN EAT RUBBISH

I asked her to keep a food diary on the days she gorged. A few weeks later Bev brought me her homework. To my surprise, on some of the days she consumed 25,000 calories. I could not believe it and worked it out again with the same result. I know that the average American consumes 8,000 to 11,000 calories at Thanksgiving, but this amount? I had to be convinced.

I interrogated her about the validity of her records. Further research also revealed recorded instances of people consuming up to 28,000 calories a day. Bev was eating high calorie, dense, adulterated junk. If she attempted to consume the same calories with nature's formulae, she would have to literally force-feed herself until her stomach ruptured.

I admitted her and force-fed her on nature's formulae for a month. She stayed in remission for many months, but relapsed. Luckily, it was nowhere as bad as in the past. Then I lost touch with her. Years later she surfaced again, this time "cured". I was delighted for her. She said that she just had to grow out of it and all she needed was time.

Then she did say something that made sense to me: "If I'd lived in hunter gatherer times I couldn't have binged. The food supply wouldn't have allowed that. Our modern environment brought it out in me. When you compelled me to eat only nature's formulae it left me with a powerful message. I realised I had wasted my youth."

This realisation was probably not the only factor in her recovery, but she did make a very valid point.

Nature's formulae versus present day food

Let us return for a moment to the dawn of nutrition. There was no agriculture and no processing of any kind. Plants and animals are products of nature's laboratory too. We eat these natural products and, since we are made for it, we get all the nutrition we need from them. What is also important is that the nutrients come in neat packages in the right ratios.

Zoos in the past made mistakes with the nutrition of lions and tigers for instance. They fed them steak that we would eat, because it was thought if it was "good for us it should be good for them". The lions loved it. It was easy to eat and probably tastier for them. Sadly, human naivety about nature's formulae made them lose condition and die.

We know now that big cats need to eat whole free-range animal. Wild game has a very low fat percentage and some of the fats are omega 3 fatty acids. Additionally, big cats also need other nutrients that are found in organ meat, cartilage, bone, bowel - the whole works need to be eaten for good health. This was the laboratory in which the lion's metabolism was created. Giving it anything else is like giving ice cream and hamburger to your pet canary.

Nature did not invent refined sugar and white flour.

The decision needs to be made: Am I going to leave my health and happiness in the hands of so-called food scientists and gurus, for them to formulate, adulterate and chemically change my food to something that never existed in nature... or am I going to trust formulations that evolved in nature's laboratory? Disrupting the relationship between nature's formulae and our metabolism leads to **GOFES** and disease.

"If God didn't make it - don't eat it."

The fifth lesson of nutrition is: it was not necessary in the past, but know a bit about nutrition in the present day.

We need over 50 nutrients just to survive. The Stone Age diet had them all. We did not know what they were. We just hunted, gathered and ate. Alas, in the third period of nutrition the food became so adulterated that we now need some education to make better choices.

You do not have to be a scientist to understand the basic building blocks of nutrition. This is a book about health and **GOFES** and contains much of the basic knowledge you will need.

The illustration is largely self-explanatory.

It is important to understand that food has both a nutritional and an energy value. Modern food is packed with calories and is low in nutrition. To correct this balance is of the utmost importance for your health and efforts to control **GOFES**.

BASIC TYPES OF FOOD	
Macro Nutrients ↓	Micro Nutrients ↓
Protein	Vitamins
Carbohydrate	Minerals
Fat	Phytonutrients
Fibre	
Water	

A calorie = a calorie, but it is very important where these calories are derived from. By the end of this chapter you will have a better understanding of this.

THE FOUR AUSTRALIAN AND AMERICAN FOOD GROUPS...

fast...

frozen...

instant...

microwaveable...

"Health and appetite impart the sweetness to sugar, bread and meat."
RALPH WALDO EMERSON

Phytonutrients - food as medicine

To *survive* we need macronutrients, micronutrients and phytonutrients (from the Greek, phyton, plant). There are thousands of chemical substances that occur in food that play various roles in health. New ones are regularly discovered.

Plants exposed to the sun and UV rays had to develop their own "sunscreen" and defensive substances for protection. We evolved to benefit from these substances in various ways. These phytonutrients are often in brilliant colours such as white, lime green, orange and yellow. They play important roles in protecting us against cancer and cardiovascular disease. Most of them also serve as strong anti-oxidants.

Garlic and onion contain various phytonutrients that protect against heart disease and certain forms of cancer. Chillies can protect the cardiovascular system.

A haematologist was testing the bleeding time of a patient's blood one Monday morning and used his own blood as a control. To his concern he discovered that his blood did not seem to clot. Two days later he tested it again and found that the clotting time was normal. The next Monday, again it would not clot. When it happened on the third Monday he did some detective work. His wife had done a Thai cooking course and on weekends was cooking Thai with lots of ginger. Ginger is like aspirin - it can thin a person's blood, while additionally containing other advantageous phytonutrients.

Doctors have discovered that aspirin protects against heart disease, stroke, colon and breast cancer. Salicylates are phytonutrients occurring in plants, but our modern food supply is very low in these and doctors often prescribe aspirin as a replacement.

Apples contain various phytonutrients like quercetin. Regular apple eating can help to protect lung function. An apple a day can indeed keep the doctor away.

Green tea assists in suppressing genes that fuel breast cancer in women. Turmeric helps to inhibit genes that fuel inflammation. Broccoli contains phytonutrients that help ward off breast and colon cancer, like Indole-3-carbinol, sulforaphane and others. Broccoli, also stimulates genes that protect against heart disease.

Citrus fruit is very rich in phytonutrients and is probably the number one fruit. Various herbs and spices contain many of the phytonutrients that promote good health. Red wine - in moderate quantities - is a chemical cocktail of polyphenolic phytonutrients that offer cardiovascular protection.

You do not have to know the names. **This is the take home point:** We have thousands of years of experience with food and only recent experience with "plastic" food and protein powders. You can get all the nutrients to survive from modern food, but merely to survive as opposed to surviving *in good health* is an entirely different concept. Unless you regularly eat various phytonutrients your health will suffer.

Many of these phytonutrients are yet to be identified, so drink your green tea, eat your colours, eat your herbs and spices, fruit and vegetables. Phytonutrients protect against cancer and heart disease and slow down aging.

"I don't like broccoli and I'm glad I don't like it. Because if I'd liked it I would have eaten it - and I hate the stuff."
BROCCOLI HATER

PROTEIN

The building blocks of protein are amino acids. Our bodies need some 22 of these amino acids. Somewhere between eight and 11 amino acids are derived from food, but these are indispensable because our body uses these to manufacture the 22 amino acids needed in the healthy body. The eight to 11 are essential amino acids. The others are useful, but non-essential in our diets.

Nature presented us with two types of protein.

Complete protein: containing all the **essential** amino acids, as well as some other amino acids.

Incomplete protein: do **not** contain all the essential amino acids.

COMPLETE (ANIMAL)	INCOMPLETE (PLANT)		
	LEGUMES	GRAINS	SEEDS/NUTS
Eggs	Beans	Barley	Almonds
Fish	Lentils	Buckwheat	Brazil
Fowl	Peanuts	Corn	Cashew
Meat	Peas	Millet	Pumpkin
Milk	Sprouts	Oats	Sesame
Milk Products		Rice	Sunflower
Poultry		Rye	Walnuts
Venison		Wheat	Wild Rice

The best single protein source

The only complete absolute protein, all in *one package*, with the optimum amino acid ratio and balance is eggs.

Even if only one amino acid is missing, or not in the optimum quantities and ratios, it can constitute a limiting factor which can impede the assimilation of other amino acids leading to protein malnutrition. Therefore, except for eggs, animal and plant proteins must be combined to create this essential balance.

An egg is probably the single healthiest food available. Some 21 days after it is laid a little chirping, breathing, lively chicken comes out with bones, flesh and feathers. This little creature was created out of what was once the egg yolk and white. If put in a position where a single food must be chosen to survive on, the best option would be eggs. For human consumption we may become Vitamin C deficient, since we are not like most mammals which have the ability to produce their own Vitamin C.

It is true that egg yolks contain saturated fats and that we need to be careful about the over-consumption of eggs in our present day circumstances. Nevertheless, egg yolks do contain a number of essential nutrients in a natural form. Pritikin, sadly, gave the egg an unwarranted reputation. Egg consumption can actually improve your cholesterol levels.

Egg whites are fat free. A neat way of getting your nutrients and limiting some saturated fat is by fortifying a whole egg with a couple of fat free egg whites. The left over yolks can be used for other purposes, like giving it to your dog - it is good for its coat.

Eggs reach the consumer in the same form they leave the hen, with zero processing, so the large companies show little interest in merchandising eggs. You are better off buying eggs and separating the yolks and whites yourself, rather than buying commercially packaged egg whites.

Since eggs are the only complete protein, they are awarded a biological value of 100. All other proteins are compared to eggs, although whey from cheese production, when purified, contains protein of a higher biological value than eggs.

A whole commercial industry has sprung up around whey protein powders and not all the products are as they seem. This is unfortunate because whey protein powders can be a valuable part (only) of a nutritional program, particularly for athletes.

The protein you eat cannot be stored. Today's deficiency will be cannibalised from your organs and muscles. If you eat too much, it will be converted into energy and/or fat.

There are a lot of other things to know about protein, but the above is about all you need to know for the purposes of staying healthy. The following points may also be useful.

Protein
- Has a high thermogenic response. This means it encourages your metabolism to burn calories. Fat has a low thermogenic response and lowers your metabolism's calorie burning.
- Promotes satiety and helps control **POD**. Inadequate protein makes it hard to control your cravings.
- Protects your lean body mass (LBM). Your LBM is largely protein. When you are on a calorie deficit diet to lose weight, your LBM can be quite vulnerable to loss as well.
- The main purpose of excess fat loss is body composition change. Excess fat should reduce while your LBM increases, and not just proportionally. Having

an adequate and high quality protein intake throughout the day is the first requirement to achieve these goals.

- Protein, amino acids and combinations of amino acids are absolutely essential to your immune system. Any disturbance here and the immune system is compromised.
- Blunts the insulin stress of carbohydrates. Good news.
- Good protein sources like meat, fish and eggs have a zero insulin response because they slow down stomach emptying.
- Lowers bad cholesterol and increases good cholesterol.
- It is mood enhancing. Protein is important in brain chemistry.
- Protein and carbohydrate ratios have hormonal effects. Get it wrong and the effects are negative, get it right and your metabolism is enhanced.

Recommendations

There are roughly 20-30 grams of protein in 100 grams of chicken, fish and beef. If the whole day's protein requirements are eaten in a single meal, the body cannot assimilate the sudden influx and the residue will be burned as calories. Protein has to be spread over the day for optimum advantage.

If you are in the process of getting rid of superfluous flab, you need the best quality protein you can get, at least twice per day, five or more hours apart. Once you are on maintenance you need it three times a day on average. Athletes, especially body builders, need protein up to six times a day. For the average person just trying to be healthy, three times a day is ample.

Protein intake needs to be fairly consistent.

Combine protein sources for the same day. If just chicken is eaten for the day you may be short on one essential amino acid, Lysine. Body builders have discovered this and they will not rely on chicken as their only source of protein for that reason. Just as plant proteins must be combined to get complete protein, except for eggs, animal proteins also need to be combined. Plant and animal protein can also be combined to improve the completeness of protein for the day. This is usually done in traditional diets anyway.

Vegetarian protein

Reducing animal proteins in the diet and replacing them with vegetable sources will increase vitamins, minerals, fibre and phytonutrients, while reducing cholesterol, saturated fats, nitrates and some agricultural chemicals. Studies continue to prove that these dietary changes will aid in protection against cancer, cardiovascular disease, diabetes, gastro-intestinal disease, osteoporosis and premature aging.

Recent studies indicate that probably the healthiest diet is a vegetarian diet that contains fish - pesco-vegetarian.

Warning: A strict vegetarian diet needs to be well planned and some knowledge of nutrition is essential.

We did not evolve as vegetarians... look at our incisor teeth. It is difficult to balance protein well on such diets. There are various reasons why we are taller than in the past, but one is better protein nutrition. Nowadays a vegetarian has to eat too many calories to get enough protein and, for Polar Bears, this can lead to **GOFES**.

At one stage I became a vegetarian. When I went back to my previous diet I felt better. I seldom see healthy vegetarians. At a nutritional conference the question was asked: "Do you know any healthy vegetarians?" No hands went up. Please do not misunderstand me. A well planned vegetarian diet can be very good for a very disciplined and knowledgeable person. For the average person it is not recommended unless you are part of a community where it is practised for cultural or religious purposes.

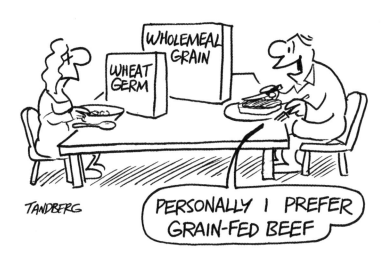

MIXING & MATCHING OF VEGETARIAN PROTEIN

	*No Limiting Amino Acids	Low in Lysine	Low in Sulphur-Amino Acids	Low in Tryptophan
Eggs	Eggs			
Grains	Wheat Germ *(Not limiting in Lysine, sulphur and Tryptophan)	Barley Buckwheat Bulgar Wheat Cornmeal Millet Oats Rice Rye Wheat	etc.	
Legumes	Soybeans Tofu (Soy Curd) Soy Milk (Fortified)	Peanuts	Beans (dried): - Pinto - Red - Black - White Black-eyed Peas Chickpeas Lentils Limas Mung Beans Peanuts	Beans (dried): - Pinto - Red - Black - White Chick Peas Limas Mung Beans Peanuts
Vegetables			Asparagus Beet Greens Broccoli Brussel sprouts Green Beans Green Peas Mushrooms Parsley Potatoes Sprouts	Beet Greens Corn Green Peas Mushrooms
Nuts	Walnuts	Almonds Brazil Nuts Cashews Coconuts Filberts Pecans English Walnuts	etc.	
Seeds		Pumpkin Sunflower		
Dairy Products	Cheese Cottage Cheese Milk Yoghurt			

To get the necessary amino acids from protein can be difficult. Combine different foods from any two columns to achieve a better amino acid ratio.

260

CARBOHYDRATES

As with protein, your body cannot store carbohydrates. The excess you consume will be converted to FAT. If you don't consume enough food, your body will burn fat.

More people fall victim to **GOFES** from consuming too many carbohydrates than from consuming too much fat. Since being told to eat less fat, we have become fatter. As the fat is reduced in yoghurt, for example, the difference in calories is offset with refined carbohydrates. This has negative metabolic consequences. We got fatter than ever before, resulting in - among others - a diabetic epidemic.

Generally carbohydrates fall into two main groups.

COMPLEX CARBOHYDRATES (Eat these)	SIMPLE CARBOHYDRATES (Cut These)	
	Naturally occurring	Processed
All vegetables Whole grains (eg. Barley, Oats, Rice, etc.) Legumes	Fresh Fruits Honey Lactose (Milk)	Cakes, Donuts, etc. White & Brown Sugar, Corn syrup, etc. All Alcoholic Drinks ("Carbohydrate Like")

Advice from our experts

Our nutritional experts have taken us on a roller coaster ride. Latest "trends" are often just an attempt to correct the previous bad advice. The "carb versus protein" debate, for example, has become uncontrolled.

In time, present advice will be proven to be inadequate or simply wrong and a new trend will surface. To change the minds of so-called experts is often an exercise in futility.

The temptation to interfere with nature's formulae is enormous.

There appears to be a number of reasons for this.

- Food scientists believe they know best. They have become control freaks over our food supply.
- There are strong commercial reasons for processing.
- At an individual level we hold out hope for a wonder food product that can do magical things.
- There are potent comfort reasons why we like fast and instant food.

It is important to remember that all vegetables and fruit are carbohydrates. However, there is a carb group that is starchier that the rest. These, especially in the refined form, can cause us a number of problems in modern nutrition. These should be eaten with care and caution.

- White bread
- White rice
- White pasta
- Potato - especially processed and mashed.

Remember, in nutrition White is not Right.

These should be eaten only in small amounts and in the unprocessed form.

The Insulin Response of foods

Carbohydrates have potent effects on insulin and blood sugar metabolism. Insulin Response or stress is somewhat incorrectly referred to as the Glycaemic Index (GI) of foods. Foods do have powerful metabolic and pharmacological effects.

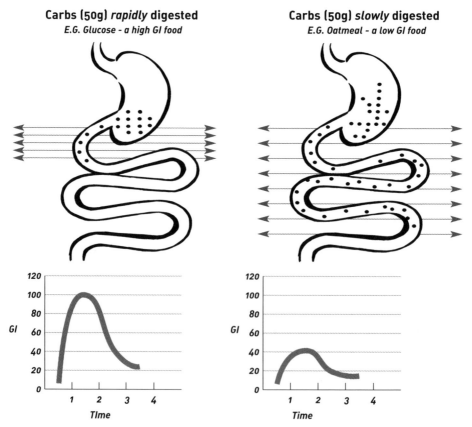

Carbs (50g) *rapidly* digested
E.G. Glucose - a high GI food

Carbs (50g) *slowly* digested
E.G. Oatmeal - a low GI food

If 50g of one carbohydrate is compared with the same weight of another carbohydrate it will be noted that they have different effects on insulin metabolism. The rate at which it is absorbed into the blood stream affects how much and how quickly insulin levels are raised. Different food and food ratios can have powerful effects on the endocrine system. Given that our metabolisms are still in Period One - hunter gatherer, Period Three food plays havoc with our metabolism and wellbeing. Fast food causes insulin levels to rise fast.

Some health writers advise us to reduce the sugar risk by using unsweetened bread and cereal products. They fail to realise that processed starches are absorbed by the body just as quickly as sugar, and are immediately converted by our bodies to sugar!

50g of Glucose is the standard and is given the value of a 100.

You can see that oatmeal is a relatively low GI food by comparison.

But GI only tells you how rapidly a particular carbohydrate source is turned into sugar.

Point: For good health and successful weight maintenance you must keep insulin levels low. Processing increases the GI of food. Baked potatoes have a lower GI than mashed potatoes.

Do not spike your insulin.

INSULIN RESPONSE OF FOODS (GLYCAEMIC INDEX)

	Under 30% EAT MOST ✓✓		30 to 60% EAT MORE ✓		Over 60% EAT LESS ✗	
Herbs and Spices	Basil	V low				
	Garlic	V low				
	Parsley	V low				
	Turmeric	V low				
	Onions	V low				
Vegetables	Green veg	15			Parsnips	98
	Broccoli	V low			Instant mashed	
	Cabbage	V low	Sweet potatoes	44-48	potatoes	95
	Cucumber	24	Peas frozen		Potato	70
	Lettuce	V low	boiled	43	Carrots	85-92
	Peppers	V low			Beetroot	64-70
	Squash	29			Yams	49-71
Fruit					Orange juice	51
	Cherries &				Banana	58-70
	strawberries	23-32			Cantaloupe	65
	Berries	20-30	Apples (golden		Dates	99
	Fresh fruits	35	delicious)	36-38	Grapes	45-60
	Grape fruit	26	Mango	51	Kiwi	58
	Peaches	29	Oranges	33-40	Pineapple	65
	Pears	34	Pear	38	Pumpkin	75
	Plums	25			Raisins	68
					Watermelon	72
Legumes	Kidney beans	29	Baked beans (canned)	48		
	Lentils	29	Chick peas (garbanzos)	35		
	Peanuts	14	Green beans	30		
	Soy beans	15	Lima beans	36		
	Peas	22	Peas (black-eyed)	33		
Grains, Seeds and Nuts	Cashews raw	22	Brown rice	50-66	White rice	72
			Whole wheat		Corn flakes	85
			spaghetti	40-45	Millet	71
			Oatmeal	42-48	Shredded wheat	68
			Swiss muesli	6-66	White bread	80-95
			Whole grain rye bread	42	White flour	
			Whole wheat bread	40-72	spaghetti	50-65
			Pumpernickel	49	Whole wheat bread	40-72
			All-Bran	48		
			Buckwheat	51		
			Sweet corn	60		
Sugars and Snacks	Fructose	19-23	Dark chocolate	50	Glucose	100
			Figs	59	Honey	55-87
			Milk	31	Maltose	110
			Popcorn	55	Mars bar	80
					Sherbet	65
					Sucrose	100
					White Sugar	75-95

GI is only the beginning of the story. *It does not mean much in isolation.* Watermelon and cornflakes have similar GIs. What would you rather eat - a cup of watermelon or a cup of cornflakes? On the face of it, you may think that they would be the same, but on closer examination the **impact** of a cup of watermelon on insulin levels is about 8.25 times less than a cup of corn flakes.

Why? The governing factor is the amount of carbohydrate per volume of a particular food. GI is only measured by the amount of carbohydrate and not the volume. To address this deficiency, another measure was developed - the Glycaemic Load (GL).

Glycaemic Load (GL) takes the *impact and volume* of a particular carbohydrate into account. It defines the *insulin stress* of a carbohydrate.

It is this impact of insulin that has more practical value than simply knowing the GI.

Glycaemic load (GL) = GI x carbohydrate per gram per unit volume.

GL of one cup of...	GI x gram per cup	/100	GL/serve
GL of watermelon	72 x 12g	864/100	8
GL of corn flakes	71 x 94g	6674/100	66
GL of white rice	72 x 33g	2376/100	23
GL of broccoli	20 x 20g	200/100	2
GL of spaghetti	60 x 50g	3000/100	30

The following are some examples comparing the GL of different food.

GL per meal: <10 is low
11-19 is moderate
>20 is high
Aim for less than 120 per day.

You can have *4 cups* of broccoli and still have a low GL of eight for the meal. While *one cup* of corn flakes results in a high GL of 66 for the meal.

2 cups of broccoli
+ 1/2 cup white rice
+ 1/2 cup watermelon
= 19
Thus, moderate GL.

Dietary factors modifying the GI and GL

Food processing increases the GI

Instant mashed potatoes = 95

Boiled potatoes = 70

White = not right. Fast food = fast rises in insulin.

Fibre

Enzyme access - it takes longer for enzymes to access the carbohydrate in fibre. This slows down absorption considerably.

Fibrous content - high fibre slows down digestion especially soluble fibre.

Acidity

Lemon, vinegar and grapefruit lower the GI. Add these healthy products regularly to your meals.

Cooking

Starch gelatinisation - when rice and oats are over-cooked, their starch changes to a higher insulin response **GI** and **GL**.

GI of mixed meals

Adding a low GI food to a high GI food lowers the GI of the meal.

Peas = 22 and white rice = 72

$(50\% \times 22) + (50\% \times 72) = 47\%$

Peas lower the GI of rice.

Fat and oils

Olive oil lowers the GI of a meal.

The key is to keep insulin levels low,
to prevent getting fat and sick.

To lower the GI of bread - wholemeal preferably - dip it into olive oil with balsamic vinegar.

A word on sugar

When Africans follow a traditional lifestyle and diet in their villages, they do not suffer from GOFES, diabetes, coronary thrombosis, varicose veins or diverticular disease. This has nothing to do with genetics, because when people of these cultures adopt a western mode of life, they become prone to western diseases just as much as anyone else.

The Masai in Africa have a relatively high fat diet, eat a lot of red meat and drink plenty of milk and yet their cholesterol levels are low and they do not suffer from western diseases. *A common factor in all tribal diets is the complete absence of sugar, white bread and other refined carbohydrates.*

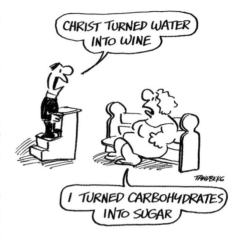

Get the connection? Their diets contain low glycaemic loads.

Sugar
* Is a drug - so concentrated, it is pharmacological.
* Decreases various hormones like GH, E2, and DHEA. These decline with aging, so it can be argued that sugar speeds up the aging process.
* Increases cortisol levels. This hormone increases with age and is called the "killer hormone". Cortisol levels increase with stress, over eating, aging and of course sugar consumption.
* Decreases testosterone. Men (and women) take note.
* Increases insulin. This is the last thing that you want because insulin is appetite stimulating and is the fat hormone.
* The average American consumes up to 80kg (176lb) of sugar a year.

FAT

The most fattening thing you can put in an ice cream sundae is a spoon.

For the last 20 years or so we've been given the run around on the subject of fat.

There are two fatty acids that the human body cannot make and has to acquire from outside sources. These are **Linolenic acid** and **Linoleic acid**.

From these the body can make other fats it needs - and those it doesn't need. As a population we are quite deficient in these two essential fatty acids. When our diet is distorted, our cholesterol level goes up. As egg consumption reduced in recent years, heart disease increased.

Going into all the details is not the purpose of *Polar Bears and Humming Birds - A Medical Guide to Weight Loss,* rather to make you aware of the issues involved in maintain your health. Each chapter is a book on its own. With so many "books" in one book, space is the obvious problem. There are follow up books in the pipeline.

The commercial fat-free-craze has hit the market by storm. The pace of life in western society is such that we choose to believe and trust our food producers and marketers. When they promote a product as 97 per cent FAT FREE - rather than saying it contains three per cent FAT - we tend to ignore the sales psychology. To achieve a FAT FREE state in processed foods, the fat-calories are replaced by refined-sugar-calories.

If you want to determine the fat content of food it is more practical to look at it in the following way. It sounds obvious, but is often ignored.

Obvious Fats	Hidden Fats
Butter	Cheese
Gravy	Chicken fat and Skin
Ice Cream	Chocolate
Lard	Donuts, Cakes, etc.
Margarine	Fried food
Mayonnaise	Milk
Salad Dressing	Nuts
Vegetable Oil	Processed Snack Foods
Vegetable Shortening	

Next look at the types of fat

In arctic animals and cold-water fish, omega 3 fatty acids act as anti freeze.

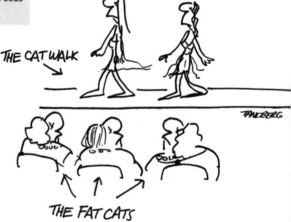

THE CAT WALK

THE FAT CATS

TYPES OF FAT	PLANT SOURCES	ANIMAL SOURCES
Omega-3 fatty acids **High in super-unsaturated fats** Help prevent inflammation, endocrine and immune problems by balancing prostaglandins and other hormones. Powerful cancer preventing effects, help prevent tumour formation and help burn fat.	Beans Flax Seed Flax Seed Oil	Mackerel Salmon Sardines Trout Tuna
Omega-6 fatty acids **Moderate and high in poly-unsaturated fats.** Essential in small amounts, but excess produces adverse effects	Corn Oil Peanut Oil Peanuts Safflower Oil Sesame Oil/Seeds Soybean Oil Soybeans Sunflower Oil/Seeds Walnuts	
Omega-9 fatty acids **High in Mono-unsaturated fats** Mostly neutral effects with moderate intake. Good for stir-frying – except olive oil.	Almonds Avocado Canola Oil Cashews Olive Oil Olives Pecans	
Saturated fats and partially **hydrogenated vegetable oils** When consumed in excess have "toxic" effects on the body	Chocolate, etc. Coconut Oil (not bad) Margarine, etc Palm Oil	Butter Ice Cream Lard Milk

The bottom line is that you only need some oils and fat. The others should be regarded as bad news. The bad ones are those that have been through numerous processes, have been heated repeatedly and contain trans fatty acids.

Stay away from:
- All commercial vegetable oils
- Margarine (the invention of food scientists)
- Modified butter
- Shortening.

Only have:

- Extra virgin, cold pressed, olive oil. We have a few thousand years of experience with olive oil. A combination of olive oil and balsamic vinegar is good for lowering the **GI** of a meal. Dip your wholemeal bread in a bit of olive oil with balsamic vinegar - just like the Italians do. You not only lowered the GI of the meal, you also satisfied your hunger by eating fewer calories. However, always beware of portion distortion.
- Flax seed oil. Unlike olive oil, it can go rancid quickly. A more complete oil than olive oil, containing lots of good omega 3 fatty acids, you have to be careful how you store it. Mixing with olive oil, and/or rosemary oil for instance, can make flax seed oil more stable. Keep it in the fridge.
- A bit of natural butter and ghee in small quantities.
- Why didn't you mention canola or pumpkin seed oil? They are okay too, but why have so many choices? Boutique oils like avocado and macadamia oil can be useful on your gourmet days, but why not stick to those that have stood the test of time?

Any oil and fat, and above all bad ones, in the presence of refined sugar or other high **GI** carbohydrates is bad news for your metabolism – and if you are a Polar Bear, helps induce **GOFES** and its consequences. Humming Birds may not fall victim to **GOFES**, but develop other ailments instead.

Fat portion distortion

Distortion occurs in two ways - large physical portions, or small concentrated portions with very high calorie density. People get caught out more on the calorie dense foods. Oils and fats, especially when hidden, fall in this category.

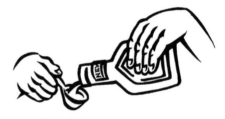

The calories in the spoon above equal the total calories in the food below.

Fat is high in calories. Good fats are essential, but beware of excess - what nourishes me, also destroys me. Fat is so concentrated in calories that a small amount may appear moderate to the eye, but is in effect portion distortion. That extra teaspoon on the salad or in

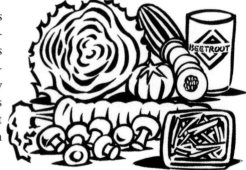

food is not noticeable, but in 10 years it can translate to 20 to 40kg, depending on your Polar Bear status.

In years gone by, European housewives would take a small bottle or container to market and buy the family's olive oil. It had to go a long way and it was used sparingly. These days food is much cheaper and consequently these housewives now buy big containers for much smaller families. Excessive olive oil is poured over everything.

When I visited friends in Paris, they ordered a "force-fed castrated cock" for a special occasion. I volunteered to go to pick it up and pay for it. At €175 it was the most I have ever paid for a chicken!

With black truffle underneath its skin, the fat poured out of it and it tasted quite nice. The French do eat butter, fatty things, drink wine and have desserts, but in spite of it, they are some of the leanest people in the industrial world. We need fat, but our total food intake needs to be moderate. How much you eat is just as important, perhaps even more so, than what you eat. Even so-called good food is bad for you in excessive quantities.

FIBRE

"Eat fibre and prunes and get a good run for your money."
OLD SAYING

Until relatively recently, humans consumed much more fibre than they do today. Fibre is relentlessly removed from our food by processing and so-called refinement. I have trouble with the word "refinement". Refinement means to make something more sophisticated or effective, but taking natural fibre out of food is not smart.

Good quality protein and fibre in the diet decreases blood pressure. Soluble fibre decreases the **GI** and therefore insulin levels.

There is soluble and insoluble fibre. They are both essential. Soluble fibre such as oats, forms a gel like substance in the gut.

When it became clear that some of our diseases were actually caused by the lack of fibre, the food industry reacted by selling us the bran they used to throw away.

This created the flatulence epidemic. The latter is so common, we now have flatologists who specialise in its treatment! Even on a very good diet, the average person will produce at least two litres of flatulence a day. Fibre additives can keep you embarrassed all day. Heavy fibre supplementers take in too much phytic acid that binds with minerals and may result in a mineral deficiency. If you do take fibre supplements, take them in moderate quantities in the mornings only, because minerals are better absorbed in the evening.

How do you know you have enough fibre in your diet?

Large stools. Village school children in Africa who eat traditional food have much bigger and heavier stools than children on a typical western diet.

Word of warning - not all constipation is due to a lack of fibre. If you have self-treated with fibre supplements without any success, it is time to consult your doctor. A tumour or other problem in the colon may be the cause. If your car is not performing the way you anticipate what would you do? Your body needs more care and cannot even be compared to a car in this respect.

Nothing should be taken away from food - nothing should be added

By taking the fibre away, you have destroyed nature's formula, causing a chain reaction. Glycaemic load increases, the bowel transit time decreases, constipation can develop, as well as diverticulitis and many more problems, including **GOFES** and its consequences.

If you must supplement your diet with fibre

- Adopt a natural, traditional diet with all the natural fibre still in the food.
- Do not supplement every day, unless there are compelling reasons. Courses of supplements may be better until your diet has rebalanced.
- Supplements should be taken in moderation.
- Only take them at breakfast.
- While taking supplements, eliminate anything that is white and therefore not right.
- Eat your vegetables and fruit.
- Your exercise regime should include abdominal training.
- Increase your water intake.
- Eat Asian and/or Mexican spices and herbs with some of your meals. Some stimulate bowel action.
- Eliminate refined sugar.

LIQUIDS

"The problem with some people is they not only drink to excess, they drink everything."
ANONYMOUS

While our bodies are mostly water, you still have to drink it regularly. Not only will drinking water help you to lose weight, it will moisturise your skin and put into solution those waste products that we need to excrete. Water is the best solvent - dilution is the solution to pollution.

A teaspoon of salt dissolves in a cup of water. If you add more and more salt, a point will be reached where the salt cannot be dissolved, because the amount of water has become saturated with salt. The excess salt will just sink to the bottom where you can see it as crystals. Uric acid in the body needs to be kept in solution or it will crystallise, forming agonising kidney stones or razor sharp crystals in the joints. Typically, we do not consume enough water.

You will never control your **GOFES** if you do not develop the love for pure unadulterated water. High cholesterol suffers who drink enough water on a regular basis have less heart attacks than those who do not. The glut of soft and carbonated drinks in today's society is a major contributing factor in tooth decay and a number of other illnesses, including the genesis of **GOFES**.

The doctor says: "Take the green pill with a big glass of water when you get up. Take the blue pill with a big glass of water after lunch. Then just before going to bed, take the red pill with another big glass of water."

Startled to be put on so much medicine the man stammers: "Hey doc, exactly what's my problem?"

Says the doctor: "You're not drinking enough water."

The sixth lesson of nutrition:
don't drink your calories - eat your calories.

Condiments

"What is safe eating? Eating with condiments."
ANONYMOUS

There is some truth in that. Herbs and spices do not just enhance taste, but help unlock nutrients from food. Additionally, they contain anti-oxidants and a whole army of phytonutrients. Even gorillas in the wild will come out of the forest into open spaces and eat a variety of herbs for good health. Mankind has fought wars over condiments, like the spice wars of the sixteenth and seventeenth centuries.

Condiments also give flavour and spice to otherwise dull food. If you need to lose excess fat, be careful how you spice up your food. You can inadvertently stimulate **POD**. Sufferers of anorexic nervosa often try to make food as dull as possible to over-ride POD and restrict their food intake.

Learning from anorectics and body builders

When it comes to **POD/POEx** control in the extreme, these people have unwittingly developed various techniques to achieve radical weight loss, or muscle gain and low fat percentages.

Herbs and spices play a big role in your nutrition if used properly.

Eating Fresh

Until recently, humans consumed mainly fresh, tree ripened fruit and other produce. Until some 35 years ago most French households did not have a refrigerator. Food was purchased fresh each day at the local market.

Most fresh food requires preparation to aid digestion, but on the plus side it contains more nutrients, less preservatives and other chemicals, and tastes better. Actually, for GOFES sufferers, preparation is a plus too, because it *delays eating*. Instant foods are not only bad for Polar Bears, but can have serious consequences for the health of Humming Birds as well.

The seventh lesson of nutrition: eat as fresh as you can.

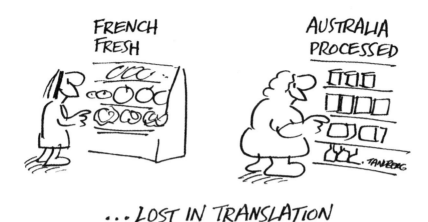

FRENCH
FRESH

AUSTRALIA
PROCESSED

... LOST IN TRANSLATION

The variety and diversity bandwagon

We are constantly told to eat a wide variety of foods. In principle there is nothing wrong with this, but it is not necessary to go overboard. In fact, it may even be bad for you if you are a Polar Bear. The greater the variety, the more difficult it is to lose weight.

We get all we need in a balanced diet. Just one item, like a piece of fish, contains a variety of nutrients. Eggs contain virtually all the nutrients you will need. If you eat a good traditional diet, such as the Mediterranean diet, you will have all the variety and all the nutrients you'll ever need, even though the choices are somewhat standardised. You do not need to achieve variety in any one day. The nutritional cycle is often completed over a couple of days. Your body copes well with this. With fresh foods, there's seasonal variety too.

A steak with condiments, a few pieces of fruit and vegetables gives you plenty of diversity. Our ancestors had nowhere near the variety and choice we have today. We suffer from chronic-choice and variety-fatigue, often leading to a rampage on a variety of junk.

The following is the rationale behind variety, but don't go over the top.

Food intake should be varied, because

1. Complete optimum nutrition is not found in only one food or food group.

2. Most food contains toxic substances. By eating a variety you dilute and counteract these substances.

3. Anti-cancer and disease prevention properties are spread over a number of different foods working in synergy.

Your condiments, spices and herbs also count for variety in your food supply. The more different things you eat in one day the more you tend to eat in calories. Spread your variety over a week.

Bali

A patient once told me she frequently returned to Bali to eat only locally grown foods. After two weeks she felt rejuvenated. She initially thought it was the break that made her feel good, but eventually realised it was the food. Balinese crops tend to be richer because of the high nutrient content in the local volcanic soil.

A change in eating from time to time can hit the spot, but don't have all your variety in a single day.

The eighth lesson of nutrition is:
have a variety of foods, but do not go overboard

Special days and special meals

You might want to refer back to Chapter 17 and the section on Sin Days.

The ninth lesson of nutrition is: *sin days*

MEAL FREQUENCY AND BIORHYTHMS

"Wait a minute, I thought you were on a diet?"
"I am. But I have had my diet and now I'm having my dinner."

How often should we eat?

Once a day? Five times a day? Grazing and nibbling all day? How long should we go without food in a 24 hour day?

There are conflicting correct answers to this. We evolved to eat during the day and our metabolisms synchronised with these rhythms. Period Three food supply and its lifestyle have thrown these natural biorhythms into disarray.

In days gone by we normally ate small in the mornings, had our biggest meal around midday and seldom ate anything in the early evenings, other than left-overs from lunch. During the night, various hormones like melatonin and others are secreted at maximum levels. This formed a unique rhythm of hormonal secretion linking into our metabolisms.

This also meant that we had a long period, every day, where we fasted. This stimulated the production of other hormones associated with digestion and assimilation. It also gave our bodies time to tend to "house keeping". In the "just eaten" state, our bodies have little time to do anything but attend to digestion.

As discussed earlier, the body and the digestive system need rest periods every day for optimum health. Fasting mimics our eating of more primitive times, giving your body time to tend to the "house keeping" and to ready itself for the next eating cycle.

The no-dinner diet and breaking the fast

A combination of, moderate breakfast, lunch and no dinner, followed by a long period of fasting, is an excellent combination for our metabolism. Then the fast is broken with a "cautious" meal, followed at midday by the largest meal of the day. The word breakfast literally means "breaking the fast".

The larger the meal before the fast and the shorter the duration of the fast itself, the more rapidly degenerative diseases set in. A huge late dinner and an early "break-fast" also speeds up aging.

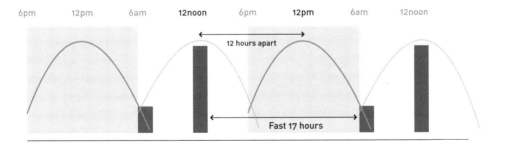

This illustration shows the food intake during the day, peaking far away from the nocturnal peak of hormones. There is a 17 hour fast, which combined with the two peaks at maximum distance apart, is the best way to synchronise our eating with our metabolisms for optimum functional health and controlling **GOFES.** We developed this way.

277

Typically nowadays our eating and hormonal peaks are too close together and the fasting period too short.

Combine this typical eating habit with the adulteration of our food supply and lack of physical activity and what do you get? You guessed it - **GOFES** and all the diseases caused by this condition.

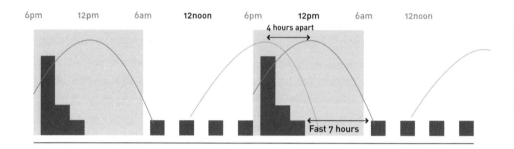

In this diagram the eating peak is encroaching on the nocturnal hormonal peak and the fasting period is too short. We get home late, having eaten little or nothing during the day. We then consume a huge meal and a few drinks plus nibbles until it's almost bedtime.

Experts, know-it-alls and five small meals a day

There are always experts who seem to know and mean well. These experts love making recommendations - this is the correct way and that is wrong. Their latest recommendations are that we should eat small meals during the day to keep insulin stable. Supposedly, you'll be much less hungry and you'll lose weight more easily.

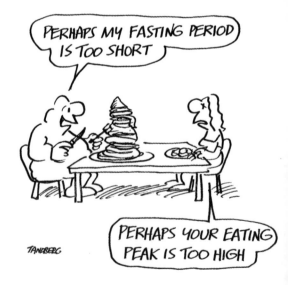

Do not believe them. **The more often you eat during the day, the more calories will be consumed by day's end.** Eating like this won't satisfy **POD** and there is no scientific evidence to support the theory. Nevertheless, eating five small meals a day is fashionable, just as low fat diets were once equally fashionable.

The theory sounds good, but in practice it is a disaster. For **POD** control it's better to have one large meal a where you can eat to contentment (**POE**), rather than five small *unsatisfactory* meals.

"One is too much and a thousand is too little."
ALCOHOLICS ANONYMOUS

As you can see the peaks are close to ideal, but the eating is too low and spread out. This eventually leads to eating more. Unless you are a diabetic on insulin, or an elite athlete, you will not benefit from this practice.

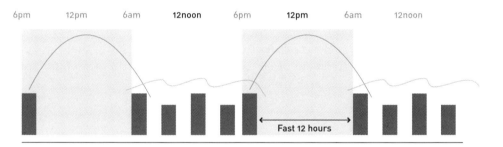

During excess fat loss, you can get away with only having two good quality main meals a day. Main meals meaning those that draw on good quality protein sources and with nothing in between.

The less often you eat the less you will eat for the day, unless you have one humungous meal after dark.

No-dinner-diet
Your two main meals should always be five hours or more apart. You would be even better off trying the *"no-dinner-diet"*, where your two main meals are breakfast and lunch. That means fasting for 15-18 hours - perfect. This allows for the two peaks to be the maximum distance apart, facilitating excess fat loss and other beneficial metabolic changes. This approach mimics the eating habits of our ancestors.

"I don't eat breakfast, because I don't like to eat on an empty stomach."
ANONYMOUS

Recommendations for maintenance and day-to-day

Throughout this stage, three good quality main meals are recommended, simply to ensure protein balance. It is better to get a bit too much protein than too little. No snacks in between. Remember what the French say: "Yes I am hungry, but what's the point in eating now when I'm having lunch in two hours."

As a general rule; lunch should be your biggest meal of the day and dinner considerably smaller. Nowadays we call our evening meal "tea" - perhaps we should call it a banquet.

The once popular expression talked of "eating breakfast like a king, lunch like a prince and dinner like a pauper". We really should change this to: *eat breakfast like a prince, lunch like a king and dinner like a pauper.*

On the whole it is not a good idea to skip breakfast. A small snack is okay, but it should always contain some good quality protein, either animal or vegetable.

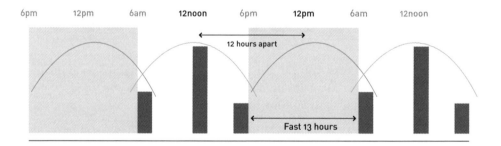

The above may not be as ideal as what we evolved on, but for modern times, it's about as good as we're going to achieve. The peaks are further apart, there is no constant snacking, the fasting period is more than half a day, and meal sizes range from lunch as the largest to dinner as the smallest.

Athletic

If you are very active, you may need four protein meals a day. Athletes and body builders may require protein up to five or six times a day. Unless you are training 18 hours a week or more, you don't fall into this category. Eating like this without significant physical activity will simply result in you accumulating fat.

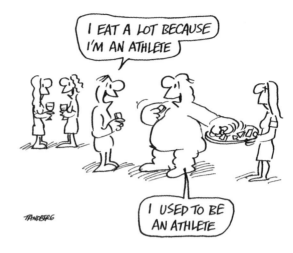

Athletes need specialised advice. Their primary concern is not optimum health, but optimum athletic performance.

The tenth lesson of nutrition is: frequency
- three main meals per day with nothing in between

Behavioural modification

Failure to plan is planning to fail... good nutrition should be planned. If you do not have a plan, in a moment of confusion you will convert to fast and furious food. It is not only the nutrition you put in your mouth, but how and under what circumstances you do it.

More on this in a later chapter.

The eleventh lesson of nutrition is: eating habits
and behaviour modification

"No matter what I eat - it's bad for me."
ANONYMOUS

The million dollar question: what is the best diet ever?

Food is an essential part of any balanced diet. True or false?

On the Internet:
For those of you who watch what you eat, here's the final word on nutrition and health.

It's a relief to know the truth after all those conflicting medical studies:

1. The Japanese eat very little fat and suffer fewer heart attacks than Americans, Australians, British, or Canadians.

2. Mexicans eat a lot of fat and also suffer fewer heart attacks than Americans, Australians, British, or Canadians.

3. The Japanese drink very little red wine and suffer fewer heart attacks than Americans, Australians, British, or Canadians.

4. The Italians and French drink large amounts of red wine and also suffer fewer heart attacks than Americans, Australians, British, or Canadians.

5. Germans drink a lot of beer, eat lots of sausages and fats and suffer fewer heart attacks than Americans, Australians, British, or Canadians.

6. Ukrainians drink a lot of vodka, eat a lot of cabbage rolls and perogies (dough rounds filled with potato, bacon, cheese and sauerkraut then dropped in boiling water for five minutes) and suffer fewer heart attacks than Americans, Australians, British, or Canadians.

CONCLUSION: Eat and drink what you like. Speaking English is apparently, what kills you!

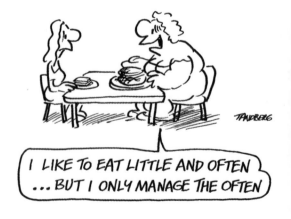

I LIKE TO EAT LITTLE AND OFTEN ... BUT I ONLY MANAGE THE OFTEN

Hurry up. What is the best diet ever?

Eating a traditional Mexican diet you will get all the nutrients and nutrient ratios that are needed for optimum health. If you are not allergic to legumes you can live healthily on this diet for the rest of your life. It contains the right amounts of calcium, vitamins, proteins, fatty acids and the rest of what we were designed to consume. It also contains a good source of phytonutrients for an even higher level of health.

Traditional French cuisine is completely different food, yet it contains the right amounts of calcium, vitamins, proteins, fatty acids and the rest of what we were designed to consume. It also contains a good supply of phytonutrients.

Off to Tokyo. Surprise, surprise completely different cuisine but the same nutritional facts, and you can follow this process to numerous other destinations across the world.

Who designed these healthy and complete diets - so diverse, but each good for you and balanced in their traditional form?

Well, definitely not food technologists, dieticians or other experts. These time-honoured diets may have been studied in the laboratory, but were definitely not created in one.

These unique cuisines were created in a very different type of laboratory - the laboratory of generations passing tid-bits of practical information and observations on to the next generation. These cuisines evolved over thousands of years. Trial and error played its part to derive the ideal formula for the local environment. Because it was good, people stuck to it and thrived on it.

Maggie

As a student I stayed in the university's student accommodation. At one time during renovations we had to move into alternative lodgings. A fellow student and I found an old widowed lady, called Maggie, in the same neighbourhood, who was willing to take us in during this time. Until that time I had to look after my own food. Breakfast was mostly cereal. Lunch was what I bought in the student canteen and dinner was a sandwich or a meal bought at the student accommodation. The latter was typical dormitory food with over-cooked, tasteless vegetables.

For "energy" I would buy the odd chocolate or other dessert. Weekends we drank beer and stout. Cola drinks and other soft drinks, once or more a day. Sometimes I skipped meals because I was too busy or didn't have the energy to bother. I probably had one piece of fresh fruit a week - if that. I must have been showing signs of malnutrition because one of my classmates invited me over for a meal.

I still remember the meal. It looked too much like good food to me. Not only did I enjoy it, I felt better the next day. What I learned academically at the time certainly did not apply to nutrition. The very next day, I was back to my old ways again. The lesson had not sunk in.

Maggie insisted that part of the deal was that she supplied breakfast and dinner. Perhaps she needed the extra money. We certainly didn't object because this would save us time and effort. I played squash several times a week at the time. I often felt tired and exhausted, and my concentration suffered. I naively thought that my studies were too demanding and that I needed a holiday.

After a week or so at Maggie's I started to feel better - much better. I experienced new vitality. I could not believe the difference. My studies seemed all of a sudden too easy. If we were not too late, Maggie ate most dinners with us. Initially we found her company a bit uncomfortable due to the age and interest difference, but before long, we looked forward to these dinners with Maggie. Occasionally, due to student activities, we skipped dinner with Maggie and reverted to beer, soft drink and overcooked, fried food.

It was years later that I realised Maggie knew much more about nutrition than any expert. She didn't even attend high school - the knowledge had come from her mother and her mother and so-on. As Maggie would say: "Not too much of this or that... a bit of this... and boys don't complain... you know I do not have white bread in my house."

She provided fresh food that was in season and followed time honoured recipes.

Raw or cooked vegetables?

I noticed Maggie would "overcook" some vegetables, have others raw and some in between. I was of the opinion at the time that overcooking vegetables in water was not good.

"Maggie..." I asked, "...why do you overcook the vegetables?"

Her reply: "Some vegetables need to be cooked well to unlock the goodness, others don't. My mother and grandmother taught me."

Years later I realised she was right. Today we are obsessed with eating raw and often miss out on the nutrients. Cooking is a biochemical and pharmacological process and some foods do need it.

Eating with the chef

Instinctively, Maggie also knew "eating with the cook" had health benefits that complimented the food. I often wonder how our modern way of eating on the run and not eating together is affecting our health.

Portion sizes

She knew about portion sizes too. A relative brought her a pot of farm honey every so often. When she took one of her wholemeal breads out of the oven she would offer us some of this honey and fresh butter to put on the fresh, warm bread. She would help herself to just half a slice and only one small spoon of honey, but would let us have as much as we liked.

"Maggie, why are you having so little?" we asked. "You are young and active..." and here it came again, "My grandmother said, as you get older, enjoy, but eat less."

To my knowledge she was not on any medication or suffered any ailments.

I realised in hindsight, after we returned to university accommodation and I lost condition again, that it was food related, but I did not realise all the implications until I studied nutrition much later on. Thereafter, we often visited Maggie for a good, home-cooked meal.

Even though the French eat white bread - which they should eat less of - and cream, eggs and so forth, their diet is still very healthy and complete. Over all,

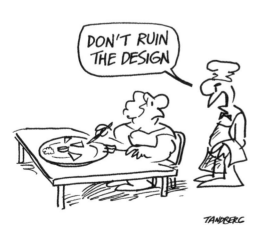

they eat less in calories than most other western countries, and somehow balance their "decadence". Their rate of heart disease is 25 per cent of the British, who have largely abandoned their traditional diet.

In the region of France where they produce foie gras and grow walnuts, the heart disease rate is half that of the rest of France. That is only 12 per cent of the British. Why? - because foie gras and walnuts contain good fats, and they know about portion distortion. In small quantities most food plays an important role in health, but in larger quantities: "What nourishes me also destroys me."

Maggie made soup for us with fresh vegetables and cream. "Isn't cream bad?" I asked. "No," she said. "There are good things in cream... and I only used a small amount. Besides, it goes with my grandmother's recipe."

Once I helped her carry new plants to her spice and herb garden. Most of her meals contained fresh herbs and spices. I didn't show much interest in such things at the time and was of the opinion it was just to keep her busy. I realise now how important these ingredients were to her instinctive nutritional knowledge and skills.

She often said: "I just know" or "From my mother" or "...grandmother", unlike scientists who refer to this and that study and typically come up with bizarre notions about nutrition. With Maggie's traditional diet you didn't have to make decisions about how the number of calories of fat, protein or Glycaemic Index. As humans we are not designed to follow artificial rules and regulations when it comes to food. *We want and need to draw on deeper instincts for our food intake.*

Acquiring nutritional knowledge

Animals in the wild learn from generation to generation what to eat and what to avoid. Zanzibar's red colobus monkeys have somehow learned that they can eat toxic plants, provided they also eat charcoal gathered from human fireplaces. This charcoal neutralises the poisons.

How on earth did they discover this? Just as we discovered over many generations what is good and bad for us. However, these days we are caught out because bad food is marketed as "good" food at a rate that exceeds our ability to determine by trial and error what is good and bad.

Nutrient ratios

Excluding a very obsessive person, any attempt to dictate how to eat, what to eat and what proportions is bound to fail. So-called reputable sources tell us what percentage of our diet should be protein, fat and carbohydrate, but they never give us the tools to calculate the recommended nutritional proportions. Even if we were given the tools, we'd soon get frustrated and leave it to the commercial food industry to determine the proportions for us instead. We are spontaneous and opportunistic eaters. To work out calories and ratios and arbitrary rules is doomed to failure. Tradition and culture is easier to follow.

To solve our food problems we need to "think outside of the lunchbox". What we have been trying for the last 50 years has done more harm than good.

Traditional means traditional

Traditional means just that. For example, if you want pasta, you should eat it as traditional Italians ate it - not like it is eaten today. Until 40 years ago, mostly wholemeal pasta was eaten and pasta was an entrée, not a huge main course.

Sauces and stock

Traditionally, sauces, stocks and extracts were not just to add flavour to a dish, but to enhance the nutrition. Large quantities of food are condensed into a small flavoursome amount. This also concentrated the nutrients, serving as a vitamin, mineral and phytonutrient "tablet" or supplement.

Some food is not all that nutritious, but extractions of it can concentrate the nutrients. In some cases it can also concentrate calories and this needs to be taken into account if you are serious about controlling **GOFES** - for example, concentrations of sugar cane produce white sugar which is highly undesirable.

Fermentation

Lots of foods contain too many toxins to be good for us. Fermentation can sometimes reduce these toxins - for instance, fermented milk is better for us than modern raw milk. The Chinese only started using soy in the Chou dynasty around 300BC, when they found out how to ferment soybeans to produce foods like tempeh and tamari. You may find it worthwhile to learn more about fermentation of foods.

The French paradox

A big fuss is made about why the French live long, drink wine, eat sugar and cream, smoke and have a significantly lower heart disease rate than many other western peoples.

Many reasons are given. The wine companies love the prominence that has been given to wine. All this commotion is missing the point. There are three main reasons for the French paradox and the so-called "other reasons", including wine, are *distant* fourth and fifth reasons.

1. The French eat less, having developed cultural habits to bring this about despite being in the midst of plenty. They culturally control their supply - **DES**. It is not politically enforced on them. French culture talks of "a little too little".

2. French cuisine is based on quality broad-spectrum nutrition.

3. As a result, they have a low incidence of **GOFES**. This translates to a low incidence of the diseases caused by **GOFES**. The French live longer because they control their **GOFES**.

Good quality nutrition in lesser amounts prevents **GOFES**.

Please do not stray
Keep excess fat at bay.
AUTHOR

There are other factors about the French lifestyle that are not as important and don't necessarily apply in this order:

1. Tend to walk a lot.
2. Eat fresh and seasonal.
3. Eat slow.
4. Main meal is lunch.
5. Drink red wine - the most sensationalist claim and given too much prominence, but I do not discount it altogether. It's so chic. A cardiologist friend told me: "You cannot argue with the studies - red wine is good for you." My view: too much credence is given to single item studies instead of looking at the whole problem in an overall perspective.
6. Sleep dark - discussed in a later chapter.

Ask yourself the question

Do I want the food industry and their paid scientists to dictate my diet for me, or am I going to rely on eating practices instinctively worked out over many generations?

The choice is yours.

The twelfth lesson of nutrition is: eat traditionally

STAGE 3 - MEAL PLAN DURING MAINTENANCE

Use one of your Stage 2 meal plans as the basis, and gradually add to it.

Quantity

How much? This depends on your bathroom scales and on your daily metabolic weights as we have discussed previously. Adjust until a steady state is achieved - it usually takes about two weeks to stabilise, however true stability can take one or two years to achieve. Do not consume the same amount of calories every day. For instance, deliberately eat less on Mondays and Thursdays and eat more at weekends. It will even out and mimic Palaeolithic times.

Variety

Gradually increase variety until you feel free to use any fresh fruit and vegetable.

Be very careful with variety because we are constantly attracted to food that is easy to over eat, and that may be not as good as other foods.

Eating foods that are not necessarily to your liking, but are good for you, is a very important health strategy. Often in the past we had to eat more of what we had, rather than what we preferred.

Today we have the luxury of not necessarily eating what is on our plate... "I don't like broccoli..." We have too many choices and it is making us fat and sick.

If you start liking a certain food too much and overdoing it a bit, it's time to fill - not stuff - yourself with some other types as well. Eating only what we like is self-indulgent **POD** and not a healthy strategy in modern **DES** circumstances. Adapt with the times.

Quality

Do you want less than the best?

Customer in sleazy restaurant: "Er... what's the catch of the day?" The reply: "Hepatitis."

The 12 lessons of nutrition

1. We eat too much - develop the eat less habit.

2. Keep it simple.

3. Understand food evolution and degradation.

4. Take nothing away - add nothing. Eat food that fills you up, instead of foods that fill you out.

5. Basic food knowledge was not essential in past, but now it is - but beware of paralysis by analysis.

6. Eat your calories, don't drink your calories.

7. Eat fresh.

8. Variety is important, but don't go overboard.

9. Have planned "Free Days" - Sin Days.

10. Meal frequency - stick with only three meals per day, unless different circumstances apply. "Fast" every day for at least half a day - 12 hours.

11. Behaviour modification - planning and eating style.

12. Eat traditional cuisine.

Meal composition

Wherever you are - actually there you are. We live in the real world, in a Period Three food supply. In the long run it will be difficult for the average person to avoid eating rubbish from time to time. But because you want to be healthy, ultimately *you will be eating from all three periods*. In making healthy choices you should eat least from Period Three foods.

Choose most of your food from Period One

Period One food is all you really need. It contains *everything* that you need. No need to go further. Use traditional recipes to put it together. Eat simple.

"I am so hungry I could eat a vegetable."

AUTHOR

PERIOD 1: PALEOLITHIC

1. Vegetables - Low GI/GL, root veg, eat your colours...

2. Protein (animal) - Fish, Turkey, Whey, Eggs... Low GI, High Thermogenic response.

3. Fruit - Fresh

4. Herbs, Spices, Condiments, oils - Safe eating.

5. Nuts

Period Two

Choose much less from the following in quantity and frequency. Choose unprocessed, or make it a Sin Day. Some good cuisines regularly use these, but if you want to control GOFES, stick more to Period One.

PERIOD 2: AGRICULTURAL

6. Legumes & Grains - Good fibre

7. Starches - Breads, Pasta, Rice, Potato - Higher GI and GL

Period Three

Very rarely choose from the Period Three junk. Only occasionally for Sin Days.

These are trap foods. Stimulating appetite, instant, fast, frozen and microwavable. Low thermogenic response, low phytonutrients, high **GI**, high in contaminants, high in calories and hormones. Wait a minute - do you want to control GOFES and be healthy? **Do you really need any Period Three foods at all?**

PERIOD 3 - MODERN

8. "SINS"

Important point

Nutrition is of the essence. We are what we eat.

The relatively new science of nutrition has gripped the imagination and some people mistakenly see it as a panacea for things it cannot do.

Nutrition is vitally important and indispensable to health, but it does not operate on its own - it is one part of a system of health principles that are just as important. A chain is as strong as its weakest link. Nutrition is just one of the cogs in the wheel that determines health or disease. In the following chapters we discuss nine health principles that are just as important as nutrition.

The magic really only manifests itself if they are all operating in harmony.

Synopsis:

1. The most important thing in nutrition is to develop the eat-less-habit. Aim for a third less calories than the average person in western countries.

2. Choose good quality protein, vegetables, fruit, nuts (moderate) and condiments. This is all you need. The others are just add-ons.

3. Do not bother about analysing, counting and calculating anything. Just know what is bad for you and know the approximate calorie value of your portion sizes. Our traditional food and recipes are already balanced and nutritious - why waste your time with a calculator?

4. Eat food that fills you up rather than fills you out. We need food that is high in nutrition, high in fibre and high in protein.

5. Foods must only be eaten at meal times.

6. **Just before you put food (or rubbish) into your mouth - consider the following:**
   - Does it look as if it was alive at some recent stage, coming from a plant or animal? **RULE:** if you don't know what it is, don't stick it in your mouth!
   - What nutritional value am I likely to derive from these calories?
   - **Do I NEED it for my metabolism or do I just want to satisfy self indulgent POD?**

7. **Basic criteria of what to eat and drink:**
   - Relax and enjoy your food.
   - Memorise the nutritional lessons - and apply them.

8. Relax and enjoy your food. Bon appetit.

CHAPTER 20

2. SUPPLEMENTATION PROGRAM

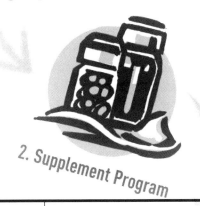

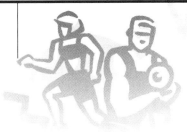

2. Supplement Program

2. SUPPLEMENTATION PROGRAM

Take a block of butter and leave it on the kitchen table. The next day it will still be there, virtually unchanged. After another day it will become darker yellow. Scraping the yellow off will reveal a lighter yellow underneath. A few days later the whole block of butter has collapsed in a rancid mess.

Put a head, legs and arms on the block of butter and you have a human. Being exposed to air and oxygen the butter "decomposes" until it has used up its anti-oxidants. In part, as we age, humans also oxidise away. Just as iron oxidises or rusts, we too "rust away" over time.

"Aging does not come about by a clock, or a number of years, but by detrimental changes in cells. Cells age and eventually die from damage. This primarily occurs by uncontrolled oxidation. The same process by which metal rusts, and apples brown, oxidation produces free radicals. We now know that free radical damage is a major cause, if not the major cause of cardiovascular disease, many forms of cancer, diabetes, pulmonary diseases, liver and kidney disease, Parkinson's, Alzheimer's and other forms of brain degeneration. The injurious effects of radiation, air pollution, pesticides and other poisons also occur mainly because of free radical damage".
DR MICHAEL COLGAN

Humans would oxidise very quickly if we didn't have anti-oxidant defence systems to slow the process down. Although we have an internal anti-oxidant system, we need plenty of external help in the form of various and numerous anti-oxidants in our diets.

A number of vitamins and minerals act as anti-oxidants. Numerous phytonutrients are also powerful anti-oxidants. We have to get these from what we eat. A poor or inadequate diet will lead to premature aging.

The Anti-Oxidant Defence System - is a bit leaky and although the body tries to plug all the holes, we still oxidise away over time as we age. Aging is in part an oxidation process. A baby with a clean nappy is fresh smelling. Get near your old grandparents and you cannot miss the "rancid" smell of old age. At one stage I was the surgical assistant to a vascular surgeon. One of his operating theatre tricks was to make us smell the arteries of old people as we cut through. The smell was reminiscent of rancid fat.

These oxidation processes in our bodies are continuous. Various diseases are caused by a lack of anti-oxidants or malfunction of the defence system. During oxidation, an oxygen molecule can lose one of its electrons forming a so-called "free radical".

Free radicals are not hippies from the '60s. They are very reactive and can only exist for a fraction of time. Free radicals bind with anything they can find and can do tremendous damage to tissues and cell membranes. They're like a tiny hand grenade in the body with the pin pulled out.

All this creates DNA damage, accelerating aging, degeneration, cancer and disease. We need to strengthen our internal anti-oxidant defence system, minimise our exposure to circumstances that result in free radical damage, and obtain adequate amounts of anti-oxidants from external sources.

Internal free radical creation

Various metabolic reactions, for instance cellular inflammation, can cause a chain reaction of free radical damage in tissues and DNA. Some of these radicals, such as the hydroxyl free radical, can be quite vicious.

External free radical creation

Air pollution, ionising, UV radiation and smoking all create free radicals and accelerate the aging process. Due to these mostly modern sources of extra free radicals, we need more anti-oxidants in our diet than ever before. People who smoke, consume excess alcohol and have a poor diet, are free radical "factories".

Near the Sudan in Africa, there are regions where people eat diets very low in antoxidants. Twenty five year olds often look and behave like 50 year olds.

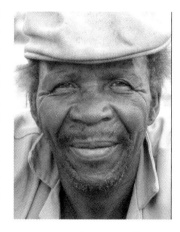

29 year old on a low anti-oxidant diet - life expectancy seldom higher than 45 years.

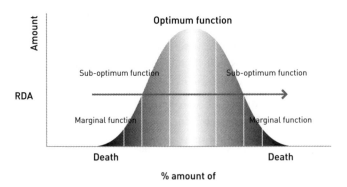

Micronutrients - how much do we need? - do we get enough in our modern diets?

Take ascorbic acid - Vitamin C - for instance and let's apply it to the above illustration.

Death - with very little Vitamin C in our body we will die. Vitamin C is vital to life. Most animals, like dogs, actually manufacture it in their bodies. Guinea pigs are like humans in that they must obtain Vitamin C from outside sources.

Marginal function - with marginal levels of Vitamin C the body can only *marginally function*. Scurvy is the likely outcome.

Then at some almost magical point, according to food technologists, we get enough Vitamin C to prevent scurvy. This point is the Recommended Daily Allowance or RDA. The problem is that all the Vitamin C we are consuming to this point is simply preventing scurvy. Then there are RDAs for other nutrients to prevent other classical deficiency diseases like the Vitamin B3 deficiency characterised by dermatitis, diarrhoea and dementia.

Suboptimum function - at marginal or RDA levels a person will be alive, but not necessarily in good health. We need even more Vitamin C than the RDA to be in good health since other functions of Vitamin C, such as its anti-oxidant qualities and immune stimulation, are manifested at higher levels.

Optimum levels - at these levels all the benefits of Vitamin C manifest themselves. When you cut a slice of apple, within minutes it will brown as it oxidises. You can considerably delay this oxidisation by using a strong anti-oxidant. Apply a few drops of lemon juice - Vitamin C - and, like magic, the apple stays fresher much longer. Our bodies use Vitamin C in a similar way.

Any nutrient in excess, including Vitamin C, will become toxic to the body. Function will again decrease and a disease state will develop. Eventually death will be the result. In general, nutrients are very safe, even in fairly large quantities, but all nutrients have toxic levels.

Let's look at the role of selenium. At one stage it was noted that the cancer rate in sheep was the highest in the world in Australia and New Zealand. Veterinary surgeons worked long and hard to find out why. Eventually they narrowed the cause to selenium deficiency in the soil. With selenium supplements in their diet, the cancer rate became comparable with other countries.

It also became clear that the human cancer rate in Australia and New Zealand was much higher than for instance Japan, where the diet includes higher selenium levels diet. It was also noted that where there were higher selenium levels in the soil in parts of the United States, the cancer rate was lower than in other areas of America with lower selenium levels.

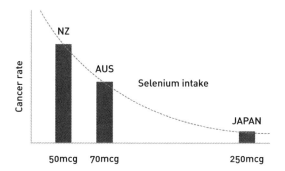

Selenium is a strong anti-oxidant, especially in the presence of other anti-oxidants like Vitamin E. Garlic and grains are generally good sources of selenium. Brazil Nuts are quite a rich source. However, grow garlic in a selenium deficient soil like New Zealand and the garlic will be selenium deficient.

A word of caution - selenium is one of the most toxic substances and has a narrow window of effectiveness. You can take large quantities of Vitamin C before it will become toxic, but I would NOT recommend that you supplement your diet with more than 200mcg selenium without medical supervision. Eating large quantities of Brazil Nuts may lead to selenium toxicity, especially if you take additional selenium supplements.

NUTRIENT LOSS FROM FARM TO TABLE (foods aren't 100% anymore).

Soils today are generally devoid of minerals and essential nutrients

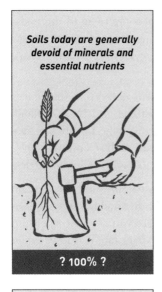

? 100% ?

Further 20% loss

Chemicals, Pesticides, Early green harvesting

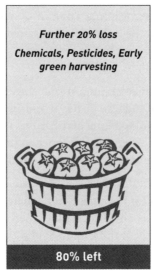

80% left

Further 20% loss

Storage, Freezing, Milling, Preservatives

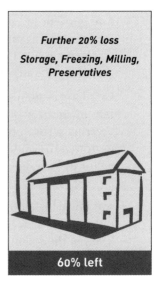

60% left

Further 10% loss

Shipping, Shelf life, Home, storage, Refrigeration

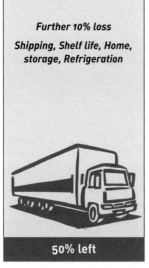

50% left

Further 20% loss

Washing, Peeling, Baking, Boiling

30% left

A good well balanced meal?

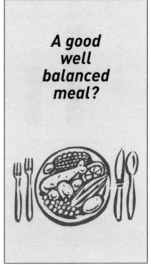

THE DEGENERATION OF FOOD LEADS TO GOFES AND DEGENERATIVE DISEASES.

Rule of nutrient supplementation

More is not necessarily better. But too little is even more harmful. All nutrients can have toxic effects, but generally they are relatively safe.

It is a fallacy to believe that if the food looks good it must be good. Modern agricultural practices do not put all the minerals back in the soil that the plants take out. Minerals do not grow in the soil. If it is not in the soil, it is not in the plant and it is not in you. To obtain the same level of minerals from a bowl of spinach of 60 years ago would require 20 bowls today.

The previous illustration illustrates how food goes through a nutrient depleting process before you get to eat it.

A word on microwaving

A microwave should only be used occasionally, in spite of the fact that it is so convenient. In general terms, according to some studies, microwaving can remove up to 90 per cent of the phytonutrients, anti-oxidants and vitamins in vegetables. Boiling removes less and steaming the least.

Advanced supplementation

Other substances in food and those manufactured in the body can also be supplemented for optimum health and function, like acetyl-L-Carnitine, alpha lipoic acid, carnosine and many more. In a later chapter we discuss time and how these substances can play important roles in suppressing aging. This is a specialised field and will be covered in subsequent books.

Synopsis:

1. Be careful of single nutrient supplementation. Use complete multi-supplements. A chain is as strong as its weakest link.

2. It is virtually impossible to get all the nutrients you need from a modern Western diet nowadays, and supplementation is your only option to stay in optimum functional health.

3. Over-consumptive malnutrition is fattening and can result in obesity.

4. We need supplementation for a number of reasons:

   - Our modern diets do not contain sufficient micronutrients.

   - Modern society has introduced high levels of free radical-producing pollution and pesticides.

- The average person eats a distorted macronutrient diet with, for instance, large quantities of white flour and ice cream. These devitalised carbohydrates require extra nutrients for processing and assimilation.

- A number of degenerative diseases are aggravated and even caused by a chronic shortage of nutrients.

- Studies have suggested that although present-day agricultural practices yield bountiful crops, the fruits and vegetables produced appear to contain less riboflavin, iron, Vitamin C and other nutrients, than they did 50 years ago.

CHAPTER 21

3. EXERCISE PROGRAM

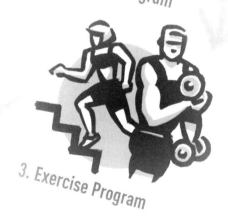

3. EXERCISE PROGRAM

The clash of **POEx** and the Effort part of **DES**.

"Those who do not find time for exercise, will have to find time for disease."
EARL OF DERBY

There is no workout more strenuous than having to push the thought of food to the back of your mind.

"We sit for breakfast, we sit on the train on the way to work, we sit at lunch, we sit all afternoon, a hodgepodge of sagging livers, sinking gall bladders, drooping stomachs, compressed intestines, and squashed pelvic organs."
JOHN BURTON JR

Disuse is deadly and sickening

"The only reason I would take up exercising is so that I could hear heavy breathing again."

A paradox

A person can have the best nutrition and supplement programs, but without exercise these programs will be to no avail. The body needs movement to "churn things around" and *stimulate metabolic processes for good health*. We evolved and were designed to be physically active. The health benefits are

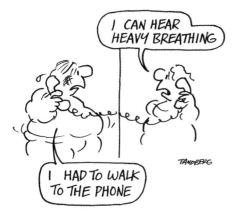

immense. But we shun what is good for us because *we were also evolved and designed to avoid exercise for survival reasons.*

This paradox, if not understood, can give rise to psychological doubt. This misunderstanding of the facts is indeed what drives many of us to over exercise in the hope that this will control **GOFES**. Wrong - it is easier to overcome **POEx** (the Pain of Exercise) than it is to overpower **POD**. Nonetheless, we shun exercise with adverse health consequences.

Exercise - meaning to get and be fit. Fit - meaning to be healthy and in shape. Exercise includes both physical and mental exercise. Many of us confine our exercise to jumping to conclusions, stretching the truth, running up bills, bending over backwards, lying down on the job and pushing our luck. Others keep fit by wrestling with their conscience.

Ask yourself - are you
1. Mentally fit?
2. Metabolically fit?
3. Physically fit?

My doctor told me that exercise could add years to my life. I have taken it up; he is right I feel older already and I have the energy of a man twice my age.

Smokers puff on cigarettes, cigars and stairs. If you are serious about exercise you must give up smoking.

1. ARE YOU MENTALLY FIT?

"The trouble with always trying to preserve the health of the body is that it is so difficult to do without destroying the health of the mind."

G.K. CHESTERSON

As we get older, even a small decline in IQ can have severe effects on our quality of life. The brain is not a muscle, but by way of analogy, it should be seen as such when it comes to exercise.

If you don't use it you will lose it, and if you lose it, you can't use it.

Train your brain

It is well established that people who use their brains regularly have a much slower mental decline than people who are mentally lazy. Engineers retain their mental acuity better than labourers, because their brains are challenged. Conversely, labourers usually have better bodies than engineers, because their bodies are challenged.

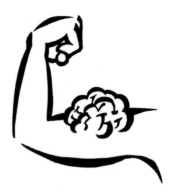

Once a person gets used to a mental task the benefits wear off. You need continually challenging exercise to protect the brain. As a young adult I was very proud of the fact that I could do difficult calculations in my head like 78 x 116, but somehow I got used to calculators and I lost the skill of mental arithmetic.

You need to stimulate the brain every day - be it reading a book, balancing your cheque book or looking for new ways to remember things. When you go on one of those lazy, boozy, sitting all day around the pool, pampering and massage holidays, you lose quite a lot of brain fitness. Just as immobilised muscles and bones decline at an alarming rate, your brain can deteriorate incredibly fast with inactivity.

"The sound body is the product of the sound mind."
GEORGE BERNARD SHAW

For those who are concerned about their brain and mental fitness there are "brain gym" products like *Think Fast*. Computer-based software, it is designed to challenge your brain. All you need is five minutes a day. The software also allows you to monitor your mental performance. As you age, your mental performance declines - "brain gym" software won't arrest the decline, but it will slow its progress. Also, and this is important, if you suddenly decline faster than anticipated, it can be an early warning sign that may warrant further investigation.

Remember this: some parts of your brain will keep growing - if they get enough exercise.

2. ARE YOU METABOLICALLY FIT?

This book is not written for people who just want to be average - it's for those who want to attain and maintain a higher degree of health. In today's world, average is not healthy. If you compare yourself with average you'll strive to be average and you'll never be better than average. To achieve Optimum Functional Health you need to strive for a set of criteria of a much higher standard.

A large number of medical investigations are designed to arrive at the lowest common denominator. Another problem is that most tests are not age adjusted. You need to aim higher than average if you want to successfully control **GOFES**.

The best metabolic exercise is experiencing **POD**. When the body is hungry and deprived, the metabolism is exercised and engages in "house keeping" that it wouldn't otherwise experience. Provided your hunger is not associated with famine or malnutrition, it is the best metabolic exercise for your body. Feeling hungry every day for a few hours is good for you. This is scientific fact - it's better than physical and mental exercise.

3. ARE YOU PHYSICALLY FIT?

A fat man had numerous unsuccessful attempts to lose weight. His doctor gave up on him. One morning at 6am there was a knock at the door. He got up and was puffed by the time he reached the front door. He opened the door to find a beautiful and sexy looking young lady. He asked her what she wanted.

She seductively replied: "If you can catch me... you can have me," turned around and started running.

He knew he was too unfit and had no chance, but because she was so attractive he made an attempt, but could not even walk to the street. Puffed, he went back to bed.

The next day she was back again at 6am with the same invitation. He tried again, but didn't get very far.

This happened every morning. He ran a bit further every day. Then one morning, he nearly caught her. He knew he was going to catch her the next day. He was very excited. He bought new runners. He got up at 4am to prepare himself - showered, brushed his teeth, shaved and at 6am came the knock at the front door.

He opened the door to find a fat lady standing there in runners. "What do you want?" he asked. She replied: "Your doctor sent me. He said that if I can catch you... I can have you."

How good is exercise for losing weight?

If I ask patients how important exercise is in losing weight they always say "very". When I enquire how far they think you'd have to walk to burn off a kilogram of fat, the typical answer is "five to six kilometres".

Unfortunately you'd have to run a marathon before burning even close to a kilogram of fat. If you need to lose 20 kilograms and you want to do it by going to the gym, it will take 20 years or never.

What comes first: you need to deal with **POD** and what you stick in your mouth. I see a lot of guys in the gym training like Trojans. They get fitter, but fatter too. These blokes will endure the Pain of Exercise (**POEx**), but they will not give up their pizzas, beer, soft drinks and hamburgers. They just do not understand **POD** or they'd rather confront **POEx** than **POD** - some people would rather do exercise than restrain their eating.

Exercise in our modern world is useless on its own in trying to lose weight. However, it is excellent preparation for the maintenance phase and will help you maintain your weight loss - plus there are all of the health reasons why you should be physically active.

Why bother exercising if we are motivated to avoid it. The list of benefits to be gained from exercise is long, but the bottom line is: "You've just gotta do it!"

POD > POEx

One study revealed that despite the proven benefits of exercise in preventing a wide range of diseases, only 34 per cent of patients were advised by their physicians to exercise.

These are just some of the benefits of exercise:

- **Exercise is a strategy for preventing disease** - low fitness levels as a young adult increase the risk of several health conditions later in life, from diabetes to high blood pressure. Studies lend support to the theory that health conditions do not have to be a normal part of aging and that what you do now can help prevent illness later.

- Exercise fights cancer and strengthens your immunity.

- Exercise keeps your bones healthy and strong. Astronauts need to exercise regularly and vigorously in space to prevent bone loss and osteoporosis. On earth gravity helps a bit, but on its own gravity is not enough - your body needs weight-bearing exercise.

- The best way of dealing with insulin resistance is, apart from excess fat loss, to exercise. Looking for a diabetic among a group of lean, fit athletes is like looking for a needle in a haystack.

- Your heart and cardiovascular system will benefit.

- Your bowels will function better.

- Men who exercise regularly retain their sexual potency for longer.

- A broken bone in a fit athlete will heal weeks faster than in a sedentary person because the body's repair processes are stimulated by exercise.

  Once, while I was working in a trauma unit, victims from a road accident were rushed in. There were only two doctors on duty and we had to call for extra help. Due to the severity of the injuries we had to prioritise patients as best as we could.

  The ones that looked as if they had no chance were "ignored". When the head of the unit arrived he asked why we weren't working on one of the victims. We responded that he was too severely injured to survive and we were working on those with a better chance. His response: "Get working on him. Can't you see he is an athlete? He will survive injuries better."

  He was right. The athlete stayed in hospital for eight months, but he survived.

- Exercise is a POD fighter. Exercising regularly will enhance your control over the pain of hunger.

- Exercise has direct fat burning effects but, don't forget, on its own you will not get very far unless you control POD and cut your food intake.

- Exercise helps build self-esteem.

- Exercise helps in the management of stress.

- Physical activity, if done regularly, slows the aging process. "My doctor told me exercise could add years to my life - I feel 10 years older already."

- In some cases exercise can be as effective as medication in controlling depression. Fitness testing should be a part of depression management, but before self-treating with exercise you should see your doctor.

- Exercise protects your brain. An enzyme, Protein kinase C, declines with age. This decline also coincides with a decline in IQ over time. Men who exercise regularly have less of a decline in Protein kinase C and less of a decline in IQ decline than those who do not exercise.

- Exercise stimulates Interleukin-6 which helps burn fat.
- Exercise does a lot of positive things for your health that are still to be documented.

Being fit now is like investing in a retirement fund for a healthy future.

No matter your age, gender, Humming Bird, Polar Bear or not, you have to exercise.

The best form of exercise to control fat

Skipping - skipping breakfast, skipping lunch and skipping dinner!

Patients and experts alike will tell you walking is the best exercise for controlling fat.

Of course walking is good for us - our hunter gatherer forefathers used to walk 60 to 80 kilometres (40 to 50 miles) a day.

But the best exercise is resistance training. Helen, one of our clinic councillors, had a fat percentage of 31. After a year of resistance training and healthy eating she reduced her fat to just 12 per cent. Her bone density was that of nearly a seventy year old due to a premature menopause. One year later it had improved to that of a thirty five year old.

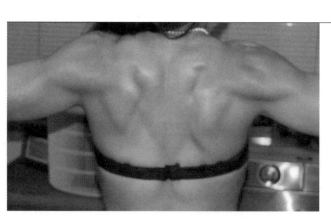

Helen.

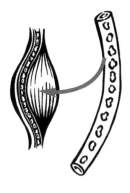

Muscles burn fat

Muscles burn fat. Working muscles constantly draw on your fat reserves. If your muscle mass is too small and inactive, then the fat will be redeposited in your fat reserves.

After weight training - or resistance training - the metabolism's ability to burn fat is enhanced for up to 18 hours. With aerobics the fat burning cycle is only maintained for one hour. Even people in old age homes benefit from resistance training. I have found that elderly patients who could not get out of bed unassisted were able to do so after regular resistance training.

From age 18 to 40, the average female loses 2.5 to 3kg (5.5 to 6.5lb) of muscle, and at the same time gains 10 to 11kg (22 to 24lb) of fat. With aging, internal fat increases by up to 50 per cent or more, while organs and muscle shrinks by 30 per cent. We have less and less muscle to burn and more and more fat. The shrinking muscle reserves can only be halted or slowed down with effective resistance/weight training.

The weights do not have to be heavy - they only have to feel heavy. You train according to your capability - the only person you are competing with is yourself.

While weight training is the best form of exercise to control fat, what you put in your mouth continues to be a governing factor. Tied in second place are walking and aerobics. Unfortunately, swimming is not very good for fat loss per se, but it is good exercise.

The SD of Exercise

What we do in our normal routine is **Subsistence Exercise (SE)**. *It is exercise we need to do to survive.* In hunter gatherer times it was at a much more energetic pace than what is necessary today. In fact, it is at such low levels today that our health suffers from lack of activity. Therefore we have to do planned or **Deliberate Exercise (DE)** to compensate for our lack of physical fitness.

The moment we increase our deliberate physical activity, of course POEx kicks in.

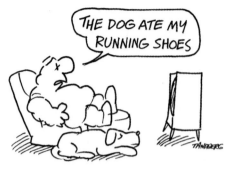

A MAN'S BEST FRIEND

Here are some excuses not to exercise - "POEx Talk"

"An earthquake drained my pool."

"My dog ate my running shoes."

"The TV at the gym is always on something I don't want to watch."

"I went to an energetic seafood disco last week and pulled a mussel."

"I am too out of shape to get in shape."

What makes our position unique in history is that it does not matter if we do not exercise, because it will not affect our survival. We can survive on incidental exercise, walking to the bathroom, flicking remote controls, shopping, raiding the pantry and getting out of the lounge chair. In primitive times we needed to exercise to survive. Today, because we have a choice, POEx will make sure we take the non-exercise option.

The best place to start is to increase your Subsistence Exercise - also called incidental exercise - by parking the car a bit further away from your destination. Exercise built into your normal routine does not always feel like exercise. There are plenty of ingenious ways to increase this type of exercise. You can keep tabs on it using a good quality pedometer. Unfortunately, you can't get away with Subsistence Exercise alone. You therefore need a regime of Deliberate Exercise, in spite of **POEx**.

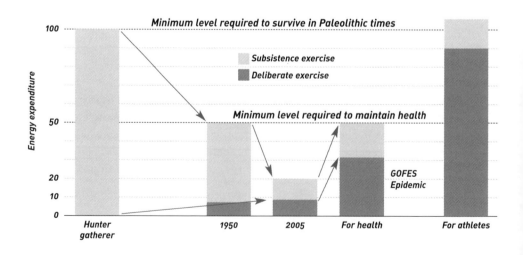

During hunter gatherer times energy expenditure was great. Let's assign an arbitrary figure to it of 100 to *survive*. Deliberate Exercise was unnecessary, in fact our ancestors had to conserve energy and rest when they could. As an example, lions rest as much as 18 hours a day to conserve their energy for hunting. No gym for them between hunts!

With time, Subsistence Exercise declined as we became more industrialised. At one point in time people felt like they needed additional exercise and so sport and games were introduced. By 1950, total energy expenditure in western countries had dropped substantially. While Deliberate Exercise gradually increased thereafter, our activity levels remain dangerously low.

Although activity levels are not the main cause of our GOFES epidemic as many experts claim, it is nonetheless an important spoke in the wheel.

What should we do?
"My wife drives me to drink."
"You're lucky! I have to walk."

Number one: confront **POEx**. Get out of your **Comfort Zone**, then increase your total activity levels to the required amount for good health.

There are three levels of physical activity.
A. Stay with the modern trend at the **GOFES** level and pay the consequences. Even if you are a Humming Bird your health will suffer.

B. Increase your Subsistence and Deliberate exercise to healthy levels. The 50 level in the illustration is enough. It is not as much as you think, as long as you do it regularly, habitually, often, frequently, repeatedly, regularly - get the message? No need to over do it. Overtraining is dangerous and will damage your immune system and speed up aging. Have you noticed how many older, over trained athletes look older than their years?

C. If you have athletic aspirations you'll need to strive for higher levels of activity than those recommended. You'll need to achieve levels of 100 or even higher. Your sleep and eating habits need to be in line with this as well. If you are aiming for level B, don't waste your time training like an Olympian - spend your time indulging in other health activities and enjoy yourself.

Some of the women at my local gym recently competed in a body building competition. I went as a spectator. The presenter announced: "Body building is the most dedicated and egotistical sport - give them a standing ovation for their devotion."

I though he was a bit unfair, but we can learn two things from body builders as far as **GOFES** control is concerned.

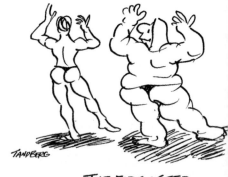

THE FIRST STEP

1. Like the Latin proverb "Many will hate you if you love yourself." However you do need be a bit selfish and somewhat dedicated when it comes to your health, but of course, not too self-centred. You cannot be nice to **POD** and **POEx**. You need to be ruthless in dealing with these instincts in our present **DES** circumstances. Remember, **POD** and **POEx** are over protective and can destroy us.

2. The body building life style is centred around shape and showing it off. In order to do this properly, they develop dietary and exercise techniques to increase their lean body muscle mass and decrease their fat percentage. This is exactly what you need in **GOFES** and health control. The level you want to achieve depends on your aspirations.

The case of two lawyers

Two solicitors were patients at the clinic. They were both very busy and decided to swap car parks, since they were working a few blocks apart in the city. A verbal arrangement was made to that effect. This meant that they had to walk about a kilometre extra each day, increasing their Subsistence Exercise.

One day one of them got to the car park to find the other had taken back his own car park, breaking the agreement. The other's excuse was that he had to rush to court, but for a while they weren't on speaking terms. All was eventually settled when the daughter of one became engaged to the son of the other!

Your exercise regime should cover the full spectrum.

1. Resistance/weight training. Free weights are better and you do not need fancy machines and equipment. With dumb-bells, barbells and a bench you can exercise most muscles.

2. Stretching.

3. Cardio - walking for example.

A follow up book is planned on nutrition, supplementation and exercise, with detailed information and programs. In the meantime, it is recommended that you seek advice from an experienced exercise therapist or trainer. In general I recommend weight training two to three times a week for about half to three quarters of an hour at a time... stretching three to four times per week... and walking three to five times a week. Take a day or two off each week from Deliberate Exercise. Incidentally, sport counts as Deliberate Exercise.

By training harder and longer you won't get any additional benefits in controlling GOFES. If your exercise regime is not producing any benefits, cut your food intake but do not increase your exercise. The temptation will be to increase exercise rather than eat less because **POD > POEx**.

Weight, excess fat loss and exercise

While you are losing excess fat, it is generally not a good idea to over do exercise. Over-fat people do more exercise and expend more energy than their lighter counterparts, simply by walking around.

Work = force x distance
200N = 100kg x 2km
100N = 50kg x 2km

If 100kg is pulled over 2km, then 200 energy units (100 x 2) are consumed. If a person weighs 50kg and walks 2km, this person has spent less energy than the 100kg person walking the same distance. Therefore, if a 100kg person loses 50kg then that person needs to double their walking distance to expend the same energy.

What this means is that as you lose weight you need to increase the intensity of your exercise, or alternatively, put the weight you have lost in a backpack and walk the same distance as before.

With all exercise the following applies:
Make haste slowly - slow is fast
Be persistent - be regular
Keep it interesting
Keep it simple
Keep it up for life.

"Fitness - if it comes in a bottle, everybody would have a good body."
CHER

Thirteenth characteristic of successful weight maintainers: *increased physical activity of incidental and deliberate exercise, leading to moderate fitness*

Synopsis:

1. Do not rely on exercise alone to control **GOFES**. You will just be disappointed.

2. Do the three types of exercise: Resistance, Cardio (aerobics/walking) and stretching. You do not have to do all three every day.

3. "Running late seems to be the only exercise I have time for", but remember: "Those who do not find the time for exercise - will have to find the time for disease." - The Earl of Derby.

4. Build movement and activity into your life. Keep fit.

5. Get expert advice.

6. We really do not have to exercise for survival. Your incentive to exercise, driven by **POEx**, will be very low. You have to override the pain - *"You've just gotta do it."*

CHAPTER 22

4. HYGIENE PROGRAM

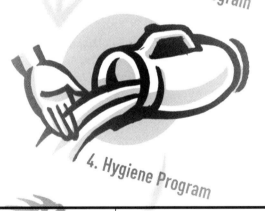

4. HYGIENE PROGRAM

"Better keep yourself clean and bright; you are the window through which you must see the world."
GEORGE BERNARD SHAW

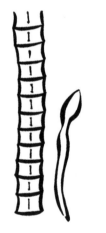

Tapeworm

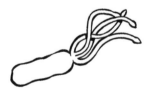

Helicobacter pylori

A tapeworm may grow to approximately 11 metres (35 feet) in length and live 10 years inside a person's intestine. If you had no symptoms but find out you were infected, would you like to eradicate it?

Similarly, Helicobacter pylori is an interesting bug that infects the stomach. At one stage it was believed that it would be impossible for bacteria to grow in stomach acid. Surprisingly, H pylori can do just that. We know now that it causes most stomach and pyloric ulcers. What is also disturbing is that in certain individuals, by affecting the gut associated lymphoid tissue, it can cause stomach cancer.

It has also been suggested that H pylori may predispose the infected individual to heart disease. H pylori can be eradicated with a combination of antibiotics. Some experts recommend eradication only in those who show symptoms, and that those who don't should be left alone. I can understand where they are coming from, but from the point of Optimal Functional Health, infections by H pylori and tapeworm constitute a noxious contamination that places an overload on the metabolism.

A married couple, Gordon and Stacy, lost weight very successfully at the clinic and have kept it off for years. They still came to see me about twice a year for medical monitoring of their health. They have become very conscientious after their excess fat loss, and their cholesterol, blood pressure, other health parameters and fitness levels, were like those of teenagers.

Their biomarkers for aging were consistently at considerably younger ages. They were pictures of good health. When I suggested to Gordon that at his age he should have a colonoscopy he rebutted: "I am not going to have that thing stuck up my back side... and besides I am so healthy, doing the right things and feeling good. You told me that yourself."

Between Stacy and I we eventually talked him around. A month later he had his colonoscopy and I discussed the report with him.

"Gordon, I have good and bad news for you... you have a couple of polyps and the histology showed very early cancer."

"What's the good news then?" a pale looking Gordon asked.

"Well, it was early and it has been completely removed. We only need to monitor the situation every two years or so. If we did not pick this up when we did, it would have progressed and spread."

What have the above three examples in common?

Even if you have your principles of nutrition, supplementation and exercise under control, it is not automatic that your health will hold up forever. This is where the fourth principle of good health comes into play: **Hygiene**.

What I mean by hygiene is not to insult you by reminding you about cleanliness, but as it pertains to the *science of dealing with the preservation of health.*

Today we have the means to identify the presence of many diseases before they become a problem. Once you are seriously ill the medical profession is not as good at curing you as you might think. The best idea is to try to avoid getting sick in the first place. The Ten Health Programs are designed to give you the best chance to achieve this.

Hygiene is the science of dealing with the preservation of health.

Public Hygiene

Bad news from scientists this morning. The chemical formula of water is now H2Yuck!

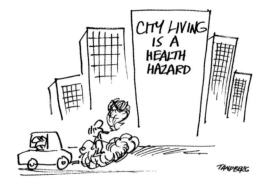

In the mid-1800s the death rate plummeted in Europe. This was not due to the medical profession or medical advances, but due to engineers designing and building sewerage systems and cross ventilation in homes. No matter how healthy you live on a personal level, you may be affected by a number of public health issues that will damage your quest for weight maintenance and optimum function.

Public noise pollution can also be just as dangerous to your health as smoking for instance. A few years ago I bought an electric shaver and noticed that it was fairly noisy. I took it to the agency that handled warranty issues and they informed me that all shavers are equally noisy. I was not satisfied and had the sound level independently tested. I was not surprised that it was higher than the recommended safe level.

I have since bought another brand, but it is still too noisy close to the ears and I use industrial strength ear protectors to protect my hearing while shaving. I get a sceptical look when I mention this to patients and friends.

I discussed this with an ear, nose and throat specialist friend who said he'd noticed a lot of women were experiencing declining hearing as he would expect of industrial workers. He had a number of hair dryers tested and found the decibels too high. He now advises people to wear earplugs when they dry their hair.

As we've discussed, our food supply is polluted and eating fast-foods and canned foods on a regular basis is a slow form of suicide. We are also burdened with various forms of chemical pollution, pesticides and acid rain. Even dogs get lung cancer in our cities. At post mortem a non-smoking person from the country has pink lungs while the city dweller has almost black lungs.

The "sick building" syndrome

According to the World Health Organization, three million people die each year from air pollution. Some 2.8 million of those deaths are from indoor pollution. In Canada, the harsh winter months mean many people rarely venture outside for months on end. They work and shop indoors for long periods. Their constant exposure to toxic fumes given off by building prod-

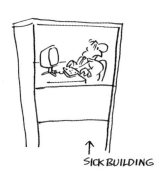
SICK BUILDING

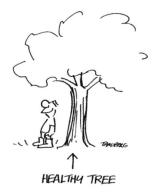
HEALTHY TREE

ucts, paint, carpets and so on results in them feeling ill - the so-called "sick building" syndrome or "cabin sickness".

Good quality air purifiers and ionisers may be a good way of limiting some of the damage and worth the investment.

Personal Hygiene

This covers in part your personal maintenance.

The teeth-obesity-heart disease connection

The mouth can be a cesspit of billions of bacteria causing all sorts of local and systemic consequences. The main thing about these bacteria is that they are not the same types and in the same ratios that previous generations experienced. These bugs invade all the nooks and crannies and also live under the gum line.

Not only do they cause cavities and bad breath, but gradually the gums inflame and the consequences become systemic. It is well established that there is a relationship between heart disease and bad oral hygiene. Pregnant women with bad oral hygiene have a much higher risk of premature birth due to the systemic effects affecting the foetus.

I have also observed a strong link between **GOFES** and oral hygiene. It appears to be a prerequisite for keeping excess fat at bay - being meticulous about what is going on in the mouth in more ways than one. Reasons I can't give you, but I do have some theories.

If the teeth are brushed and cleaned after a meal, a sense of cleanliness ensues and it is easier to control nibbling after the meal - you don't want to spoil that clean feeling. In part this is probably true, but I'm sure there are systemic factors as well.

The connection is so strong that I can claim: if meticulous regular oral hygiene does not form part of your maintenance strategy, you will not maintain your weight loss and you will not achieve Optimal Functional Health.

I recommend brushing your teeth twice a day, once with an electric toothbrush and once with an ordinary brush. Flossing at least once per day - twice may be better, depending on your diet. The odd mouthwash may also help in decreasing the bacterial load, but be careful of them as most contain debatable substances. Be careful to not brush too hard.

People without teeth live on average three years longer than those with their teeth. As we get older it is difficult to clean all the nooks and crannies and inflammation sets in. But before you rush out to have all your teeth extracted, just clean them daily.

If you love your kids, yourself, your heart and want to manage **GOFES**, keep your oral cavity clean.

14th characteristic of successful weight maintainers:
the GOFES/teeth connection - bad oral hygiene contributes to GOFES

Screening

Screening for health problems is controversial. Health departments insist that most of it is not cost effective. For readers of a book of this nature, screening can be very effective, even if your health cover or the government does not pay for it. You are opting for Optimal Functional Health and metabolic fitness.

Screening for heart disease, cholesterol and certain forms of cancer is usually sponsored. You should also be screened for aging. Screening of the biomarkers for aging can be very rewarding in monitoring health and early intervention - more on this later in the chapter on "Time".

Some people may object to treating aging as a disease, because it is a normal part of life. Pregnancy is a normal part of life, but in the medical profession it is treated as a "disease". Pregnant women are seen by medical doctors and most have their babies in hospital. As a result the maternal and infant mortality rate has fallen dramatically. Dramatic things may happen too if we formally treat aging as a disease. It should be recognised as a field of medicine with its own specialists.

Most households should have an instrument (sphygmomanometer) to measure blood pressure. Not only to detect early elevations of blood pressure, but also to monitor the effects of treatment for hypertension. Most patients suffer to a degree from "white coat syndrome" - visiting a doctor typically elevates the blood pressure and may lead to unnecessary treatment. By measuring your own blood pressure you can obtain a true reading and have a better understanding of this aspect of your health.

However, don't attempt to be your own doctor - *always consult your doctor on any medical issues.*

Eradication

Parasites and freeloading micro-organisms can be a burden on the body. Such a burden on the body and the immune system should be eliminated. Some micro-organisms, such as lactobacillus, can be beneficial and should be encouraged.

Synopsis:

1. Screen vigorously for early detection leading to early intervention and treatment.

2. Teeth - bad oral hygiene can contribute to GOFES.

3. Maintain a normal fat percentage.

4. Screen for aging and treat it as a disease.

CHAPTER 23

5. REST AND RECREATION

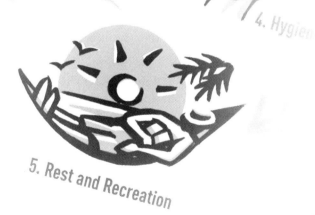

5. Rest and Recreation

5. REST AND RECREATION

"Just when I was getting used to yesterday, along came today."

ANONYMOUS

Going through a stressful event in my life, I was walking somewhat aimlessly through a shopping centre. I wanted to buy something, but didn't have anything in mind. Maybe, I thought, it would make me feel better - retail therapy.

I walked into a pet shop, browsing around without purpose. I passed a cage with a canary in it. It started singing. On my way out I passed the cage again and the canary sang even louder. Whether the singing was coincidental or not, I felt an instant bond with the bird.

Without hesitating I walked to the counter and purchased the canary, the cage and some feed. I can still remember it clearly, the canary was $20, the cage $80 and food $5. For the journey home the canary was put in a little box, which I put next to me in the car. At home, as quickly as possible, I found a spot for the cage in the TV room near the kitchen. Expecting the canary to be stressed after the journey, I was surprised when hardly back in its cage it put on a spirited song.

Every afternoon when I came home I could hear it sing. I would stop and enjoy the singing for a while, then continue my routine. One afternoon when I came home I realised that it was a she when I saw an egg in the bottom of the cage. I rushed back to the pet shop and bought a little nest. Over the next few days she laid three more eggs.

Then one afternoon when I came home, she sang slightly differently and I rushed to see if she was alright. To my surprise all four eggs had hatched - she was fertilised when I bought her.

Yet again I rushed to the pet shop to buy special feed. With her babies she sang even more confidently than usual. Occasionally when I was on the phone, the singing was so loud I lost concentration and had to go to another room. Not that I minded. Sadly, her babies died after a few days.

She was such a remarkable canary that I bought her a male companion, but she never got on with him. A second male was no better and in the end I gave the males away.

When she was about three years old she started losing some of her feathers. At first I did nothing - like we often do in medicine - watchful and waiting. She still sang beautifully and I assumed that she was starting "menopause" and maybe her feather loss was due to that. Gradually it got worse and I took her to the vet. He said that she did not have enough nutrients and sold me some expensive "medicated" feed. This made not an iota of difference and I went ahead, mixing and matching feed to my own formulae - also to no avail.

After some time she looked like a plucked chicken with just the odd feather on the tip of her wings, two on her head and a few on her tail. I suspected some serious disease, but she sang even more vigorously than before.

When I went away on conferences I usually had the neighbours come in to feed her. One time I had to go away, but the neighbours were away as well. I had no option but to take the canary to the clinic so that the staff could look after her while I was away.

Three weeks later I was back. I walked into the clinic to the room where the canary was kept. To my horror there was a new canary in the cage. My first thought was that she had died and the staff must have bought a replacement to soften the blow. I confronted the staff as to what had happened. They reassured me it was the same canary. I didn't believe them and rushed back for another look. This time she started singing and I sighed with relief.

"What did you do for her to grow her feathers like this?" I asked the staff. "Nothing," they replied, "we only gave her the feed you supplied. A few days after you left we noticed she was developing what looked like pimples on her body. On closer inspection, new feathers were coming out of the little lumps. In the last few days she became fully feathered."

I was dumbfounded. What could the reason be?

That evening I started researching this "miracle". I even asked a psychiatrist friend of mine if he had a theory. Within days at home, she started losing feathers again.

"It must be some pollution at home," I thought by myself. The next morning she was back at the clinic again. I was resigned to the fact that the clinic would be her new home. Patients liked her - it might be that the "attention" may have been good for her.

My research went on and I could not find a satisfactory answer. Then one day, quite incidentally, I stumbled on the reason. Canaries need about 10 to 12 hours a day of darkness and sleep for good health. Lack of it affects their pituitary glands in their brains with various negative consequences. That's when it dawned on me she was overexposed to light and was too close to the TV. The lights were seldom off before 1am and most mornings were back on by 5.30. At the clinic when the staff left, the lights were off at 6pm and back on at 8am. From that moment on she got her uninterrupted sleep and darkness.

She never lost feathers again.

Sleep deprivation and humans

This incident in my life set me wondering how lack of sleep affected humans. What can sleep deprivation do to us? We don't have feathers to lose, but what other damage might we suffer?

Humans need different types of sleep, like a catnap or siesta and of course deep sleep - Rapid Eye Movement sleep. Are we getting enough? Unfortunately not. An article in one of the medical journals under the sensationalist headline: "Are the British becoming Morons?" - claimed chronic sleep deprivation could lower a person's IQ by 15 points. It is also mentioned that British people sleep the least in the world. The average person's IQ is 100 - lower this by 15 points and you may reach the moron level.

Some quite intelligent students often lose too much sleep during their exams, lowering their IQs. As a consequence, their results are mediocre for their abilities. Driving in a sleep deprived state can be the same as driving over the alcohol limit and is just as dangerous.

Snooze for health and GOFES control

"Sleep is the golden chain that ties health and our bodies together."
THOMAS DEKKER

One of the most destructive free radicals, the hydroxyl free radical, is very damaging to the brain. During sleep we secrete a hormone called melatonin that is very effective against the hydroxyl free radical. More on this in a later chapter.

The science of sleep is very interesting and the full picture is still not known. It is interesting that we can survive longer without eating than we can without sleeping. Apparently no person has lived without sleeping for longer than eleven days. Sleep deprivation is a well-recognised way of torturing prisoners. Why torture yourself?

Our metabolism relies on biorhythms established in our genetic past. Not synchronising yourself as much as possible to these rhythms is not only very destructive to your health as a whole, but detrimental to your efforts in controlling GOFES.

"Sometimes I think I understand everything, and then I regain consciousness."
ANONYMOUS

Sleep deprivation is a powerful force in sabotaging a person's efforts in controlling their Obesity. It has a remarkably strong influence in a person's ability to control DES, POD and POEx. Sleeping for less than six hours or more than nine hours a night has been associated with an increased risk of diabetes in some studies. These same poor sleep habits have also been linked to impaired glucose tolerance.

"I have not slept in days. It's good I can sleep at night."
ANONYMOUS

Your sleep is just as important as your food intake.

"Sleep is such a wonderful thing. It's a shame you can't stay awake to enjoy it."
ANONYMOUS

Meditation

Meditation is not sleep. I believe it to be a very important part of a person's life. Constant high stress hormone levels can be very destructive to a person's health. Meditation is a way of lowering your stress hormone levels. Just daydreaming a bit or listening to good quality music is a form of meditation. There are much higher forms of meditation, but the average person finds it difficult to practice these regularly. For years I have suffered from sleep deprivation and when I try to meditate I just fall asleep. You need breaks in your day - every day.

It may be worthwhile for you to undertake training in meditation, but like food and exercise it is only good for you if applied with consistency.

You need every day:
- Good quality deep sleep.
- A catnap or siesta - they are very good for you.
- Some form of meditation.

Sleep and meditation should form a third of your life to make the other two thirds more meaningful. Depriving yourself of sleep will not only affect your IQ, but GOFES will be your unpleasant travel companion.

In nature all creatures go to some trouble to get good sleep. Chimpanzees built tree nests and other animals go to great lengths to find a safe, comfortable sleeping spot. We humans should not neglect our own sleeping habits. Since we spend so much time in our beds it is quite appropriate to invest in your bed, mattress and bedroom.

You should sleep in the dark. This is the time that you secrete most of your melatonin. The blind have 30 per cent less cancer because they secrete more melatonin. Noise and dark proof your bedroom. Never keep a television in your bedroom if you are at all serious about **GOFES** and your health. Read a book if you cannot sleep.

What is not realised by the general population is that alcohol and caffeine are the most disruptive drugs for good sleep. As a general rule it's worth trying to avoid consumption of these drugs after 3pm.

We are sleeping 20 per cent less than we were two generations ago. Most of us have a sleep debt. Aim for at least a 10 per cent increase. Your health, happiness and work performance depend on it.

"Faddists are continually proclaiming the value of exercise. Four people out of five are more in need of rest than exercise."
LOGAN CLENDENING

15th characteristic of successful weight maintainers: good sleeping and meditation habits. Why torture yourself with sleep deprivation? Sleep deprivation is fattening.

Stress management

Never believe that you will ever have a stress free life. Stress is a survival mechanism like the pain of deprivation. You can only manage stress.

In primitive times as a hunter gatherer being chased by a lion your stress level would be at maximum. You had two choices - be eaten or escape - *each had a clear outcome.* If you escaped your stress level would soon return to the base line for survival.

These days the outcomes are not as clear-cut. When we reach the Extreme Stress Line, we may never return to the base line for survival again. The descent is much slower because of the cumulative pressures of modern times. *Although some of our stress levels do not reach the Extreme Stress Line, we don't always return to the baseline.* The following illustration depicts this scenario.

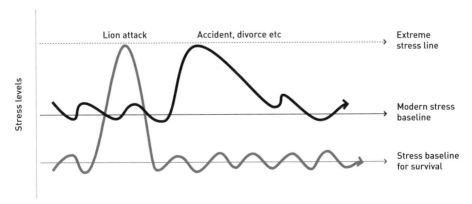

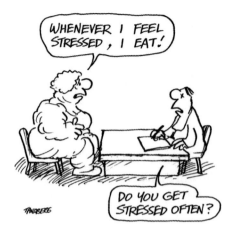

We can handle extreme stress in short bursts quite well, but in these modern times we are having to function at much higher stress levels, on average, than we are designed for. This elevation of our average stress levels affects our health. We secrete constantly higher levels of stress hormones - and the aging process and onset of degenerative diseases are accelerated.

You must do your utmost to decrease your stress hormone levels. *Higher levels make your metabolism more efficient in storing fat.* Additionally, higher average stress levels make it mentally more difficult to deal with something as powerful as **POD** and therefore **GOFES**.

Stress threshold

We all have an individual stress threshold. This threshold varies according to genetics and circumstances. It is the level we can tolerate at a particular time without showing signs of stress.

When your stress threshold is lowered, POD will sneak up on you - you over eat, and because you're a Polar Bear, you get fat.

I used to believe there were "no calories" in stress. Therefore stress cannot promote GOFES. I was wrong, because I did not take the hormonal and other metabolic effects of high stress levels into account. This makes the metabolism more efficient in storing fat.

What is stress anyway? Sometimes I am not sure the stress experts know what it really is. Normally we see stress as tension, worry, hassle, pressure and strain. **Stress is anything that makes demands on our ability to cope.** It has a lot to do with our coping skills.

Stress arises when there is a mismatch between the demands in your life, your coping skills, and your abilities.

Give this some serious thought. The demands in your life - do you know what they are? Have you clearly defined them?

Our coping skills are inborn, but can be improved by managing stress. Similarly, our abilities are inborn. The one factor you can control are the demands in your life.

There are different types of demands made on our ability to cope. **Dys-stress** is negative stress that is harmful to a person and **Eu-stress** is positive stress. The latter still makes demands on our coping skills, but is more positive.

One person's dys-stress is another's eu-stress. *John tries parachute jumping for the first time. When he lands he is excited and can't wait to do it again. Jane follows him and when she lands, is overcome by nauseating anxiety and certainly does not want to repeat the experience.* One person's eu-stress can be another's dys-stress. It depends on your make up.

A high-powered executive job can be eu-stress for some people - they thrive on it. While for that same person, a boring job could be very dys-stressful, because the person has to cope with the boredom.

Stressors are the events and things that cause us to suffer from stress. Dys-stressors are those things that make demands on our ability to cope that we perceive to be negative. They can vary. Nobody seems to have enough money and for many of us debt can be dys-stressful. Marriage and children are stressful. Hopefully, for most of us it is eu-stress. Resentment can be a heavy burden and be very dys-stressful. Sometimes stressors are vague and can only be identified in therapy or with intensive introspection.

GOFES *and its effects can be one of the most significant dys-stressors in a person's life.*

> *"I read this article that said the typical symptoms of stress are eating too much, impulse buying, and driving too fast. Are they kidding? That's my idea of a perfect day."*
> ANONYMOUS

The dys-stressors have effects on you the stressee. Low levels may merely be a small inconvenience at times, but as they build up the effects became progressively more apparent. As they build, your stress threshold drops, as does your tolerance for further stress. At first a bit of vague anxiety becomes noticeable. If the levels continue to escalate, some symptoms of depression develop. By now your body has gone through an alarm reaction and your cortisol levels are increased. This is followed by the controversial state of *burnout*. While you don't feel particularly anxious or depressed, you have lost your enthusiasm. You continue your life and few people realise the pressure you are under. You have reached a state of exhaustion.

If your stress is not managed at this point depression becomes apparent and stress hormone levels continue to climb. Organ damage and failure creeps in. If this continues you will suffer a nervous breakdown. The latter simply means that you have *run out of all your coping skills.* Your stress threshold has now reached rock bottom.

This process also speeds up the aging process. You have reached a state of total incapacity and you cannot even brush your teeth. You need therapy, medication, dys-stressor avoidance and perhaps hospitalisation. Sadly, some people will even commit suicide in such circumstances - they have had enough.

Most of us at some stage in our lives get quite close to this point, but thank goodness, we make an about turn and avert the breakdown. You cannot expect to run and run without reaching a point of collapse and exhaustion.

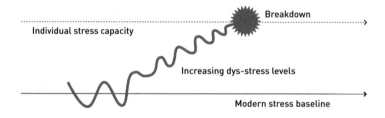

Individual stress capacity varies. It is exponential, not linear. Looking at a mathematical model it is obvious that 2 + 2 = 4. Another + 2 = 6 and so on. There is a linear relationship.

Psychologically the relationship is exponential. That is to say a dys-stressor of two plus another with the same magnitude equals for instance eight. 2 + 2 = 8 in this case. Plus another 2 = 16, etc.

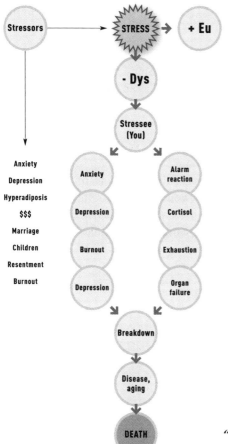

Stressors

STRESS → **+ Eu**

- Dys

Stressee (You)

Anxiety
Depression
Hyperadiposis
$$$
Marriage
Children
Resentment
Burnout

Anxiety	Alarm reaction
Depression	Cortisol
Burnout	Exhaustion
Depression	Organ failure

Breakdown

Disease, aging

DEATH

This has two very important consequences for you.

Another, even an apparently insignificant dys-stress, when added to your dys-stress total, can have huge effects on your health, mental state and performance. This one tiny dys-stress can tip the balance for you - "the straw that breaks the camel's back". The higher your dys-stress score, the more careful you have to be to avoid a breakdown.

The opposite is also true. If you deal effectively with one dys-stress your total levels will drop exponentially and dramatically.

This has great significance and you should do your utmost to deal with and manage your dys-stress levels. What a relief!

GOFES management will give you such relief.

"To live long it is necessary to live slowly."
CICERO

Who really decides if you suffer from stress or not? *You do!*

It is amazing how we worry and stress-out over little things. Worry is interest paid on trouble before it comes due.

A tree can be struck by lightning and battered by wind and still survive, but an infestation of termites will bring it crashing down. It is the small things that eat into us and often do the most damage.

We are all born with an individual tendency to anxiety. If it is high we tend to panic more often and suffer from anxiety and phobias. If it is low we are not so easily affected. To know how much stress you can take is important in dealing with your own dys-stress. Do not make the mistake of trying to change your nature - just deal with it as best you can.

One of the more effective ways of managing stress is to plan a daily routine and stick with it. "What are you going to do when you get up in the morning until you leave for work and in what order?" This schedule is important to set you in the right frame of mind for the day. You need to plan this routine in a scientific way like an efficiency engineer. Be careful of *"double-handling"* and aimlessly walking back and forth. The following is an example.

	Action	Sections and time
1	Alarm Get up	
2	Go to toilet	
3	Weigh yourself	
4	Enter it on your bio-rhythm graph	A ± 3 min
5	Grooming: shave, nail, etc	B ± 10 min
6	Exercise: physical, medication, etc	
7	Bath/shower	C ± 20-40 min
8	Break-the-fast (eat)	D ± 10-20 min
9	Clean teeth	
10	Get dressed	
11	Final touches - ready for work	E ± 5 min
TOTAL		± 60-90 min

Most of us have a morning routine, but if you are Polar Bear it is important for you to sit down, think it through and put pen to paper. Divide activities in blocks by grouping certain activities together. After a while it becomes ritual and you will be surprised how you cope better with the day.

Different days may require different routines, and the end result may be totally unlike the example, but the bottom line is - *have one!* You will thank yourself for it.

When not managed well, stress will lead to increased alcohol consumption and overeating encouraged by **POD**.

According to medical experts, being under mild pressure is actually good for you. Research shows that some stress can actually help your body to stay young and healthy. It is a survival instinct. Just like POD is good for us, but bad in modern times if not controlled, so is dys-tress.

16th characteristic of successful weight maintainers:
stress understanding and management - distress is fattening - lack of routine is fattening.

Life has certain rhythms and we have developed cultural habits that coincide with these. Unfortunately our modern frenetic lifestyles have disrupted these rhythms. The Sabbath, Sundays and religious festivals were once days of rest and respite. Today we are never given the chance to switch off.

Of course **GOFES** is less easily controlled in such an environment. You are well advised from a health and **GOFES** point of view to celebrate your own days of rest and relaxation.

Mobile phones have made us available to each other and strangers twenty-five hours a day, eight days a week, anywhere, any time. In spite of some advantages, this constant accessibility has created havoc with our biorhythms and deep rest, no doubt with further sociological change to come.

Holidays

Holidays are not just for other people. You don't have to go on expensive cruises, but somehow you have to get out of the house and out of town at least once a year. Studies have shown holidays to be an important part of a health program - *good or bad*. The latter for those who think holidays are an opportunity to over indulge!

Some people approach holidays on the basis that they paid for it and they are "going to enjoy it". Their abuse of food and alcohol starts on the plane. Suffering hangovers, they lie in the sun and feel even worse by day's end when the drinking and eating binge starts all over again. When they come back from holiday they actually need another holiday to recover.

Holidays should be seen as a change in routine, not an opportunity for abuse. For **GOFES** victims holidays are a great opportunity to resynchronise themselves.

Leisure time and special interests

If you cannot afford the time every day, then have at least some hours on a weekly basis. Interests and hobbies increase the strategies available to you in dealing with POD and, as a result, GOFES.

Massage

Touch is important for bonding. Monkeys are masters at grooming each other and it is indispensable for their wellbeing. Massage is not only good for therapy and relaxation, but also stimulates the immune system. It can do wonders if you can afford it on a regular basis.

Felicity and Eric, husband and wife team, lost their excess fat and did very well on maintenance. Eric was looking to do a course of some sort and settled on massage. He practiced on Felicity, and unbeknown to them, this had unexpected benefits. They strengthened their marriage bond and Felicity's health improved, having been prone to respiratory infections.

Noise pollution

Go to great lengths to control the noise in your life, especially during sleep time. It has been suggested that noise pollution is as bad for your health as smoking. Noise pollution will increase your stress hormone levels and make you more prone to **GOFES**.

Laughter, humour and optimism

Growing old is mandatory - growing up is optional. Enjoy life - you will never get out of it alive.

Have fun. Laughter increases your endorphin levels. Some years ago I attended an obesity conference in Hawaii. When I arrived I was informed that the conference had been postponed by 10 days at the last minute and there'd been no time to inform attendees. I had to make a decision - stay or fly home and return in 10 days. I decided to stay. Every day I watched the whales off the coast. At that time I did not realise they swam from Alaska and do not eat for this eight month trip. One night I attended a meeting of the Hawaii Comedy Club. I still have a laugh from time to time, remembering some of the jokes, and I also met some very pleasant people.

"Laughter is a tranquilliser with no side effects."
ANONYMOUS

A laugh a day keeps the doctor away.

Various studies suggest that laughing and a sense of humour contribute to good health. Conversely, depression increases your chances of cancer and heart attack. Every survival kit should include a sense of humour. And pessimists generally don't live as long as optimists.

Smell the roses

When a cynic smells flowers, he looks around for a coffin!

When did you last take time to smell the roses? If you are a modern, frenzied **GOFES** victim, chances are it's been a very long time.

Sometimes we just have to sit back and enjoy. Your health and happiness depend on it.

Things may be bad, but they'll be better tomorrow, or the day after.

Comfort zone

Our comfort zones have been shrinking at alarming rates for half a century. We have become so cocooned we can't handle straying outside of these ever contracting zones. It is survival driven for us to stay within our comfort zones hence our reluctance to confront the discomfort of **POD** and **POEx**.

Our intolerance levels can be quite exacting.

Have you ever had a passenger in your car who constantly adjusts the temperature setting because one moment the temperature is too cold, then too hot. Many people have a very narrow range of comfort and we moan and groan if we are taken just marginally outside this zone.

We don't seem to be able to relax outside our comfort zone - the slightest POD, for example, and we have to eat immediately. The thought of having to walk somewhere, rather than driving, pushes our limits. There's nothing unusual about this - after all, it is the Pain and Pleasure of Survival phenomenon - PPOS - that demands it. But to be hungry is good for the metabolism and exercise is good for our wellbeing.

The extremes of discomfort are bad for us, but a moderate amount is highly beneficial. *In fact, it helps you to expand your enjoyment of life and health.*

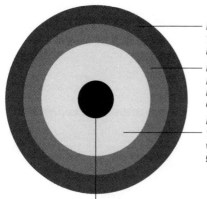

DANGER ZONE
The outer circle symbolises the danger zone. There's no need to be this uncomfortable. Stay away.

DISCOMFORT ZONE
Regular visits to the discomfort zone will benefit your health. Physical exertion, saunas, cold water and deprivation all play a role in maintaining our health.

NORMAL COMFORT ZONE
The next circle or normal comfort zone is the cocoon in which many of us choose to live - nothing ventured, nothing gained.

ABNORMALLY SMALL COMFORT ZONE
If you don't stray outside of this region of greatest comfort, you're in danger of imploding. If you don't give a muscle some exercise, it shrinks too.

Reduce the amount of time you spend in the discomfort zone, and the frequency of your visits, and your comfort zone will shrink. You need to spend time in the *discomfort zone* on a regular basis. A patient of mine who was 97 when he died, used to take a cold shower every morning, summer and winter, until his death.

We need some pain to get pleasure, discomfort for comfort, and exertion for relaxation. As the saying goes - no pain, no gain - unless the pain is in the danger zone.

Our comfort zones and tolerance shrink with age. Venturing outside our comfort zone includes saying "NO" to that last piece of cheesecake.

Synopsis:
1. Sleep hygiene is closely linked to the ability to control **GOFES**. Insomnia is fattening.

2. Manage your stress hormone levels by stress management, massage, meditation, humour and smelling the roses.

3. Take a holiday from your normal routine and surroundings.

4. If society has abandoned its traditional rest and reflection days, create your own and/or celebrate your cultural days.

5. Get off your butt and get out of your comfort zone to expand it. Build up a *comfort reserve* so that you can be comfortable over a *wider range*. Pushing our discomfort levels increases our comfort zone. Do things that demands effort.

CHAPTER 24

6. PHILOSOPHY

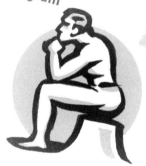

6. Philosophy

6. PHILOSOPHY

"Philosophy is the art of living."
PLUTARCH

"The art of living is more like wrestling than dancing. It is not death a man should fear, but he should fear never beginning to live."
MARCUS AURELIUS ANTONINUS

To think only of the pot of gold at the end of the rainbow is to miss the beauty of the rainbow itself. Ultimately it does not matter how long we live, but how.

If you don't have a religion, have philosophy. There is scientific proof that to understand philosophy and live by its credo will improve your health and increase your chances of living longer and healthier. Life may not be all you want, but it's all you have.

Taking time to nurture your spirit may be a path to better health, according to researchers. A study of the health perceptions of older adults revealed that the people who reported being the most spiritual are the healthiest. Non-religious people with an appreciation of philosophy recorded similar benefits. Taking care of your spiritual or philosophical health and well-being can improve your functional age by years.

There are many and varied views on this subject and I am not advocating any particular viewpoint. A philosophical outlook is also beneficial in coping with negative stress. Some studies indicate that philosophers with PhDs are often better at helping their fellow man with psychological issues than psychologists and psychiatrists.

A rabbi, priest, preacher, or elder is often able to assist more than you might think. Everyone is different, but sound philosophical thinking and its principles benefit us all.

Finally:

- The most important things in life aren't things. We are not really meant to understand life - just to live it.

- It is not only the most difficult thing to know oneself, but the most inconvenient.

- Wherever you are - there you are.

CHAPTER 25

7. SOCIAL PROGRAM

7. SOCIAL PROGRAM

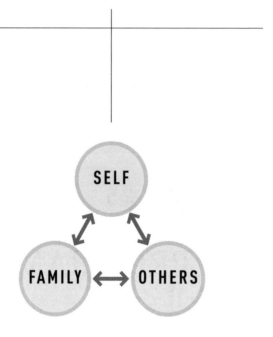

The most important thing a mother and father can do for their children is to love each other.

We do not live in isolation. We need and yearn for social bonds and interaction.

To live without love is not really to live. Like Plato said millennia ago "He whom love touches not, walks in darkness". This social interconnectivity plays a substantial role in our health. Some people focus too much on themselves, others too much on family, while others focus too much on others. For optimum health there should be a balance.

Once upon a time there was a man who asked a woman to marry him.

She said "No."

And he lived happily ever after...

According to Jean-Paul Sartre: "hell is other people." A bumper sticker: "The more people I meet the more I like my dog." Aldous Huxley: "Maybe this world is another planet's hell."

Not the right attitude to achieve success with the Social Program.

Take care of yourself

"Why are married men and women fatter then unmarried ones? Because an unmarried person goes to the fridge, sees nothing that he/she likes and goes to bed. A married person goes to bed, sees nothing he/she likes and goes to the fridge."
ANONYMOUS

Neglecting your social program is neglecting yourself. It is not suggested that you live constantly in the pockets of your friends and family - we are all different and have dissimilar social needs. What is important is to have a balance of the self-family-others equation, and to be active in this bond to the degree your personality allows.

You are only as good to others as you are to yourself

Your battle with **GOFES** and your health should be *more* important than the friend or family member you help out with *their* projects. You should even put yourself first when it comes to your children. The instruction in passenger aircraft is clear: "In case of a sudden loss in air pressure, put your oxygen mask on *first*, **before** you assist the child next to you."

Why? If you lose consciousness, due to a lack of oxygen, you will not be able to help the child. Therefore, helping yourself first is often best for our friends and loved ones.

Pets

Even a pet is part of the family. Various studies have shown that people who keep a pet are healthier and have less cancer. "A pet does not ask questions" and "a dog is a man's best friend" carry a lot of truth.

"All animals, except man, know that the principal business of life is to enjoy it."
SAMUEL BUTLER

Love and affection

This section is not meant to serve as a guide or to be superficial about relationships and marriages, but to make the reader aware how powerful these factors are in mental and physical health. Humour quite often plays on great truths and should not be seen as dismissive of the positive aspects. To laugh is therapeutic.

Since this book is about **GOFES** and **Health**, a patient brought his wife to see me and asked: "what is marriage?" Before I could reply he said: "It's a ceremony that turns your dreamboat into a barge."

Adam and Eve were strolling in the Garden of Eden when Eve turned anxiously to her mate:

"Adam," she asked, "tell me the truth, do you love me?"

Adam shrugged. "Who else?"

All people, even the arrogant, are influenced by affection. Mark Twain said: "Praise is well, compliment is well, but *affection* - that is the last and most precious reward that any man can win, whether by character or achievement." Somerset Maugham believed love is what happens to a man and woman who don't know each other. I feel that love is what's left of a relationship after all the selfishness has been exhausted.

The love and affection of a happy marriage and the close family bonds that it brings can be one of the most reassuring and health-preserving medicines known to man. Our psyche and metabolism are designed to operate in such an environment, and there is sound evidence to support this.

An exceptionally successful person I know always tells me that everything in his life revolves around his marriage and family. The glowing and endearing terms in which he describes his wife and family is like a romantic novel. At their 40th wedding anniversary you could see the mutual admiration the couple has for each other.

He told me that in the first 10 years of their marriage he worked very hard to achieve success, but she stood by him, while others would have either left or become petulant. Nowadays, people give up too quickly on each other.

I once asked a retired multi-millionaire in his eighties why he emigrated at his age? He responded: "My wife and I could not live without the children and grandchildren, even if we could just hop on a plane and visit them. Love is everything... money means nothing without it."

Failed relationships

Marriage is like a violin. After the beautiful music is over, the strings are still attached. A divorce is like being hit by a truck. If you manage to survive it, you start looking very cautiously to the left and right.

Yet failed marriages are a source of ill health and a huge cost to any community as well.

Goethe said: "Love is an ideal thing; marriage is the real thing. A confusion of the real with the ideal never goes unpunished." More recently John Barrymore uttered: "Paper napkins never return from a laundry, nor love from a trip to the family law courts."

Recently in a medical journal there was an article about failed marriages and their cost to the individual and community. It was quite pessimistic and in the last paragraph it read: "...and the secret of a happy marriage still remains a secret."

"What is the secret of marriage? When you are right, apologise fast!"

Is there any hope?

A patient recently sent me the following story off the Internet. It is a good illustration of how we can easily fail to notice and appreciate the love of a family.

The story goes that some time ago, a man punished his five-year-old daughter for wasting a roll of expensive gold wrapping paper by decorating a box to put under the Christmas tree.

Nevertheless, the little girl brought the gift box to her father the next morning and said: "This is for you daddy."

The father was embarrassed by his earlier overreaction, but his anger flared again when he found the box was empty. He spoke to her harshly: "Don't you know, young lady, when you give someone a present there's supposed to be something inside the package?"

The little girl looked up at him with tears in her eyes and said: "Oh Daddy, it's not empty. I blew kisses into it until it was full."

The father was crushed. He put his arms around his little girl, and begged her to forgive him for his unnecessary anger.

An accident took the life of the child only a short time later and it is told that the father kept that gold box by his bed for all the years of his life. And whenever he was discouraged or faced difficult problems, he would open the box and take out an imaginary kiss and remember the love of the child who had put it there.

In a very real sense, each of us as human beings has been given a golden box filled with unconditional love and kisses from our children, family and friends. There is no more precious possession.

The Social Program is profoundly powerful in a positive way and can be extremely devastating in a negative way.

This is your opportunity to work on one of the most powerful of the ten health programs.

Longest-shortest consultation I have ever had

A new patient came to my consulting room. A lady in her mid-60s, she was neatly and conservatively dressed, but was about 20 years out of fashion.

She was very composed but seemed almost sad. She had come to see me about a relatively minor medical matter in that she was trying to stay healthy for her grandchildren. As we were talking I soon realised that I was dealing with a person of substance and character. The more she talked, the more I enjoyed it. Eventually, she stood up and said it was getting late and she had to pick up her granddaughter from school. I looked at my watch and realised that well over an hour had passed. I have never had a consultation that was so long, yet so short.

She told me many interesting things, but what stuck in my mind was the story she told me about her own life. She got married at 19 to John who was 21. By the time she was 22 John was an alcoholic. She stuck by him, but by the time she was 26 and had three children she realised the time for drastic action had arrived. She told him: "John I have to leave you. I cannot live like this anymore."

Life wasn't easy for her, but she eventually bought a small house and her children were well cared for. Some 22 years later there was a knock on the front door.

The man standing there looked vaguely familiar. "I'm John and I want to come back."

She looked at him intently and asked: "Have you stopped drinking?"

He replied without hesitation: "Yes, a long time ago and I have been looking for you ever since."

Three weeks later they remarried. The next 16 years, until John died, were the happiest of their lives and they never stopped loving each other.

Gazing at familiar faces, even in pictures, may help you feel less stressed. The look of a familiar face appears to soothe nerves and dampen the stress response. Spend time with friends and family when you are feeling stressed. Keep photos on hand for times when they cannot be near.

Friends and acquaintances

People are often unclear about the difference between friends and acquaintances. Often a person describes another as a "good friend", but on further questioning cannot even remember the surname. This "good friend" is obviously an acquaintance. There is a difference between good friends, friends and acquaintances. It may be useful for you to know the difference.

Synopsis:

1. No matter the negativity and warped humour that surrounds relationships, you have to be very astute when it comes to your Social Program.

2. If it is not your disposition to be socially involved, don't force it. Forcing yourself may cause stress, but remember: if you're not prepared to push your Comfort Zone you will lose out on many health benefits.

3. In your Social Program you do not always need to be right. There are many ways to save face.

4. Mother's Day and Father's Day were invented for very good reason. They bond friends and family together. So do birthdays and other family occasions. Celebrate them.

5. Remain social and productive as you get older. Maintain the balance between Self, Family and Others.

6. "To live is like to love - all reason is against it, and all healthy instinct is for it."
   SAMUEL BUTLER.

7. Fight as hard as you can for your Social Program. Love yourself and your family. Your health, happiness and existence depend on it.

   "Happy is he who dares courageously to defend what he loves."
   OVID

CHAPTER 26

8. TIME

9. Protection and Security

8. Time

8. TIME

"He who would pass the declining years of his life with honour and comfort should, when young, consider that he may one day become old, and remember, when he is old, that he has once been young."

JOSEPH ADDISON

There's something about the age of 50. Maybe you don't consider yourself over the hill yet, but you're sure getting a clearer view of the other side. That could mean it's time to think about the steps you can take to ease into old age. What you do now could make a big difference to how you feel in another 20 or 30 years.

How long is 20 years?

The answer to this question depends in part on your age - the younger the longer, and the older the shorter.

However, if you realistically think about it, it is not too long and when "it's over it's over". Only 1,040 weekends and how quickly they go.

If you are over 40 you can probably remember what you did 20 years ago. Attending a class reunion today you soon notice how everybody has changed over this period of time. In some cases the physical deterioration of your classmates will shock you. At the same time you will be surprised at how well others have preserved themselves. We are not always so adept in noticing these time changes in ourselves. Maybe we don't want to face it.

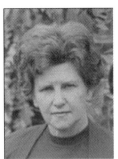

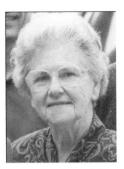

50 years **70 years - 20 years later**

We age relentlessly

Q: "Have you lived here all your life?"

A: "Not yet."

One morning a man awoke feeling miserable. The past 15 years hadn't been very pleasant and he dreaded continuing his life like this. Rather than give up, he decided to replan his life. He'd try it for a month.

Taking stock of his life and planning the future, he wanted to know how long the average person lived. This he hoped would give him some idea how long he still had left. Armed with the statistic that the average person lives only about 650,000 hours, he calculated that he had 105,000 hours left to live - 624 weekends.

He bought a big glass jar and a bag of pebbles and counted out 624 pebbles. Every Friday morning he would walk up to the jar, pick out one pebble and say to himself: "I'll never have this weekend ever again - I'll do the best for my family and myself and enjoy this weekend."

Every Friday he could see the pebbles getting less and less. Then one day he picked up the last pebble, repeated his affirmation and tossed the pebble in the garden.

For years after the last pebble he continued his Friday ritual, walking up to the empty jar. The realisation that he had to do something with the time he **had left** transformed his life.

The philosophical question we need to ask ourselves is:

"What sort of life do I want and expect to lead, as I grow older with the time I have left?"

What are you going to do with the time you have left? Isn't it time for you to start counting your pebbles?

"Everyone desires long life, not one; old age."

JONATHAN SWIFT

Time can be described in different ways. It can also be defined as a limited period during which an action, process, or condition exists or takes place - your life.

The anti-aging bandwagon

"I don't know how old you are, but you certainly don't look it."
ANONYMOUS

Rather than talk about anti-aging, we should talk about time-left - a much more dynamic approach. "Anti-aging" may make good sense, but what do you want out of it? Life extension? Extending it for what reasons? Life span or health span?

All these concepts have merit, but there are philosophical and ethical issues. The concept of *time-left* and age-retardation are more appropriate concepts in the philosophical wisdom of aging. Anti-aging is often promoted as a commercial concept but is merely part of what Functional Medicine is all about. *It's about the maintenance of health - for as long as possible.*

The bottom line - I've called this Health Program simply **"Time"**, because of its truth-seeking connotations.

Gerontology is the study of aging and old age. Anti-aging is the active treatment of aging as a disease in order to slow it down or even reverse it.

In 1796 life expectancy was 25 years. The primary causes of death were influenza and infection.

Today's life span is 74 years. The primary causes of death are degenerative diseases of **GOFES**, over consumptive malnutrition and aging.

At age 60: 50 per cent of people suffer from major disease.

At age, 80: 75 per cent suffer major disease. The rest have suffered minor diseases, as well as the illness called aging - but they are diseased nonetheless.

Catabiosis: aging

"The best way to tell a woman's age is not to."
ANONYMOUS

Youth is an anabolic (building) process and age is a catabolic (breakdown) process.

Catabiosis is the medical term for aging. In a scientific way it can be seen as a slow form of decomposition and putrefaction. It is a distinct and unyielding progression with a known ending.

I propose to discuss catabiosis under four headings: The negative effects of aging / The consequences of aging / The causes of aging / What can we do about it?

Many of us cope with aging in part through humour. It is normal for us to ignore or choose not to "see" the negative consequences of aging. Most of us don't want to be burdened with the so-called unpleasant aspects of life. In particular, we do not want to be reminded what we may look like as we grow older. That said, from a health viewpoint it is important to examine the affects of aging at least once in our lives.

"Growing older is mandatory. Growing up is optional.
Laughing at yourself is therapeutic."
ANONYMOUS

There are powerful reasons why we should pay more than just a bit of attention to aging. If you want to grow older you have to anticipate what to expect, the good, the bad and the ugly. In this way you can avoid some of the pitfalls of aging and still enjoy a full life. Like an investment account, if you start early and invest regularly you will have more to live on later in life. Growing old is worthwhile if you make the investment. It is like an insurance policy for the future.

We should not complain about growing old - *Many people are denied the privilege.*

1. THE NEGATIVE AFFECTS OF AGING

"Old people have fewer diseases than the young, but their diseases never leave them."
HIPPOCRATES

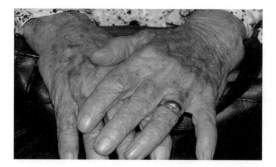

There is no tissue or organ in the body that aging does not affect. The only way to prevent the affects of aging is to die young. The only thing that becomes easier as you grow older is getting tired.

Skin

Time is a good healer, but a poor beautician.

Our skin and its structures like hair and nails never stop growing during our lifetime. The facial cartilage also keeps on growing. Long after we have completed our growth the skin is still marching on. Gradually, the combination of continued skin growth, a reduction in supporting structure and gravity, and our skin starts to hang loose.

The cartilage of the nose and ears continues to grow, and facial features become coarse. A picture speaks a thousand words - compare your 80 year old grandfather with a picture of him in his 20s.

The skin coarsens and thickens in some places and in other places it becomes paper-thin. Combine this with the loss of collagen and elastin and wrinkles appear in places where you don't want them to materialise.

Two old ladies sitting in the garden of an old age home. One of the other residents decides to cause a bit of excitement and streaks naked through the garden. "What was that?" said one of the old ladies. "I don't know," said the other, "but whatever it was it needs ironing."

A lady told her husband; "You don't look anything like the long haired, skinny kid I married 25 years ago. I need a DNA sample to make sure it's still you."

Hair

Your hair is getting thinner. So, who wants fat hair?

With aging, your hair greys, becomes brittle and deforms. Hair falls out in some places, and becomes coarse and more vigorous in others - those pesky nose, ear and eyebrow hairs that twist and turn at odd angles.

By the age of 70 many women need to shave or at least remove coarse facial hair.

A man asked his hairdresser: "What do you have for grey hair?
Came the reply: "Just the greatest of respect, sir."

Nails

The nails form ridges with age, become brittle and disfigure. Their growth slows with time and they infect more easily.

Eyes

The eyes tend to become drier and sink deeper into their sockets as the supporting tissue diminishes. Meanwhile, your arms stretch further and further as you struggle to read the newspaper.

Also with age, our eyes become less transparent and less sensitive to light. A person aged 60 requires twice the light of a 20 year old for maximum visual efficiency. Poor light can contribute to eye fatigue, headaches and nervous tension.

Vision decline is a bio-marker for aging and a very certain one at that.

Teeth and jaws

You may be meticulous with your dental hygiene, but with time your teeth start to yellow and discolour. They also start showing signs of wear. And your jaw structure loses some of its fullness. Gums retract and bad breath is more common.

A young nurse on her first night on duty at an old age home - checking a resident's medication she noticed a bowl of almonds next to his bed. Knowing he had no teeth, she helped herself to an almond. "Who gave you almonds when you don't have any teeth?" she asked. "Well," he said, "they were covered in chocolate before."

Elephants have four sets of teeth. As one set wears out, it is replaced. It is not unusual for an otherwise healthy elephant to have worn out its fourth set of teeth and die of starvation.

Lips

The lips lessen and lose their sensuousness with age. No wonder it's fashionable to have the lips injected with collagen for a more youthful look.

"Inside every old person is a young person who wonders what the hell has happened!"

ANONYMOUS

Hearing

Hearing declines the older you get, and can make life difficult. I have heard the odd person say "I'd rather be blind than deaf". Deafness leads to almost total isolation.

Bernard Shaw was reputed to have said: "I'll never make the mistake of being 70 again."

Brain

"That judges of important causes should hold office for life is not a good thing, for the mind grows old, as well as the body."

ARISTOTLE

I used to be young once. What a memory!

"Where are the keys??" This is usually the first sign that a person's memory and orientation is suffering. In most cases our IQ declines with age, significantly impacting many of us. Parts of the brain atrophy with age, just like other organs. The incidence of confusion, senility and Alzheimer's increase as we get older.

You know you are getting old when your doctor diagnoses you with A.A.D.D. - Age Attention Deficit Disorder.

By age 70 we have learnt everything there is to know, then we spend all our time trying to remember what it was we learnt.

There are only four things you need to know about Alzheimer's disease: you can hide your own Easter eggs, you meet new people every day, you can buy your own surprise presents and... and... you can hide your own Easter eggs.

A local politician was electioneering at an old age home. He walked up to a lady in a rocking chair, shook her hand and asked: "Do you know who I am?" "No," she replied "but you can find out at the front desk."

An elderly patient once complained to me about the pains and aches of old age. Trying to reassure him I said: "At least we get wiser as we get older." His reply: "I'd rather be young and stupid."

Psychology of aging

Depression and isolation are common problems with aging.

The problem with old age is that when you have finally lived to make the most of it - most of it is gone.

A few years ago a couple consulted me together. She was 39 and he was 41. They'd left and I was making some notes in their files when the wife knocked on the door: "Doc, I just want to tell you I'm actually 49, but my husband doesn't have to know it - okay?"

A personnel manager asked a new applicant for her birthday.
"September 30th," she said.
"Which year?" he asked.
"Every year" she replied.

Breasts

The breasts become less full and start sagging, while the risk of breast cancer increases dramatically with age.

Pamela Anderson once said, or it could have been Dolly Parton: "What the Lord has giveth, gravity has taketh away"

What does a 75 year old woman have between her breasts that a 25 year old does not? A belly button.

Gut

Just as there are visible signs of aging, so there are the invisible. The gut also ages, gets thinner, becomes more fragile and becomes less efficient in handling absorption and excretion processes. This is one of the reasons why older people are more bloated and "gassy".

An octogenarian once remarked once to me: "Nobody listens *until* you fart."

Taste and smell also diminish with age and many older people suffer malnutrition because they simply do not feel like eating.

Glucose metabolism

The body's ability to process glucose declines progressively with age, forming Advanced Glycation End products - known by the acronym AGE.

Bones

Bones and joints, like other organs, deteriorate with advancing age. Osteoarthritis and osteoporosis are rife. Even a large proportion of older men suffer from bone thinning and osteoporosis.

Muscles

Muscle mass can decrease by as much as 40 per cent and strength fades. The quality of the muscles also deteriorate so that, even if the muscle mass does not decline, it functions less effectively.

At a BBQ children play and run around with boundless energy. Adults stand around with their drinks. Old people sit in chairs.

You may say: "But I know old people with lots of energy." Unfortunately, these people are in the minority. The elderly can never compete with a younger, healthy person.

A number of our organs deteriorate and shrink by up to 30 per cent and the gaps soon fill with fat. Fat seems to be the only thing that thrives with advancing age.

Loss of balance unsteadiness and dizziness are also common among the older generation.

Immunity and endocrine system

The decline of the immunity and endocrine system with age also increases the risk of cancer and disease among the elderly. If we live long enough we will all get some form of cancer. There is no youthful output of hormones anymore.

Catabiosis can be seen as a *deficiency disease* - a youth deficiency.

Menopause

Q: "Do you wake up bitchy in the morning?"
A: "No, I let her sleep."

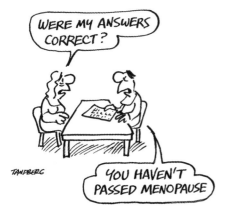

It is normal to suffer from menopause. Many people and doctors alike try to trivialise menopause, describing it as natural, with nothing to worry about. Death is also natural and so is snake poison. Menopause is part of the aging process and can have unpleasant consequences. It does not only signal the end of the reproductive period, but is accompanied by a proliferation of unpleasant symptoms and signs. Occasionally I see 25 year olds with menopause. If this is not a disease I do not know what is.

"Going into menopause at the normal expected age should not be seen as a disease," you may argue. I would say it is not synonymous with good health. Without sounding crude, anything that rots your bones, suck the collagen out of your skin, dries up the vagina, sags your boobs, doubles your chances of heart attack, triples your chances of contracting Alzheimer's and fattens you up in places you didn't even know you had, cannot be healthy.

This touches on an important point. Menopause is a disease and so is the whole aging process, of which menopause is a symptom. Aging should be treated as a disease, even if it is a normal progression of advancing age. I cannot see how anyone can argue that aging is healthy.

In my opinion, menopause starts at about 35 and has three distinct phases. The first, when fertility and hormones start declining, while body fat and weight increases. Women can still fall pregnant during this phase, but often their progesterone levels have dropped and maintaining the pregnancy may require these levels to be supplemented.

If you tick off six or more of the following Yes, you probably suffer from menopause

	YES	NO
Itchy		
Scratchy		
Bitchy		
Sweaty		
Gassy		
Bloated		
Forgetful		
Sleeplessness		
All dried up		

The second phase sees a sudden, almost overnight plummeting of oestrogen levels. This sudden event can be quite unpleasant for some women. Most describe this phase as menopause. I describe it as the *second phase* of menopause. It is certainly not as subtle as the first phase.

In the third phase hormone levels become so low that women are often described as post-menopausal as they get used to these low levels.

If aging is to be treated as a "normal disease" these three distinctions in menopause are important.

Many patients say "I've gone through menopause". Fact: you never get rid of menopause - it is for life. There is no way that you will ever produce the deficient hormones naturally again. If you want them at youthful levels, you will have to top them up from external sources.

Men are also afflicted by menopause. Perhaps in men it should be called "womenopause" - *think about that one for a while!* It is more usually known in men as viropause or andropause. This also has three phases, but these phases present quite differently. It is associated with lower testosterone levels. The second phase can be even more devastating in men than women.

Unlike women, men do not usually talk about their health problems and as a result this was never really seen as a problem in men until women started talking on their behalf.

Sexual activity

Libido dwindles and can drop away completely with age. Men quite often find they are good neither in the boardroom nor the bedroom.

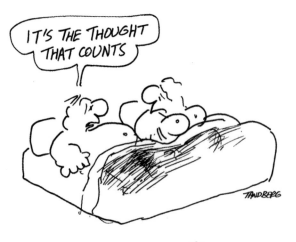

Old age: our strongest survival instinct, **POD**, operates at a higher level, while our second strongest survival instinct, reproduction, wanes. It would almost be better the other way around.

An elderly couple was sitting downstairs watching TV when she suddenly felt amorous and suggested: "Darling, let's go upstairs and make love." He thought for a while and responded: "Well you better make up your mind, because I can't do both."

You know you are old when:
- Work is less pleasure and pleasure is more work.
- It takes all night to do what you used to do all night.
- At a restaurant you look at the menu instead of the waitress.
- You remember when the air was clean and sex was dirty.
- Don't worry about avoiding temptation, as you grow older, it starts avoiding you.
- Old is when: "getting lucky" means to find your car in the car park.
- All girls look alike.
- You think less of passion and more of your pension.
- You proposition a girl and you hope she says "No".
- A long distance telephone call tires you out.
- You have an off day after your day off.
- It takes you longer to rest than to get tired.
- You feel like the day after the night before, and you haven't been anywhere.

Fun is like life insurance - it costs more as you age.

"As my years keep on advancing, this fact comes to the fore: my opinions carry lesser weight, while my body carries more."
LEONARDO DA VINCI

Reflexes

Our reflexes age and slow down too. As a result, old animals in the jungle cannot escape predators. Predators get old too, and lose the reflexes to hunt. They in turn are eaten or die from starvation. This is the reason why there is no old age in the wild.

We are all born with primitive reflexes. In babies these include the startling reflex, the suckling reflex and the groping reflex. If you tickle the side of a baby's mouth it will start to suckle your finger and if the palm of a baby's hand is tickled, it will grope your hand and hang on tightly. As we age, these primitive reflexes reappear. When an old person is asleep in his rocking chair, tickle the side of his mouth and he will start sucking on your finger. Or you tickle the palm of his hand, at which he starts groping your finger.

In Greek mythology there was once a prince who asked Zeus for his blessing. Zeus said the prince could wish for what ever he wanted. He asked to live forever. His wish was granted. He became older, his skin wrinkled and he contracted all the diseases of old age. Eventually, his flesh started rotting off his body, but he did not die. He'd asked Zeus to live forever - he should have asked to stay young forever.

"We come onto this earth meek and weak and we go the same way. What we do in between is up to us."
ANONYMOUS

They say "life begins at 40", but so do heart disease, cancer and the habit of telling the same story three times over to the same people.

"Aging is not beautiful - it is an unpleasant, painful and unattractive affliction."
ANONYMOUS

What a difference 30 years makes
1975:   Long hair
2005:   Longing for hair

1975:   Acid rock
2005:   Acid reflux

1975:   Moving to Perth because it's cool
2005:   Moving to Perth because it's warm

1975:   Trying to look like Liz Taylor
2005:   Trying NOT to look like Liz Taylor

1975: Seeds and stems
2005: Roughage

1975: Going to a new, hip joint
2005: Receiving a new hip joint

1975: Rolling Stones
2005: Kidney stones

1975: Passing the drivers' test
2005: Passing the vision test

By now you must be feeling like slitting your wrists. I do not blame you, but there is hope, however growing old is definitely not for the faint hearted.

Bette Davis put it bluntly: "Growing old is not for sissies."

"The only thing worse than old age is not achieving it."
DAVE WEINBAUM

2. THE CONSEQUENCES OF GROWING OLD

"I want to live forever, or die trying."
ANONYMOUS

"There are many virtues to growing old... I'm just trying to think what they are."
SOMERSET MAUGHAM - AT AGE 80

Where does old age lead?

"The goal is the same - life itself;
and the price is the same - life itself."
JAMES AGEE

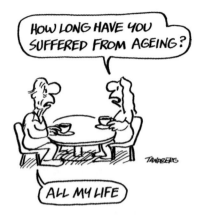

Aging is a terminal disease with a known outcome. It should be viewed and treated as such. It is natural and part of our journey through life. We have been given the means to alleviate the pain and modify its course for a better quality of life. Nobody really dies from "old age". There is always a specific ailment or a combination of illnesses that bring us to the end of our days.

The traffic is all one-way; from the cradle to the grave.

"Growing old isn't so bad if you consider the alternative."
MAURICE CHEVALIER

3. THE CAUSES AND MECHANISMS OF AGING

There are many theories around why and how we age. Nobody has yet put the complete puzzle together. I am of the opinion that **GOFES** is a major player in catabiosis and should be the first priority in treating aging as a disease process.

As chronological age progresses there is a decline in physiological functions.

When declining organ function reaches a critical level it is incompatible with life and results in death. With age, our organs and metabolic processes decline in function - that is one of the reasons we like to use the concept of Functional Age rather than Biological Age.

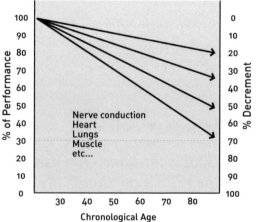

Adapted and modified from Dr Ward Dean MD - Biological Age Measurement - with permission.

366

Decreasing Functional Capacity

- and the minimal level required for sustaining life.

When declining organ functions and reserve reach a certain critical level it is incompatible with life and results in death. With age, our organs and metabolic processes decline in function and that is one of the reasons we like to use the concept of Functional Age rather than Biological Age.

The Death Threshold (DT) can increase from time to time due to, for example, disease, stress and lifestyle. When a person is young there is still a big difference between the DT and their Functional Capacity (FC). In the case of an older person the FC and DT are much closer. An increase in the DT, due to say pneumonia, can impact the Functional Capacity, resulting in death.

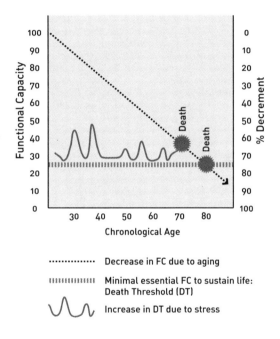

Chronological Age

·············· Decrease in FC due to aging

||||||||||||||| Minimal essential FC to sustain life: Death Threshold (DT)

∿∿ Increase in DT due to stress

This is one of the reasons why pneumonia is deadlier in older people than in the young whose lungs typically enjoy a higher Functional Capacity. Consequently, if the FC decline is slowed down, life expectancy could be longer and healthier. If on the other hand the FC decline is accelerated, so is the aging process and disease.

In combination, the first three of the Health Programs namely Nutrition, Supplementation and Exercise programs are enough to keep the body in good shape *until* age 35 or thereabouts. This also marks the start of the first phase of menopause. Advancing age sees further changes take place in the body. From then on the metabolism is unable to produce enough of these chemical messengers for optimum function and we are in decline.

Conversely, if we top up these chemical messengers - resupply them - we can slow the aging process. As a result, aging is sometimes described as a deficiency disease.

In the wild

As a wild animal's Functional Capacity decreases, the hunter becomes the hunted. Putting a wild animal into captivity doubles its life expectancy, shielding it from its predators while ensuring an ample food supply.

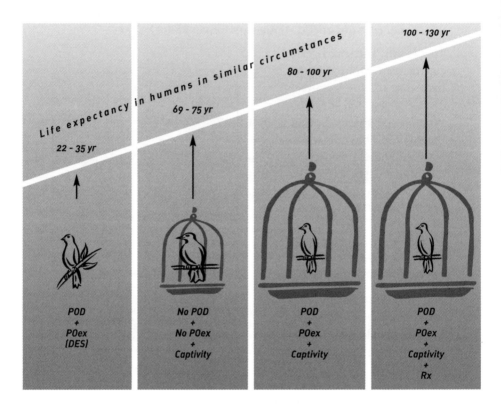

The canary on the left is still in the wild. **DES** operates such that **POD** is intense, the effort to find food is also intense and the supply is limited and erratic. There is no old age among the canaries in the wild. Extrapolating this to early man when humans were in the wild, we lived to be between 22 and 35 years depending on the community.

The second canary is in captivity and **DES** operates differently. **POD** is just as intense, but the food supply is virtually unlimited and the effort to find it zero. However the canary has fallen victim to **GOFES**. In addition, with no predators, the canary's life expectancy has doubled. In human terms we have also doubled our life expectancy but have become over fat thanks to our Polar Bear genes and changes to **DES**.

The third canary has a therapeutically controlled food supply and has been placed in a larger cage to ensure more physical activity. It is now destined to live longer and healthier than canary two. Extrapolating this to humans, improved metabolism, no GOFES, no insulin resistance and a life expectancy potential of 80 to 100 years plus. The best of both worlds seems to be the only possible outcome, but...

A paradigm shift

The final canary has the best of both worlds with *very* specific treatments administered for aging. This results in a paradigm shift. In the case of humans life expectancy could theoretically be increased to 130 or more years.

A word of warning: anti-aging treatments will never be of much use if you do not control **DES** - you must deal with **POD** and **POEx**. You must be metabolically fit if you want your body to perform to above ordinary expectation. You cannot suffer from **GOFES**.

Formula

DES Controlled + Captivity + Specific Treatments = Age Retardation and Health maintenance.

Cell duplication

If you make a photocopy on an old copier you will notice the first copy is good. If you make a copy from this copy, the quality diminishes. Repeat and you'll soon reach a point where the copies are illegible.

It's the same with cells. For example, constantly damaging the cells through exposure to UV rays eventually damages the DNA genetic material. The next copy of the damaged cell is made from an already defective "copy", in this scenario leading to accelerated skin aging.

UV damaged skin seems to recover, and it can be many years before the true damage is revealed.

Glycosylation

When bread is baked the crust forms when the sugars and the protein bind - they caramelise. This process also takes place in the body forming Advanced Glycation End products (AGE). Under certain conditions it becomes *RAGE* - *Reactive Advanced Glycation End products.*

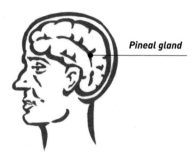

Pineal gland

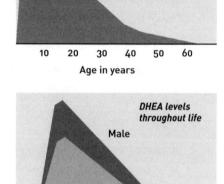

Melatonin decline

Onset of age-related diseases coincides with the decline in melatonin production

10 20 30 40 50 60

Age in years

Hormones - neuro-endocrine theory of aging

In the brain there is a gland, known as the pineal gland. Its function was unknown for a long time. It produces a hormone called Melatonin that is excreted mainly in hours of darkness, during sleep.

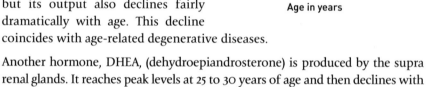

DHEA levels throughout life

Male

Female

10 20 30 40 50 60

Age in years

It not only has a rhythm of excretion, but its output also declines fairly dramatically with age. This decline coincides with age-related degenerative diseases.

Another hormone, DHEA, (dehydroepiandrosterone) is produced by the supra renal glands. It reaches peak levels at 25 to 30 years of age and then declines with age. DHEA and Melatonin serve as two of the many biomarkers for aging.

Excess body fat has undesirable consequences on DHEA levels. It *drops* as body fat increases, while middle age spread shuts down DHEA production.

Oxidation

Progeria is a disease characterised by accelerated catabiosis. We are in essence similar to a 12-year-old with this disease, except we live six times longer. Progeria is a pathological cause of accelerated aging. With sufferers of progeria, their bodies oxidise faster due to increased free radical formation and a defective anti-oxidant defence system.

Inflammation

Inflammatory processes and diseases in the body also play a role in catabiosis. Some researchers believe that inflammation is a significant part of aging. A large number of diseases that we associate with aging are inflammatory in nature.

Excessive inflammation in the body is due to high levels of sugar intake - about 75 to 80kg (165 to 175lb) per person in the USA. The resultant high insulin levels and insulin resistance, when coupled with a deficiency of essential fatty acids, *and* **GOFES** *as well*, is enough to signal to the body "age fast... fast".

Telomeres

Telomeres are the genetic material at the end of chromosomes that become progressively eroded with age and oxidative stress. A report published in the American Heart Association journal *Circulation* demonstrated that weight gain and increased insulin resistance result in greater telomere shortening over time. Telomere length has been proposed as a marker to assess biological aging, as opposed to chronological aging.

Each of us has our own genetically programmed lifespan. This lifespan can be prolonged or reduced, but our social environment and way of life play a major part.

> **Good Genetics + Favourable Environment = Age Retardation**

4. WHAT CAN WE DO ABOUT AGING?

I don't want to be young again, No; I just don't want to get old.

No skill or art is needed to grow old: The trick is to endure it.

Life is to be enjoyed. We will never get out of it alive.
ANONYMOUS

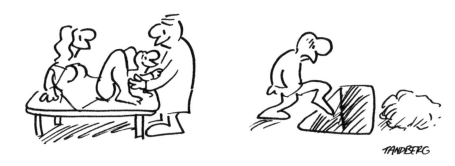

TANDBERG

The goals in achieving age retardation

- To die as young as possible, as late as possible.

  "Longevity is only desirable if it *increases the duration of youth*, and not that of old age. The lengthening of the senescence period would be a calamity."
  ALEXIS CARREL

- **CA > BA** - which means your chronological age is greater than your functional age. In other words, you are younger than average.

- Health-span rather than life-span would be a sounder philosophical approach to aim for. With proper care the human body will last a lifetime.

- Maintaining a youthful body composition and function. In our society it is acceptable that our blood pressure, cholesterol and fat percentage increase with age, while our lean body mass decreases. In communities where people live longer and healthier, these parameters tend to stay at youthful levels.

- To maintain the highest quality of life and then make a "clean, quick exit" - like an alkaline battery that delivers high output and then suddenly dies. Not like the old style batteries that start dying the moment you switch them on. Some people slowly die from the age of 40, just like these old style batteries.

A friend told me that his grandfather was still doing head stands with the grand children at the age of 88. On his 96th birthday the family came from far and wide for the occasion. Then at the end of the meal he said something a bit out of character: "I have had a good life and helped you all to get on in life. I think I am now ready for better things."

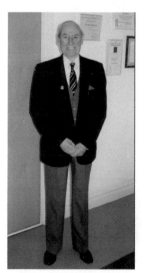

They looked at him somewhat perplexed. A week later they received the call that he had died in his sleep. He lived a full life and when his time came it was quick and clean.

Bill

Bill is an example of successful aging. Good posture and always neatly dressed. I have noticed that the majority of successful and healthy old agers tend to dress and groom themselves neatly. In this photo Bill was 95 years old. Neglect of personal appearance is often indicative of dementia, depression or another painful illness of old age.

Bill often walked the six kilometres to come and see me. He really enjoyed it when the reception staff commented on how good he looked for his age. Bill went through both world wars and he felt if he could survive that, he could survive a bit longer.

Should we do something about aging in the first place? Isn't death the natural conclusion to life?

Maybe, but snake poison is also natural and so is disease. It is not natural to drive a car, take antibiotics or eat chocolate bars. As humans we have been given the ability to manipulate our lives for better or for worse. Choose your poison.

Over the years there have been reports of exceptional life spans of people in remote, mostly vegetarian societies - none of these has proven factual.

The oldest properly documented lifespan was that of Jeanne Calment. She lived on a typical Mediterranean diet, did little exercise, and made no attempt to extend her life. She died in her home in France in 1997 aged 122.

In France they have a custom where you can buy an old person's home at a reasonable price, but the old person can stay for life, rent free in the home and have some cash to survive.

The gamble is that if the person dies soon, you make some money, but if they live a long life you could wait a long time for a return on your investment. Jeanne Calment's lawyer must have thought she was getting old at age 90 when he bought her house in such an arrangement. However, the lawyer died before she did.

We need to do something about aging

- We are getting older than ever before, but our aging is not necessarily healthy. The *increasing* incidence of the "Terrible D's" - declining, diseased, disabled, demented, deteriorating and dependent - makes huge demands on the *ever-decreasing* younger and productive portion of the population.

- It would be more desirable to have healthy, older people who are able to retire a few years later.

- Our present situation will be unsustainable in the future. We need to age more successfully such that our health bill decreases.

- Old age without intervention is not beautiful.

Grey power

There is a concern that age retardation will lead to selfishness, a pool of old people, and general community decline. The unacceptable alternative is, of course, to recycle humans faster by dying younger.

Life Extension

*"Age that lessens the enjoyment of life increases
our desire for living."*
OLIVER GOLDSMITH

The following summarises our attitude towards growing old gracefully and healthily.

*"The reality is that giving up wine, women and song may
not help you live longer. It'll just seem longer!"*
ANONYMOUS

The POD, POEx and CZ motto:
You can live <u>much</u> longer, if you give up everything that
makes you want to live longer.

Doctor to patient: "I want you to give up *wine* and *women*,
but you can still sing."

Most animals live just long enough to reproduce. Once this has been achieved, there is no need for them anymore. The human situation is more complicated, but a little of nature remains in some of us who appear to have a death wish. It's almost as if they have achieved their genetic goal of reproduction, and so what else is left? They neglect their health and their bodies and are soon on the path to rapid catabiosis.

In the interest of survival, we are genetically programmed to shun whatever seems to be good for us (give in to POD and POEx).

*"If you want to be lean and healthy, whatever you want to
eat and do you should not and whatever you do not want to
eat and do you should."*
MARK TWAIN

An attitude change is mandatory if you want to retard catabiosis. You cannot buy it, even if you are a billionaire. You have to earn it directly - you need to make the sacrifice to obtain the benefits.

"Those who enjoy the large pleasures of advanced age are those who have sacrificed the small pleasures of youth."
EARNEST ELMO CALKINS

Extending your lifespan

Research by longevity researchers Kenneth Manton and Eric Stallard of Duke University in the United States indicates that application of current anti-aging science could extend lifespan to 130 for men and 136 for women.
JOURNAL OF GERONTOLOGY 1996

STEP ONE

The key to the treatment of aging is the treatment of GOFES - to lose excess-fat. Without a healthy fat percentage your efforts to delay aging will be largely pointless.

1. Nutrition

"The secret of staying young is to live honestly, eat slowly, and lie about your age."
LUCILLE BALL

Eat less - Caloric Restriction with Adequate Nutrition - CRAN - *under nutrition, not malnutrition.*

This strategy is perhaps the single most important aspect of slowing the aging process. There are CRAN clubs in the US and the adherents are lean with very favourable metabolic parameters. They may be hungry and suffering the demands of **POD** - but this is good for them. For over 70 years we've known that if you take two groups of laboratory animals, allow one group to eat freely and cut the diet of the other group by half, the diet-controlled group will live twice as long. However, it is not just about eating less, the consumed food must be high in complete nutrients to produce the desired results.

Studies of the elderly have confirmed this discovery - *the higher the calorie value of their food, the greater the pathological changes in their cardiovascular systems.* The opposite is also true.

I once had a dog that became very sluggish so I took her to the vet. After a thorough examination he informed me that there was nothing wrong, except I was over-feeding her. He gave me a plastic cup and said I should only feed her once a day to a level he marked on the cup. No more and no less.

I protested, but his reply was straight to the point: "You're not doing her a favour by over-feeding her. Do what I tell you and she will be more attentive and lively... in fact, she will live longer too."

I did as I was told. Within days she was full of energy. She lived two years longer than was expected of the breed. The same applies to humans. One of the main causes of tiredness and sluggishness in our society is over eating. **POD** is there to help us survive, but in certain **DES** circumstances it kills us sooner than is necessary.

One of the best treatments to make many people feel better is to get them to eat less. My dog had no choice - as humans we have a choice: control **POD** and we control **GOFES** and aging.

Since our bodies use glucose less efficiently as we age, older people often find that a diet high in protein and good fats, and lower in carbohydrates, helps stabilise energy levels. It also tends to reduce body fat and cholesterol levels.

Over eating messes with your hormones and accelerates aging.

2. Supplementation

As discussed in depth in Chapter 20, multiple antioxidants supplemented in a scientific way are essential, like vitamins, minerals, and phytonutrients. Oxidation accelerates, as we grow older.

3. Mental and physical exercise

Rule: too much exercise speeds up aging - as does too little exercise. As discussed in Chapter 21, it's about getting the balance right.

Exercise is one of the best and cheapest ways to hide your age. It enhances growth hormone production, improves glucose tolerance and restores hypothalamic sensitivity. If you want to prematurely age, give in to **POEx** and don't worry about exercise.

4. The 10 health principles

Following **all** the 10 health principles, which form the basis of many treatments – but they form a chain that is only as strong as the weakest link.

Step One needs to have been firmly in place for at least three and preferably six months before you move on to Step Two.

STEP TWO

Focusing on Step One will serve you well until age 40 - thereafter you need to consider a range of other measures.

A.   Stimulation, replacements and enhancements

"You never really get old - what happens is you suffer from a youth deficiency".
ANONYMOUS

Catabiosis is sometimes seen as a deficiency disease and in part it is. If your car has an oil deficiency, what would you do?

1. Hormonal secretion

a. Secretagogue stimulation:

Secretion can be stimulated to youthful levels, provided the functionality still exists and that there is no undue aging of the pituitary and hormonal axis. Nutrition and exercise can help to stimulate the secretion of human growth hormone, while Niacin (vitamin B3), Arginine, Ornithine, Lysine and Glutamine serve as secretagogues in promoting human growth hormone production and secretion.

b. Caloric restriction:

Caloric restriction with adequate nutrition - CRAN - also stimulates growth hormone production.

c. Stimulation by exercise:

Exercise, especially resistance training of the thighs and chest, can restore flagging testosterone levels and is one of the best age-retarding activities.

d. Other means of stimulation:

The anti-hypertensive drug clonidine or Catapres has growth hormone stimulation properties that can be useful in some cases.

2. Direct hormonal replacement (HRT):

The time will come when your pituitary and endocrine system is not as responsive to stimulation as it was when you were younger. This calls for alternate strategies.

If your car's engine and brake fluid levels are low, what do you do?
Top up one or both?
How much do you top them up - to just right the right level? Perhaps a bit extra... or a little less?
Will you continue to check the levels from time to time?

The answers to these questions may seem straightforward, but when it comes to replacing hormones, the answers are not so clear-cut.

If you are considering replacement, you also need to consider the following checklist:

1. Is it necessary?
2. Do you want hormone replacement?
3. Do you need complete replacement?
4. How do you feel about hormones derived from horse urine or from a synthesised chemical process rather than a natural process?
5. Are the levels to be replaced to youthful levels or pharmacological levels? Or perhaps under-replaced?
6. Will the replacement mimic the natural hormonal rhythms?
7. Are the levels going to be periodically monitored and adjusted, as they should be?
8. Is your overall health going to be monitored as part of the process?
9. Will your aging processes be monitored to ensure HRT is beneficial and not detrimental?
10. Will you be following all the 10 health principles, especially Nutrition, Supplementation, Exercise and Hygiene programs?

Once you have addressed each of these points you'll be ready for HRT.

HRT - the meaning:

HRT is normally understood to be the replacement of oestrogen and progesterone. This is not correct. It is a blanket term and refers to any hormone replacement. Men may be on testosterone replacement while both men and women could be receiving thyroid hormone for an under active thyroid. Each of these is HRT.

Most hormones decline at varying rates and differing times in your lifecycle, disrupting the body's biorhythms and the unique synchronisation that normally exists between hormones. *These should be mimicked as closely as possible with replacement therapies.*

In the following schematic presentation for example, a 55-year-old female can achieve balance simply by topping up on oestrogen, DHEA, melatonin and other hormones to the average level of a 25 to 30 year old.

Worth noting

It is not the purpose of this book to give a detailed account of the various hormones and if you are considering HRT you should consult a medical professional who is experienced in this field. In my next book I intend to expand on this topic, particularly as it applies to our experience with weight loss programs.

There are however, some points that I will touch on. There are three main oestrogens. Doctors normally prescribe estradiol. Another is the conjugated estrogens, namely Premarin - which is an abbreviation for *pregnant mares urine*. Only prescribing one of these oestrogens is akin to topping up your car's engine oil while leaving the brake fluid low.

Progesterone is rarely prescribed to a woman who has had a hysterectomy. It makes no sense to me why progesterone and oestrogen aren't given together. Oestrogen on its own runs wild when its controlling partner is not present. Menopause is a deficiency of oestrogen and progesterone, while at the same time other hormones are declining with age. In part, aging is a hormonal deficiency disease.

DHEA is often given at doses that are too high. Hormones work together in a unique balance. DHEA can be useful for burning excess fat and I prescribe it at mild "pharmacological" levels, for a period of time, to assist in this purpose.

Primarily, the aim of any HRT should be physiological replacement. For example, testosterone deficiency in both men and women can have disastrous effects - when you are good neither in the boardroom nor the bedroom, life may take a turn for the worse in many ways. Proper replacement therapy can be very useful but should always be done in consultation with your doctor because every case is different.

Melatonin is the executive hormone in the body - like the conductor of an orchestra. HRT for women should always contain melatonin since there are melatonin receptors in the breasts and they need to be taken care of. It is very important to understand that HRT in the mildest of forms can be dangerous if the other balancing hormones are left at low levels. It needs to be the whole team or no team at all! Not only should you strive for the hormone levels of your youth, but also the *hormone ratios* of your youth.

All the following change	Change	In the following diseases
Cortisol	Increase	Aging
DHEA	Decrease	Ateriosclerosis
HGH	Decrease	Cancer
Immune function	Decrease	Depression
Insulin	Increase	Diabetes
Lipids	Increase	GOFES
Melatonin	Decrease	Hypertension
Thrombogennesis	Increase	Menopause
Thryriod	Decrease	Stress

A properly implemented HRT regime in conjunction with all the other health principles can slow down the organ functional reserve or capacity (FC) decline. By putting the brakes on FC decline we can effectively extend the death threshold or DT, therefore the prolonging life.

In the following, death occurs when the functional capacity reaches the death threshold.

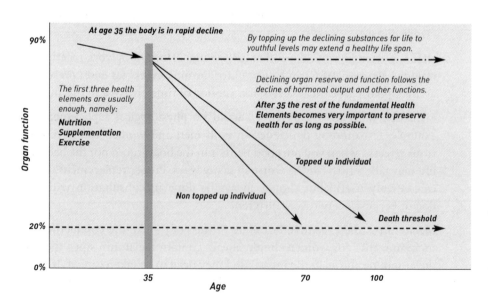

Nature has very little need for a woman's body after menopause. Bone density, cardiovascular function, muscle strength, mobility, flexibility, kidney and liver function decline dramatically, as do memory, intelligence and emotional tone - not to mention sexual function. Without proper HRT, life can be miserable for women under these circumstances.

3. *Enhancing insulin sensitivity:*
Exercise - one of the outstanding effects of exercise is the regulating of insulin.

a. *Chromium* - this aids the insulin and sugar metabolism. Correction of deficiencies often improves blood sugar metabolism.
Glycaemic index and load - as we discussed in chapter 19, consistently eating foods with a low glycaemic load dramatically improves insulin metabolism.

b. *Alpha-lipoic acid* - this anti-oxidant is also very useful in sugar and insulin metabolism and should be part of your supplementation program.

c. *Caloric restriction* - overeating raises cortisol levels and also promotes insulin resistance. Caloric restriction does the opposite.

d. *Medication* - when metformin, an anti-diabetic medication, is administered to mice, they live on average 25 per cent longer and suffer less cancer. Metformin effectively lowers Advanced Glycation End (AGE) products. Metformin in non-diabetic humans also lowers glycation and may extend human life as well. Drugs that lower cortisol levels and insulin have similar effects. Metformin has a long safety record and if you do not have kidney failure, a dose of up to 500mg twice to four times per day could be considered. However, you must first ask your doctor if it is suitable for you.

One of the world's leading anti-aging physicians, Dr Ward Dean, recommends metformin be taken from the age of 35. It also stabilises cholesterol and is used for cancer inhibition. Ward Dean describes it as one of the best weight loss and anti-aging drugs today.

A 55-year-old patient of mine with a family history of heart disease and diabetes was taking metformin as a precautionary measure, even though she wasn't suffering either of the family illnesses. When she mentioned this to her doctor he nearly exploded. She tried to explain to him that she was treating the disease of aging by, among other things, reducing her glycated haemoglobin levels.

This did not convince her doctor and I am not surprised. Orthodox medical practice plays an extremely important role but, as we have discussed throughout this book, it often has an uncomfortable relationship with functional medicine. Treating aging as a disease is not widely accepted as part of orthodox medicine.

Patients on metformin often report that they have increased energy, reduced carbohydrate cravings, a normal lipid (cholesterol) profile and an enhanced sense of well-being.

Dilantin, used in epilepsy, can also be useful in enhancing insulin sensitivity. In doses of 200 to 300mg it is quite safe under medical supervision.

4. *Balancing of neurotransmitters:*

Serotonin and catecholamines decline as we grow older. Hypericum perforatum, better known as St John's Wort, can help by raising serotonin levels. In some cases anti-depressants may be necessary.

B.   Other useful supplements:

For some people, there are a number of medications that may be useful in health maintenance and age retardation.

1. Gamma linoleic acid - as we get older the metabolism suffers from wear and tear. The body's process of converting linolenic acid into gamma linolenic acid, or GLA, becomes less efficient. Therefore, in spite of adequate essential fatty acids in the diet, GLA levels may be low. Evening Primrose or Borage oil will soon address this.

2. Aspirin - you might want to review the section on phytonutrients at this time. For most people, unless your doctor advises otherwise, it is worthwhile taking a "baby aspirin" once a day. Unfortunately, we are often not advised to take aspirin correctly - it should be taken with the evening meal and on a regular basis. Sporadic treatment does nothing for you.

The next problem is the dose. Most patients are told to break a 300mg soluble tablet in half and take half one day and half the next. Wrong. Touching it to break it in half leaves residues that, when exposed to air, will contaminate the remainder. The dose is also far too high. All you need is a baby dosage of 50 to 80mg a day.

Taking aspirin after the age of 50 has become an unquestionable rule. Why wait? Start at 30 if you like. Some of the benefits, like a reduction in colon and breast cancer, require years of taking aspirin before the benefit becomes meaningful.

3. Combinations: It is sometimes advocated that small does of an ACEI - blood pressure drug - and statins, a cholesterol drug, will prevent heart attack and stroke, even if you do not suffer from high blood pressure and raised cholesterol. There may be a place for these as a preventative measure if you have a very strong family history of these problems. I do not normally use them for these purposes because I concentrate on the primary disease of GOFES and *only then* on the secondary risk factors.

XX (Female) versus XY(Male)

A very dynamic patient of mine was the managing director of a large business enterprise. She was the one with the ideas and no one dared challenge her. As she put it: "XX can rule over XY."

One Monday morning, during a very important board meeting, the unthinkable happened. She lost her cool, became flustered and could not conduct procedures properly. Nobody took much notice of it. The next week a similar situation arose. It was then that challengers came out of the woodwork as it were. They saw their opportunity.

She consulted me for her usual health check and mentioned these episodes. I queried if this was the start of menopause in that she had an early hysterectomy.

"Doctor... I'm only 42. I had a heavy weekend and my concentration wasn't as good as usual. It is the glass ceiling and all those men want my position because I'm a woman."

I pointed out to her that she never had the problem before. Why now? She dismissed my theory completely, but I did convince her to have her hormones checked. When she saw me the next week for the results, it was quite clear she was in the second stage of menopause. Additionally, her cortisol and cholesterol levels were a little high. While her glycoselated haemoglobin was reported as normal at 5.9, in functional medicine the level should be less than five for good health.

She was reasonably fit, had a generally good diet and was on a supplement program. Her fat percentage was slightly higher than normal for her. Her bone density, however, showed early signs of osteoporosis.

I immediately prescribed sublingual DHEA, the three oestrogens and progesterone, together with aspirin and melatonin.

Over the following weeks we used blood tests to adjust the dosage rates and I added a small dose of testosterone and started her on metformin. Within a matter of weeks, apart from feeling better, she noticed that her libido had improved. However, her most significant triumph was in the boardroom where she silenced potential competitors.

Another patient of mine, a politician, could not be effective in parliament and considered giving up her beloved politics. Weeks after starting a health and HRT regime she was as effective as ever. She continued losing excess fat and was coping better than she had in years.

Oestrogen protects the brain. As oestrogen levels begin to decline during the second phase of menopause, the IQ level drops a few points each year. This is not so dramatic in men because testosterone declines more gradually. In men, testosterone is converted into oestrogen in the brain by an enzyme called aromatase. Partially for this reason, Alzheimer's disease is more common in women. As both sexes age, men start catching up as their testosterone levels decline further.

Oestrogen is a very powerful hormone and stimulates the growth of youthful tissue. I do not believe that oestrogen causes breast cancer; otherwise every 30-year-old woman with high oestrogen levels would have breast cancer. However, once breast cancer exists, oestrogen can stimulate the growth of cancer cells. Some speculate that this may be a good thing, in that it facilitates early detection and treatment. More information will be discussed in the follow up book.

Genetics and lifestyle play a significant role in breast cancer, but given that some of the *metabolites* in some oestrogens may promote breast cancer, a useful supplement to control this is Indole-3-carbinaol derived from broccoli and other vegetables in the mustard family such as cabbage and radish.

Premature aging followed by slower aging

Michael was 52 when he first consulted me. He weighed 110kg and his fat percentage was 39 per cent. He had the usual gut with a large hip-waist ratio. His blood pressure was out of control in spite of medication. He was also on medication for joint pains and gout.

Added to this, he was a Type 2 diabetic with a fasting blood sugar of 12.5. His cholesterol was 7.5, but his good cholesterol (HDL) was quite low. As a result, his risk of heart attack had risen exponentially. His liver function tests were abnormal and he was seeing a liver specialist who apparently had not considered the possibility of fatty liver. Since fatty liver is quite common in the treatment of **GOFES**, a scan soon revealed that this was the cause of his liver problem.

He was a snorer to such a degree that his wife said he sounded "like a lawnmower". He also suffered erectile dysfunction - no wonder!

As is the case with most GOFES patients, he was unfit, suffered high stress levels from owning and operating two businesses, and was suffering from depression and low self esteem. He had cut down on smoking, but was drinking alcohol moderately on most days and often to excess on weekends.

It was not a surprise that his once happy marriage was in trouble. A functional age test regime concluded that he was functioning at the level of a 72 year old.

In short, he was suffering *accelerated aging* and was an impending disaster.

His medical team did not address his primary problem, **GOFES**. Only the secondary diseases caused by his primary **GOFES** problem were being treated. He could only remember being told on one occasion that he should lose a bit of weight.

Orthodox medicine had been applied, whereas **GOFES** requires the full spectrum of medicine to be treated successfully.

I advised him to **diet or die**. His weight came down to 79kg and his fat to 14 per cent. His joint pains disappeared and his blood sugars returned to normal without medication, as did his blood pressure. He became moderately fit and stopped smoking altogether. He confined his drinking to moderate levels at weekends. He stopped taking anti-depressants and sold one of his businesses to lower his stress levels.

What was particularly important to him was that he could "do it now on average two to three times a week" - without Viagra!

Eighteen months after he first consulted me, his functional age was reduced to 46 years and today he functions at about 10 years less than his chronological age.

Conclusion - Michael is at optimum functional health and is retarding the aging process. He takes nutritional supplements and HRT comprising DHEA and a small amount of testosterone and melatonin. He also takes alpha lipoic acid, acetyl-L carnitine and some natural products for his prostate. In addition he takes 2,000mg of metformin a day, even though he is no longer a diabetic. Otherwise, he adheres to the 10 principles of good health and consults me twice a year for follow up.

Michael likes to tell me that until I made him aware of the "unpleasant" realities of life and aging, he was living in a fool's paradise not knowing about these. He was dying slowly and life was miserable. Now he is counting his pebbles and life has taken on new meaning. "I am not scared of death Doc, if it happens I know I've lived and not just had a decaying existence."

The main point about Michael is that primarily it was his **GOFES** that was tackled and treated. Everything else that followed was merely "a mopping up exercise".

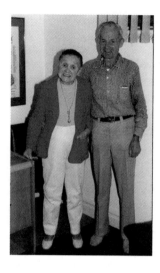

Audrey and Fred

Audrey and Fred used to come to see me very infrequently. I always thought of them as about the same age. Then Audrey suffered a stroke and I was involved on a more regular basis. I noted from her file that she was 10 years older than Fred. In the photo Audrey was 83 and Fred 73 - or so I thought.

A few weeks after I took the photograph, Audrey passed away in her sleep. Fred came in to tell me the bad news, and then told me something that left me stunned: "Doc, the day before my Audrey died I discovered she was not 83 years, but nearly 94. I was shaken for a moment, because when I was 33 I thought I'd married a 43 year old, not a 53 year old...but Doc... I realised it was the best forty years of my life and I forgave her."

All Audrey did was to try and stay young for her Fred and she lived with this lie for 40 years. Audrey never knew anything about age retardation and life extension. She used her instincts and controlled her diet. Like Maggie in the chapter on Nutritional Program, she believed in traditional nutritional combinations and methods.

Perhaps Audrey could have lived longer with her secret if she wasn't a smoker. She had smoked for 75 years. Some people have genes that protect them from some of the side effects of smoking. Nevertheless, smoking is never recommended. We should actually be kind to smokers because they don't have long to live.

STEP THREE

I classify *direct* human growth hormone (hGH) replacement therapy as step three for a number of reasons. Requiring injections daily and costing between $10,000 and $20,000 a year, it is out of reach for most people. It also puts a lot of stress on the pancreas to produce insulin. As a side effect diabetes may develop, especially in the aging population. Most people who practice the 10 principles of health have fairly normal hGH levels.

My patients on hGH replacement are watched like hawks. They have to sign comprehensive consent forms and if they do not turn up for monitoring they are contacted immediately or taken off therapy. It is a very potent hormone and can be worthwhile in selective cases. That said, I have seen good results in a select group of patients.

"First do no harm" should be the overriding consideration. The best treatment in medicine often is to *do nothing - just wait*. I think this applies to hGH therapy for most people but, underlying this, the theory suggests it may have a role to play in treating the disease of aging.

STEP FOUR

This step is the future. I believe there are therapies that will change the way the disease of aging will be treated. We just have to wait patiently and, if still alive by then, make use of these therapies. Ultimately, genetics generally determines how long a person will live. You can either live to this potential or accelerate the aging process and die before your time. To live longer than your genetic potential will take revolutionary genetic manipulation that is beyond what is available today.

Cells are programmed to die and they do. Genetic manipulation in the future may change this, but in the meantime you have two choices:

1. live a life style that induces premature aging and you will die well before your genetic potential

2. live a healthy life as we have discussed throughout in *Polar Bears and Humming Birds - A Medical Guide to Weight Loss* and reach your genetic potential in a pleasant way.

SUMMARY OF AVAILABLE OPTIONS

Step one

1. Nutrition and diet
2. Supplementation
3. Exercise
4. The rest of the 10 health programs

Step two

A. Stimulation, replacement and enhancement of declining substances and metabolic processes, as we grow older.

1. Hormonal secretion stimulation (provided the pituitary and hormonal axis has not aged too much yet. You can't flog a dead horse.)
   a. Secretagogues
   b. Caloric restriction
   b. Exercise
   c. Other means eg. clonidine

2. Direct hormonal replacement - HRT

3. Enhancement of insulin sensitivity
   a. Chromium
   b. Alpha-lipoic acid
   c. Exercise
   d. Low GI and GL
   e. Caloric restriction
   f. Medication - metformin and Dilantin

4. Balance neurotransmitters
   a. St John's Wart (hypericum perforatum)
   b. Some anti-depressants

B. Other useful additions

1. Aspirin
2. EDTA
3. Gamma linoleic acid
4. Combinations

Step three

Human growth hormone

Step four

The future. Watch this space. Stay up to date.

In many ways we are recycled and one generation rolls into the next.

"It is terrible to grow old alone".
"You're not alone. What about your wife?"
"My wife hasn't had a birthday in 10 years!"

"Growing older is not so bad...
...if you do it with someone you love."
ANONYMOUS

The Clock of Life

The clock of life is wound but once, and no man has the power
To tell just when the hands will stop, at late or early hour.

To lose one's wealth is sad indeed, to lose one's health is more,
To lose one's soul is such a loss as no man can restore.

The present only is our own, live, love, toil with a will;
Place no faith in tomorrow for the clock may then be still.
ETTA JOHNSON

*"Live this day as if it were your last, but at the same time,
live as if you are going to live forever."*
ROMAN SAYING

This is where the philosophy of time impacts. We do not know how long we have left; one day or a long time?

Planning for both is of the essence.

Synopsis:

1. Count your pebbles.

2. By the time you are 40 you should give serious consideration to time.

3. Only a brief overview is given here on this subject. And a medical doctor experienced in this type of medicine should closely monitor any protocols. This chapter is not intended as a do-it-yourself. A follow up book in the series will deal specifically with this topic. *Polar Bears and Humming Birds - A Medical Guide to Weight Loss* is a good starting point.

4. A report published in the May 3 2005 issue of the American Heart Association journal *Circulation* demonstrated that weight gain and increased

insulin resistance result in greater telomere shortening over time. Telomeres are the genetic material at the end of chromosomes that become progressively eroded with age and oxidative stress. Telomere length has been proposed as a marker of biological, as opposed to chronological, aging. Another reason you should not deposit excess fat. **GOFES** speeds up the aging process.

5. Be aware of the anti-aging bandwagon. Just as much good emerges, just as many falsehoods have been uttered. If you study healthy old people you will notice they stay lean - no **GOFES**, they eat breakfast, they consume vitamin and phytonutrient-rich foods and they remain active. They also resolved issues. Once you have all the basics in place, then you can begin to treat aging

6. Investigate credentials first.

7. "My uncle lived to be 100 and he owed it all to smoking - he never smoked!"

8. Never assume your life is over. I have observed, and it is borne out by studies, that creativity often peaks in later years.

9. *The best years of your life should always be the ones you are living right now.*

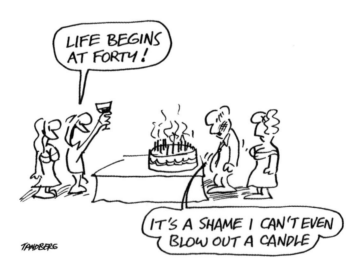

LIFE BEGINS AT FORTY!

IT'S A SHAME I CAN'T EVEN BLOW OUT A CANDLE

TANDBERG

CHAPTER 27

9. SECURITY

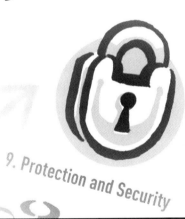

9. SECURITY

Life is full of risks. We can't do much about the unpredictable but we can manage, or at least influence, the predictable. This chapter is not about "wrapping yourself in cotton wool" - it's about risk management. If you choose to jump out of a perfectly good aircraft with a parachute strapped to your back, far be it from me to discourage you, but please do take every reasonable precaution - there are no prizes for being foolhardy. This chapter is intended to encourage you to develop an awareness of your safety and security, with a view to increasing your statistical chances for a healthier and longer life.

"The will to win is worthless if you do not have the will to prepare."

THANE YOST

What have the following in common?

1. Welwitschia plants.
2. Galapagos tortoise
3. Yellow stone rock fish.
4. Bristle cone pine
5. Melanoma
6. Motor vehicle accidents
7. Taking your safety for granted.

They all point to security and safety as will be explained next.

The following plaque was in a hospital corridor:
"The first five minutes of life are the most dangerous."
A student wrote underneath:
"...and the last five minutes are pretty dodgy too."

You can be healthy, happy and become over confident regarding your own security. If you are not vigilant and taking your safety for granted, by not *"looking over your shoulder"* your life and good health could be short lived.

I will tell you about Max. He was 32 years old and had a lot going for him - good looking, kind, a loving partner, a professional career, enough money in the bank to last him a lifetime. He was a good squash player and eager rock climber. He had a keen interest in his health and that is how I met him.

"Doctor, I have longevity genes on both sides of my family and I want to capitalise on it. Can you tell me what to do?"

I was impressed by his interest in health medicine and preventative health. The usual tests revealed he was completely normal and healthy. His functional or biological age was in the 20 year old range - at 32 he was functioning like a 20 year old and was metabolically fit.

I congratulated him and pointed out that health is only on loan to us and that he must maintain it just like he would maintain his house or car.

"Max, you cannot buy good health, even if you are a millionaire - you must earn it."

He understood what I meant, and arranged his six-month follow up appointment that same day. For this follow up consultation he brought his fiancé, Kate. Actually, she insisted on coming and the reason became clear with her first sentence.

"Doctor.." she said in an anxious voice, "please tell him not to buy a motor bike. I had a brother who was killed on one. He won't listen to me... I know he has a lot of confidence in you and... please tell him not to..." she pleaded.

I did my best to dissuade him, but a few days later Max bought a bike and all the associated paraphernalia. Four days later a driver in an overtaking car failed to see Max and he is a paraplegic as a result.

In a wheel chair he married Kate, but the marriage lasted only four years. He no longer has the use of his bowels and bladder, and he is incapable of maintaining an erection. Kate remarried after being awarded a significant portion of the estate that Max had brought into the marriage. I still see Max occasionally. I never remind him of Kate and my warnings - there is no point.

Max was always confident and may have become over confident when I gave him the good news about his health. It was indeed short lived. He must have thought he was invincible.

Melanoma - one of the most devastating cancers. Most of these cancers are caused by a genetic predisposition and not being careful with sun exposure. Do you have a skin protection policy? By the time you are older and wiser it is too late to stop damage done a long time ago.

Welwitschia, Galapagos tortoise, Yellow stone rockfish and the Bristle cone pine.

What all these fauna and flora have in common is that they have found an *environment free of predators*. The Galapagos giant tortoise has no natural enemies. The Bristle cone pine grows very high up in the mountains where it is too cold for insects to eat it. The oldest trees are some 5,000 years old. The Yellow Eye Rock Fish are 200 to 300 years old. They live so deep they have no predators of note. Welwitschia plants live for thousands of years in the Namib Desert - they too have no predators.

Security as a health concept

Some people are surprised that I regard security as part of health.

If you follow all the advice in this book you have a real chance of living longer than might otherwise have been the case. What will kill or maim you prematurely would be an accident, some other violent event, carelessness or mental abuse. Even if you are not killed your health will suffer.

Risk *age* - RA is determined by comparing an individual's chances of dying with others in the same chronological age - **CA** group, based on identified risk factors.

RA is not related to BA - functional or biological age.

In an age delaying program *every* potentially *unsafe action and habit* should be identified and eliminated.

It is a "jungle" out there today, even if we are "civilised". We do not live in a carefree environment like the Bristle cone pine or the Galapagos tortoises and we should not be carefree and casual with our safety and security. Even a momentary dropping of your guard can have disastrous consequences.

The ecological balance between the **Predator** and the **Victim**, the Hunter and the Hunted, is in some ways now more precarious than ever before. Potential victims are lulled into a false sense of security as is the man not looking over his shoulder.

Physical Protection and Security

There is a raft of potential physical events that can impact your health and life.

Road crashes

There is a tendency not to call these accidents because most are due to human error. Why would you, like Max, want to have a motorbike? A vehicle faster than a car without protection?

Most motorbike riders are probably safe, cautious and responsible, but what cannot be argued away is that motorbikes are unstable and afford no protection. They are often "invisible" to other drivers on our roads.

Duruing the Vietnam War more people died on the roads in the United States, than soldiers died on the battlefield. Cars are getting safer, but you still have to drive safely. Speed maims and kills. Some scientists believe that the average brain is only capable of responsible driving from the age of 25.

People would demand action if jumbo jets crashed every three days killing all their passengers, yet this is the rate at which people die on European roads. Currently the number of deaths worldwide from traffic accidents is 1.2 million per year. It is predicted that this will have risen by 65 to 75 per cent by 2020.

"The accident wasn't my fault. I had the right of way. Unfortunately, the other guy was driving a bus." Always think for the other drivers too.

Home security

Every time you hear about someone being killed in a home fire, mark it off on a calendar. You will be shocked to learn how many it adds to in one year.

Better still, to fast track the process find out from your local Bureau of Statistics what these figures are. It will spur you to develop a home fire policy - from smoke detectors to fire blankets and extinguishers. Most local fire departments are willing to help with advice. Fire causes possibly the most horrific of injuries.

Assault
Especially for females, walking in the dark in certain areas on your own is looking for trouble. Seek and you will find. Every major city has one or two potential serial killers. "Stranger danger" doesn't just apply to children.

In some cities piracy has extended from the high seas to the roads.

Terrorism and wars
Our circumstances are all different, but often we can avoid trouble. Stay out of the crossfire if you can.

Mental Protection and Security
Depending on your personality type, intimidation and bullying may be very unnerving and lead to stress-related hormone disturbances.

White-collar crime
Identity fraud has become a major problem. In some places it accounts for 40 per cent of all criminal cases investigated by the police.

It is easier to be alert to physical assault than the mental trickery of white-collar crime. A higher, unaccustomed level of vigilance is required. Our genetic programming alerts us to physical danger rather than these more subversive dangers. *To live more safely in the 21st century we need to adapt to "invisible" danger.*

Frivolous legal action
There are various ways to settle arguments. In days of old they were typically settled physically with duels and skirmishes. This is not politically correct any more and so we resort to the courts - "Don't get mad - get even". No-one wins... even if you think you've won, you've not only spent a lot of money, but you've also put your body under significant stress.

Talk is cheap until you talk to a lawyer.

Once I met a guy in the gym who is a well known multi-millionaire. He told me that he employs a staff of eight full time lawyers to keep him out of "trouble". As soon as you have something of value, predators appear like vultures for the pickings.

For your own health and wellbeing you must pre-empt these predators and not allow them to gain so much as a toehold. If you are not ready, the mental and physical costs can be immense. When your mental health and physical health are stressed, you are not in a position to control POD... and that's when GOFES makes a dramatic appearance.

Plan:

1. As a first step - contact your local Bureau of Statistics and ascertain your Risk Age.

2. Cultivate a sense of awareness, preparedness, protection, precaution, security, safety, caution, watchfulness and vigilance - heed the Scouting movement's motto: Be Prepared.

3. Work out an *A Plan* and a *B Plan* to minimise risk as much as you can. Who are your potential physical and mental predators? Hopefully you will never use your defence plans, but it is best to have them in place in case you need them. By being pre-emptive you can avoid a lot of health and wealth problems. Pre-emption also makes you more aware of your country's laws, such that you do not do something stupid and inadvertently break vague or obscure laws. It may be one of the best investments you have made in your life.

4. Follow this up with some philosophical thinking. Don't live in a constant state of anxiousness and paranoia. Do your best to relax. If in spite of your preparation, you do come to grief, it was an act of God. However, statistically you now have a real chance to maintain your health longer - life extension by health extension.

"Si vis pacem, para bellum" -
if you want peace, prepare for war.
LATIN SAYING

CHAPTER 28

10. FINANCIAL PROGRAM

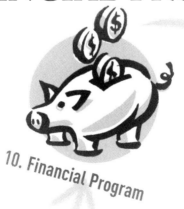

10. Financial Program

10. FINANCIAL PROGRAM

It's a little glib to say that your health is your wealth and your wealth is your health - to coin a pun, man cannot live on health alone. Throughout this book we've spoken of the external factors that impact GOFES - from the ready availability of food to the quacks and fraudsters who try to convince us that weight loss is easy. To successfully combat GOFES requires confidence in self-worth, and a factor that can impact personal confidence is financial security. While this is not within everyone's grasp, I have observed that patients who are successful in controlling GOFES are also financially aware.

Reading this chapter won't make you rich, but it might provide some hints on controlling one of those external factors that can impact your health - in particular, your GOFES.

"A good salesman is one who can convince his wife that she looks too fat in a mink coat."

S. MORRIS

"Many people take no care of their money till they come to the end of it, and others do just the same with their time."
JOHANN WOLFGANG VON GOETHE

Long-term patients of mine, John and Judy, initially came to see me to lose weight. They were well to do. Both lost their excess fat very successfully and kept it off. John lost 22kg (48lb) and Judy 28kg (62lb). Like they always said: "We lost 50 kg (110lb)!"

They became quite health conscious, *which is the overriding characteristic that I notice of successful maintainers of health and normal fat percentage.* For years they adhered to their functional health program and consulted me twice a year to screen for aging and other diseases. I was impressed with how good they looked and felt.

Said Judy: "Doctor, I have never felt this good. Life is getting better all the time. John and I discovered a new life that we didn't know existed. We can't go back."

Every year they bought a new car or two. I remember John saying: "Doc, we've just traded the Jaguar in for a Mercedes 500 SE - wanna go for a spin?"

A number of times I went for a spin in their new cars. I particularly liked the Ferrari he bought Judy for her 60th birthday. It was a bit low to the ground for my personal liking, but what a car. They regularly went overseas for holidays and the odd business trip.

At 62 Judy had a facelift and John had some other cosmetic procedure. They prided themselves on the fact that they looked much younger than their respective ages. Biologically they were indeed much younger, energetic, enthusiastic and healthy. Judy even took part in a marathon walk, out-walking women 15 years her junior. John had the latest joke to tell each time we met at the clinic. Judy's infectious laugh could brighten even the dullest joke. Their sense of humour contributed to their health, as it would do for most people.

One Monday morning, after a hectic weekend, I was a bit tired and needed a bit of cheering up. I saw that they had booked in for one of their follow-up visits and I was looking forward to John's jokes and in general their uplifting presence. Maybe they had another car that I could take for a spin?

When they arrived, I was taken aback to see two glum faced individuals. When I asked what was wrong, Judy broke into tears: "Doctor, we have just retired..."

I thought to myself, what is so bad about that?

"...and... we only have $25,000 in the bank, the house and a car. We will never be able to live a decent life with this money"

John chipped in: "We will have to take up smoking, drinking and get fat again to shorten our lives now. You made us so healthy we will out live our money."

I still see John and Judy from time-to-time. Their lives have changed a lot. They had to sell the house and make various unpleasant adjustments. *The biggest change, however, was in their health.* They lost the enthusiasm and inspiration to stay healthy. They did not have the money to afford their gym fees, supplements and replacements, holidays for rest and recreation, and they lost the general positive feeling of financial security.

"The only certain way to reduce the cost of living is to drop dead."
GOLDBLATT

"A financial program as part of a health strategy? - you gotta be joking?"

I have seen numerous instances of how mental and physical health is connected to financial health. *The connection is so strong* that I had no choice but to incorporate this as the tenth of my health principles.

I don't mean money for the sake of money, but enough wealth to give you some financial security.

The following statistics apply in most western countries.

Of 100 teenagers living today, at age 65:
40 will be dead
60 will be alive

Of the 60 alive:
40 will be dead broke
15 will still be working to make ends meet
4 will be retired on a reasonable income
1 (or less) will be well off

It appears that only five per cent will eventually be successful to a degree and one per cent or less will be thriving.

These aren't good odds.

Do these statistics sound familiar when it comes to weight loss?

What are your chances of losing excess fat and keeping it off for five years or longer?

Of 100 obese people on the best treatment available, only 20 will reach an ideal goal weight. Within five years only one of those 20 will have kept their weight under control. A depressing one per cent success rate!

The odds aren't good for maintaining either your wealth or your health.

Questions:
- What is the most popular labour saving device?
- What is the answer to many questions?
- When you come right down to it, almost any problem eventually becomes what type of problem?

Answer: Money

Anyone who says money doesn't buy happiness doesn't know where to shop. All I ask is for a chance to prove that money can't make me happy. In the end your health is your wealth, but your wealth is also your health.

The worst place in all the world to live is just beyond your means.

Just as **POD** can be difficult to control, so can it be very difficult to save and manage money. Saving can be a pain - the Pain of Saving (**PO$**). Just as a person can have an *eating disorder*, so can they have a *spending disorder*.

"I am working on my second million -
I gave up on the first."
ANONYMOUS

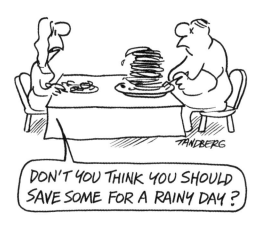

DON'T YOU THINK YOU SHOULD
SAVE SOME FOR A RAINY DAY ?

A colleague of mine almost ruined himself by having ten credit cards with a combined debt of $100,000. Just the interest payments were enough to drive him to distraction. By the time you are financial enough to eat, drink and be merry, the doctor limits you to a glass of milk! Time flies.

He said: "What have you been doing with all the grocery money I gave you?"

She said: "Turn sideways and look in the mirror!"

A lean healthy body and a fat bank account
or...
A fat body and a lean bank account.

Money worries are also fattening

One of the first things Judy did was to gain weight.

This is not unusual in western countries, because our food supply is abundant and cheap. High stress levels create high stress hormone levels, which in turn make your metabolism more efficient in storing fat.

Lower socio-economic classes are often fatter than the well-to-do for various reasons. As a strategy for dealing with the **GOFES** epidemic it has been suggested that people in lower socio-economic classes should be paid more!

Most people itch,
To join the rich,
There's just one catch,
They lack the scratch.

Over the years I have consulted to scores of financially successful patients. The following is a collection of simple advice that they have given.

- The poorest person is one with nothing but money.

- Do not outlive your money - let your money outlive you.

- Never be without any money.

- It is not how much you earn; it is what you do with it. If you just spend it on things that lose value you will end up with no value.

- Invest first, spend later. You will quickly get used to it and see your money and net worth grow exponentially.

- If you do not use your legs you will lose them - if you do not use your money you will lose it. For some, keeping money under the bed may be an option, but you should get expert advice. I have often been warned by financially successful patients to be careful who you consult.

- "Never buy that you cannot afford." CHINESE PROVERB

- Live within your means. Prepare a budget and stick to it. **POD** versus **PO$** - both difficult to manage - both very rewarding when you achieve success. If you have champagne tastes and only beer money, don't buy champagne - yet.

- Beware of retail therapy. If you are depressed or need excitement, there are other ways of dealing with it. Impulse buying and retail therapy do not solve problems, just as food does not solve problems, except malnutrition.

- Assets earn money - liabilities destroy it. Liabilities are like treading water while waiting to sink.

- You can try and pay your debts with a smile, but you will find that your creditors will still want money.

  John and Judy used debt to finance their extravagant lifestyle. They were naive and did not look over their shoulders. At least they were still alive, but when the chickens came home to roost, like they always do, they didn't have the money and the means to enjoy the best years of their lives and stay healthy. Their "financial metabolism" was unfit.

- It is easier making money than keeping it. *A fool and his money are easily parted.* A patient told me about her uncle who used to be quite a wealthy man. After three divorces he lost everything and now his children have to look after him, while his former wives are well off.

- Don't marry for money: you can borrow cheaper. *(just kidding)*

- It is always better learning from the experience of others rather than your own. This does not only apply to money, but other areas of your life as well.

- Financially successful people borrow money for things that increase in value. Those who are financially unsuccessful borrow money for things that lose value.

- Just as the first rule of nutrition is to eat less, so the first rule of your financial health is to spend less on things that do not have intrinsic value.

- People are funny, they spend money on things they don't need, to impress people they don't like.

- With money you can:
  Buy a house, but not a home,
  Buy a clock, but not time,
  Buy a bed, but not sleep,
  Buy a book, but not knowledge,
  Buy a position, but not respect,
  Buy blood, but not a life,
  Buy sex, but not love,
  Buy a doctor's consultation, but not health.

- As soon as financial or health trouble appears on the horizon, take immediate remedial action. Almost daily the financial pages reports on businesses that have traded while technically bankrupt. Most reasonable people would agree with the value of detecting cancer early so that a cure is possible. Why not apply this to finances as well?

- When I asked, Blanche, a patient: "How's business?" she replied: "Not good at all - we are having a tough time."

  As I arranged a follow-up visit with her, she remarked that she and her husband were going overseas. "For business?" I asked. "No," she replied, "just to relax a bit in the south of France. We love the lifestyle there and I may even do one of those cooking courses while there."

  "But," said me, "I thought business was bad?"

  She looked me in the eye and said: "Doc, when we started our business we didn't change our lifestyle for a long time. We didn't pay ourselves big directors' fees, nor did we buy luxury cars and all the trappings. We've suffered business downturns before. We know from experience we will trade out of this one too, *because we have enough fat to live on.*"

  Long after Blanche left, her words were still ringing in my ears: "*...because we have enough fat to live on.*" Hmh...

Seventeenth characteristic of successful weight maintainers: financial management and control.

Synopsis:

1. Remember, just as **POD** can be difficult to control, **PO$** can be even *more* difficult.

2. Money Worries = Fattening = Powerlessness

3. "You can never be too thin or too rich." THE DUCHESS OF WINDSOR

4. Apply the hints in this chapter.

5. *Money has a lot to do with the level of health that you can afford to maintain.* Your health is your wealth and your wealth is your health.

6. "The only way for a rich man to be healthy is by exercise and abstinence, to live as if he were poor." WILLIAM J. TEMPLE

7. "Money by itself has no value and never forget: *Money is a terrible master,* but an excellent servant." P.T. BARNUM

8. The real measure of your wealth is how much you'd be worth if you lost all your money. Bernard Meltzer (1914-) American Law Professor

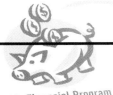

10. Financial Program

1. Nutrition Program

2. Supplement Program

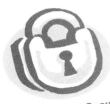

9. Protection and Security

CHAPTER 29

JUGGLING IT ALL TOGETHER

3. Exercise Program

4. Hygiene

8. Time

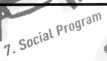

7. Social Program

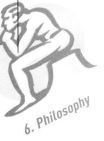

6. Philosophy

5. Rest and Recreation

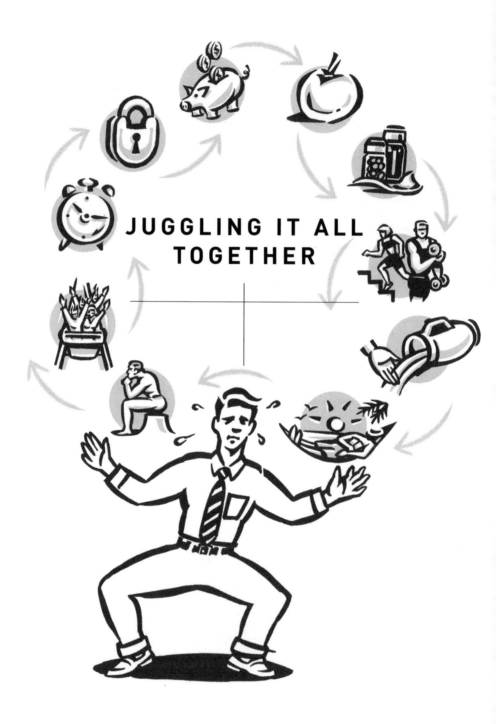

JUGGLING IT ALL TOGETHER

"I finally got it together,
but forgot where I put it."
ANONYMOUS

"He conquers who conquers himself."
LATIN PROVERB

When it comes to your health, which really is the basis of your quality of life, it doesn't hurt to be a bit Machiavellian in your approach.

"A man too busy to take care of his health is like a mechanic
too busy to take care of his tools."
SPANISH PROVERB

Action and enthusiasm

"The end of all knowledge should be virtuous action."
PHILIP SYDNEY

There is a right and a wrong way, and the wrong way always seems to be more attractive. Do not feel guilty, we are merely designed to think and act this way.

So much to do - so little time. Some of the 10 health programs detailed in this book need daily attention - others occasionally. The first step is to develop an *awareness* of the *integration* of all the programs. A neglect of any one of them can have ripple effects to your detriment. Thinking about your programs won't do it for you - you need to put those thoughts into action. Never worry about action - only inaction should concern you. You are nothing really without enthusiasm. *The deed is everything.*

Unfortunately, patients often tend to favour one or more of the 10 programs - exercise being a classic example. Exercise overdone will be detrimental to you, even if you eat and sleep correctly.

If you overdo a link, you may break the chain. The opposite is also true. Handle the chain with care - synergy and balance are at stake.

An electricity grid is made up of many interconnections and varying voltages. Sometimes specific areas need more electricity than others and power is diverted to the areas in need. Occasionally, the grid cannot cope and there are power blackouts. View your health plan as a grid. You cannot always spend equal time on all 10 programs. Learn to divert resources to areas in need. *You cannot do everything all the time, but you must do all of it some of the time.*

Decree #1
Recognise the interconnectivity and synergy involved in all the programs. A chain is as strong as its weakest link. View your health programs as an interconnecting grid.

The human body evolved from an ancient chemistry that shaped our metabolism, which has changed little since the Stone Age. Nature functions on various rhythms that range from generational to seasonal and daily. While our lives have fallen into the 24 hour or circadian rhythm, we should think in biorhythms where patterns extend beyond 24 hours.

Every aspect of our bodies functions on biorhythms. Our bodies respond to these rhythms every hour of the day. For optimum function, health and metabolic fitness we should live within these rhythms, especially if you are serious about controlling **GOFES**.

Our sleep patterns, moods and performance all rely on these biorhythms. Your hormonal cascade, for example, is controlled by daily, monthly and yearly rhythms. Genetics is also a major factor in how we respond to these life patterns.

Oscillations and boundaries

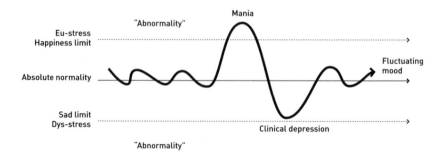

412

If the straight line represents "absolute normality", you can see that nobody can live according to a normal regime. Genetics, cultural and environmental circumstances all draw us away from "normality". How far we move depends on a range of factors, but inevitably we fluctuate and oscillate about this line. Society sets *limits* to how far we can move away from this line and still be considered normal. Our bodies also set metabolic limits - at a certain point we deviate into the abnormal.

Everything has boundaries and beyond these lies "abnormality".

As in the illustration, if we take mood for example, a person starts in the happy range but is not so elated as to be abnormal. The person becomes a little sad, but still within the range of what is normal and functional. However, if the person is too happy performance will be compromised. Conversely, too sad and morbid, then depression is the result. This can be applied equally to many other behaviours and metabolic processes. Stress is a good example.

Understanding these cycles and the range of normality is very important in your endeavours to control **GOFES** and have a meaningful health program. Your mood and metabolism will oscillate and respond to these biorhythms. Depending on your individual make-up and environmental circumstances you will at times lose the plot (or the **POD**), as it were, and embark on a path of destruction. These fluctuations, especially those in close proximity to the extremities of normality, impact heavily on **POD** and **POEx**. Maintaining normal biorhythms will be difficult at times. **POD/POEx** will, for the sake of survival, exploit and take advantage of our weaknesses as we approach these boundaries.

Remember, we are not programmed to control **POD** and **POEx** naturally. This control was always imposed on us from outside. The internal control that is now required is alien to us. Practicing this inner control can be challenging at times. It takes time, motivation and patience to acquire this skill.

The first thing to understand is that you cannot live on a line of absolute normality, thus controlling POD and POEx perfectly. To believe you can control **POD** perfectly is Alice in Wonderland stuff. We live in modern society with Stone Age metabolisms and so you cannot expect to completely escape damage all the time.

Faltering is not failure

If your performance is not always optimal, do not panic. Regroup and attack. Your ability to control performance will improve with time. In my experience it takes an average of three years to learn to control **GOFES**. Above all, do not allow the Stop Start Syndrome to take hold, or you will tread water and eventually drown.

A good place to start is with your sleeping and eating habits. Make sure these follow the patterns we have discussed.

Decree #2
Realise that all of life is a bit up and down. Ride the waves and make use of them. There is a lot of power in a wave. Roll with the punches. "Everyone of my failures contributes to my success."

Give your health principles a moral and philosophical code. Let this become your personal code to achieve wellbeing. Your nutritional Sin Days can be part of this overall plan. Your aim should be to live on the line of "absolute normality", even though this will be impossible at times.

Decree #3
Develop a health code that you stick by.

Understand your health vulnerability.

If you have a family history of heart disease and your own cholesterol readings are not optimum, you have an increased risk of cardiovascular disease. Minimising your own individual risk - your vulnerability to artery disease and stroke - can serve as powerful motivation in adhering to your health programs.

Download vivid pictures of clogged arteries from the internet and tape these to your fridge door as a constant reminder. If you do not want to make it that obvious, place them on the inside of the pantry door. Dino, a patient who suffered a mild heart attack, had a picture of himself lying in the intensive care unit, together with images of his coronary arteries. He had them laminated and put some on the fridge and others in the pantry.

"Doctor, that ICU picture of me is powerful... I just love my junk food... but these pictures of mine remind me like none of you doctors can."

The 10 health principles and how they interconnect, can also be displayed in the pantry, fridge and bar. In fact, any place that may trigger **POD**. Annette, a successful **GOFES** patient who was a graphic artist, individualised the 10 health principles. On each she put something of herself, reflecting her strengths, weaknesses and vulnerabilities. In the exercise frame she had a picture of herself in the gym, in the social frame she had a picture of her family.

In doing so, she gave thought to her health program and devised a process of constant reminder. It is now nine years since she lost all her excess fat and she is going from strength to strength.

Decree #4
Devise vivid reminders of your weaknesses, as well as what you aspire to be. Display these in strategic places as constant reminders. Remember: A chain is only as strong as the weakest link.

"I want it all...NOW"

Something as comprehensive as your health programs is not going to fall into place instantly. Remember, it takes time to refine - on average three years, 36 months, 156 weekends, 1,095 days, 26,280 hours... do you want the minutes as well? You will go from strength to strength as you renew your perspective on life. It is never a straight path and you will stray from time to time, but these deviations should also form part of your overall plan or they will degenerate into destructive holes.

When I was young I had the impatience of youth and complained to my father about medical school taking seven years. He went through medical school himself - his response: "You will never know how quickly it will be over." When I qualified I was shocked how fast it all went. In fact, the years since have gone even faster. What is three years to remodel yourself?... to effectively control your **GOFES**?

"When prosperity comes do not use all of it."
CONFUCIUS

Decree #5
Be patient, but persistent. You need a three year apprenticeship to get on top of GOFES. Rome was not built in a day.

Establish a check list incorporating these steps.

Step 1: Preparation and assessment

At this stage focus on health programs two: Supplement Program, three: Exercise, and four: Hygiene

Step 1: Preparation and assessment

✓ off

1	Diagnosis	a GOFES	- Type	
			- Degree	
			- Causes	
		b Diseases caused by GOFES		
		c Other diseases		
2	Measurements/Calculations	- Functional (Biological) Age		
		- Risk Age		
		- Risk profile		
3	Medical examination	- Full medical		
		- QT interval		
		- Other investigations		
4	Preparation for Stage 2	- Increase water intake		
		- Start Supplement program		
		- Commence exercise program		

More of the 10 health programs come into play at this point.

Step 2: Losing excess fat

✓ off

1	Treatment of GOFES	- Nutritional	☐
		- Supplement Program	☐
		- Exercise	☐
		- Other Programs introduced	☐
2	Treatment of the GOFES induced diseases		☐
3	Treatment of other diseases		☐
4	Follow up and monitoring of treatment		☐
1	Recording of weight, Fat % and individual patterns		☐
2	Behavioural Modification		☐
3	Emphasis on all the 10 Health Programs		☐
4	Monitor	- BA (Biological Age)	☐
		- Other tests as is necessary	☐
1	Continuation of Step 3, but more full on and refinement		☐

Step 3: Maintenance of normal fat percentage

✓ off

1	Recording of weight, Fat % and individual patterns		☐
2	Behavioural Modification		☐
3	Emphasis on all the 10 Health Programs		☐
4	Monitor	- BA (Biological Age)	☐
		- Other test as is necessary	☐

Step 4: Continuation of Step 3 with refinement

✓ off

1	Continuation of Step 3, but more full on and refinement		☐

Decree #6
Tick off the various steps as you go, to make sure you are adhering to your plan and have not left out important steps.

Sometimes we have to read things over and over again, not only to fully understand the meaning, but also to serve as a reminder. We all need mantras when it comes to health and survival.

Understand the impact of Quality, Quantity and Variety on **POD**, **POEx** and **GOFES**.

Decree #7
Repetition is the key to controlling GOFES. Re-read sections of this book, make notes and summaries. Understand GOFES.

There is no such thing as a free lunch. This is especially true when it comes to your health and genetics. Your efficient Polar Bear metabolism, **DES**, **POD** and **POEx** will make sure of that. Lunch will always come at a cost to you - no-one else can deal with **POD** and **POEx** on your behalf.

It's up to you. Sounds so straightforward, but **GOFES** sufferers need to be constantly reminded that only they hold the key to success. The main problem with the majority of **GOFES** treatments is that the therapist tries to be too "understanding and nice". As a result they give in to the patient who is spurred on by **POD**.

"Doc, can I have some champagne on my wedding anniversary? I'll only have a small piece of ice cream. I'll be good again the next day."

Typical therapist's response: "Okay, but just make sure you go back to your program the next day. A bit of champagne won't cause too much of a setback."

Experienced therapist's response: "You are undergoing medical treatment and you are expected to stick to it. Your question is POD driven. Get Stage 2 over and done with and your next anniversary will be a different story."

Three reasons for yearning for effortless and easy solutions:

1. We naturally look for easy solutions, which unfortunately do not exist when dealing with **POD/POEx/CZ** and **GOFES**.

2. Easy solutions may have short-term benefits, but they have poor long-term results.

3. We are exploited by the promise of easy solutions that pander to our innate survival instincts of laziness when it comes to physical activity and a propensity to overeat.

An ancient Arabic proverb: "What comes with ease goes with ease." The fact of the matter is that halfway measures just do not work when it comes to health and **GOFES** management. You either do it or you don't. Remember the metabolic versus mathematical logic that we discussed?

I have yet to see anybody successfully control **GOFES** without total commitment. I often hear and read about such people, but I have yet to meet them. POD does not respond favourably to weak and meek attitudes and behaviours. It is after all a brutal and profound survival oriented force. In our present **DES** circumstances, if you let **POD** run loose, your health will lose out. Effort applied now and over these next three years is a cheap and insignificant price to pay for the gigantic benefits you will achieve.

Sometimes it is not pleasant to accept "unpleasant facts", but a fact is a fact. Therefore, if you want to be successful in controlling **GOFES**, the following rule applies:

During Stage 3 - Maintenance - it is not what you do 20 to 30 per cent of the time, but what you do 70 to 80 per cent of the time, but during Stage 2 it is what you do 100 per cent of the time.

Decree #8

There is no such thing as a free lunch when it comes to GOFES and health. You cannot buy good health - you have to earn it!

Martin is the chief engineer for a large mining company. He never wanted to live the **GOFES** lifestyle again after he lost 30kg (66lb). Working in his back yard one weekend he picked up a bag of cement weighing 20kg (44lb) and realised he had lost the equivalent of one-and-a-half bags of cement. He put one of the bags in an old backpack and went for his usual walk. When he came back his knees were sore and he felt quite ill. "No wonder I felt so bad when I was carrying all that extra weight, with its impact on my organs and joints."

Unfortunately, Martin had trouble keeping his weight off. His work involved a lot of travel. I suggested to him: "Martin, why don't you have a checklist on your laptop of all the health things you have to do. You are clever and you can design something that can really work."

Pilots use check lists. Even though experienced pilots know the procedures by heart, the checklist is there so that nothing is left to chance.

Martin designed a sophisticated checklist that included his daily weights, Sin Days, No Exercise Days, and various other information. He divided his exercise into stretching, resistance and cardio, then allocated days for each component. He also decided to meditate up to five times a week.

With all his travel there were times when he didn't even get a chance to brush his teeth. So he included dental hygiene in his checklist.

Eventually the checklist not only embraced everything he needed to do, but it also revealed interesting patterns and predictions about his lifestyle behaviour. Martin's checklist started out on a spreadsheet, but was later transferred to an advanced database program.

"I feel compelled to do all the things on it, just like I do a good job in my profession. I handle my lifestyle as just another mining project - with excellent results."

Martin also developed a list of "commandments" that he read, as a pilot's checklist, most days.

This sort of planning is not for everyone, but for anyone who wants to control **GOFES** you cannot afford to be casual or sloppy with your approach to health. Martin has agreed that I can include his program as a CD in one of my follow-up books. I have also used it myself and found it very useful after I factored in the issues that are important to me as an individual. We are all different.

Decree #9
Use a checklist system, especially during the first year of maintenance.

Decree #10
Stay in contact with your doctor and develop a partnership.

New Year resolutions last on average just one month. By Easter all is abandoned. This is the case for the great majority of people. It may apply to you as well. What are you going to do about it?

Well, knowing it is probably going to happen to you, and that you may fall victim to the Stop Start Syndrome, why not change your attitude? If you know your enthusiasm will wane at some stage, be prepared for it and deal with it. It is part of life. Sin Days are part of such an approach, to give you little "breaks in between" so that you do not feel too deprived and discipline-fatigued and end up in an eating frenzy.

Occasionally you need more than Sin Days - you need Sin Weeks. As long as you deliberately plan them and get back on track again they may be very good for you. A bit of give and take. You will probably find that a significant lifestyle or seasonal change will require a Sin Week. If you do not take it and control the situation, you may end up in a Sin Semester, Sin Year or worse - combined with all of the consequences.

Stay in control. Plan and ride the waves and you will be successful in the long term.

Decree #11
Have a New Year resolution with a difference!
Get a coach to monitor you.

CHARACTERISTICS OF SUCCESSFUL MAINTAINERS

1. Well-informed
2. Active participant - not a passive recipient
3. Acceptance of the fact that they are Polar Bears and proud of it
4. Fully understand **POD/POE** and have developed the eat less habit
5. Know that scales are useless for excess fat loss, but good for maintenance
6. All reach a normal fat percentage for their gender and genetic body type
7. Develop a positive attitude
8. Standardise their eating habits and behaviour, often based on cultural concepts
9. Fat proof their homes and workplace
10. Adopt a maintenance program for at least one full year - often longer
11. Very health conscious
12. They eat their calories - they don't drink them. Water and tea are their main source of liquids
13. Moderately fit because they exercise regularly
14. Meticulous dental and oral hygiene
15. Pay a lot of attention to good sleeping habits
16. Know that if stress is not managed **POD** will get the upper hand
17. Work hard to avert money worries.

THE 12 LESSONS OF NUTRITION

1. We eat too much - we need to adopt the eat less habit
2. Keep it simple
3. Understand food evolution and degradation
4. Take nothing away - add nothing
5. Basic food knowledge was not essential in the past, but now it is - beware paralysis by analysis
6. Eat your calories don't drink your calories
7. Eat fresh
8. Variety is important, but don't go overboard
9. Have planned "Free Days"
10. Meal frequency - stick with three meals a day - "Fast" every day for at least half a day
11. Plan your eating style
12. Eat traditional cuisine.

Decrees #1 - #11

1. Understand the interconnectivity and synergy involved with all the programs. A chain is just as strong as its weakest link. View your health programs as an interconnecting grid.

2. Realise that life is full of ups and downs. Ride the waves and make use of them.

3. Develop a health code that you stick by.

4. Develop vivid reminders of your weaknesses, as well as what you aspire to be. Display these in strategic places as constant reminders.

5. Be patient, but persistent. You need a three year apprenticeship to control GOFES. Rome wasn't built in a day.

6. Tick off the check list as you go, to make sure you are doing everything correctly and that nothing is left out.

7. Repetition is the key to controlling GOFES.

8. There is no such thing as a free lunch when it comes to health and GOFES control. Your genetics - Polar Bear, POD and POEx - and DES make sure of that.

9. Maintain a checklist, especially in the beginning.

10. Stay in contact with your doctor and develop a partnership.

11. Have a New Year resolution with a difference.

"The ladder of life is full of splinters, but they always prick the hardest when we're sliding down."
WILLIAM BROWNELL

Murphy and O'Toole

"What will go wrong, will go wrong at the worst possible time."
MURPHY'S LAW

"Murphy was an optimist."
O'TOOLE'S LAW

You're fooling yourself if you expect a smooth run at all times. That is simply not realistic. Failure is not falling down - *failure is NOT getting up*. Adapt, roll with the punches and you will surprise yourself.

Success

If at first you don't succeed
- Don't try skydiving
- You are doing better than average
- Destroy all the evidence that you even tried
- Try to shift the blame - criticise the book
- Try and try again - just **DO IT!**

If at first you do succeed
- Try to hide your astonishment
- Look as though it was intended
- Keep on doing it!

If all else fails

Ways to stay fat and unhealthy...

1. Eat anything you like and get fat
Eat and over eat as much as you like - **POD** is your friend. If cigarette smoke and tar can't cleanse your system, a balanced diet isn't likely to. Work hard at staying at least 10 per cent over your recommended fat percentage. More is even better. Yes, the faster, more instantaneous and processed your food the more enjoyable. What are two standard drinks anyway? Just an attempt to control us. I know when I have had enough to drink.

2. Do not worry about supplementing your modern diet
It is just for sissies. Ignore all the evidence about antioxidants and phytonu-trients. Take plenty of stimulants instead. The old standards of caffeine, nicotine, sugar and cola laced with sugar will continue to do the job just fine.

3. Never exercise

What a joke. Besides I don't like it. It is not good doing things you do not like. Henry Ford used to say: "The only exercise I get is walking behind the funeral processions of my athletic friends." If it is good enough for him, it is good enough for me. Hey, I don't have the time anyway.

4. Never have a medical check-up

Why worry. My blood pressure is not up otherwise I would have felt it, in spite of all the evidence that I may actually feel good on high blood pressure and not even know it. Also, I will not allow "that thing being stuck up my backside" to check for colon cancer. Doctors are just quacks and commercial these days - why waste my time and money?

Smoking moderately is not really as bad as doctors claim. I know this 95 year old who has been smoking for 84 years.

Clean your oral cavity only once in a while - if ever. In the old days it wasn't necessary to clean teeth. Why now?

5. Never ever relax

Only go to bed if you are really sleepy. Why sleep if you can do other things you enjoy?

Throw out your sense of humour.

Worry about things you cannot control - worry about earthquakes, the stock market, the approaching ice age, the next world war. All the big issues.

Procrastinate - get high on the stress of putting things off to the last minute.

Never develop routine.

Personalise all criticism. Anyone who criticises your work, family, dog, house, or car is mounting a personal attack. The best form of defence is attack - retaliate!

Put work before everything else and be sure to take work home at evenings and weekends. Keep reminding yourself that vacations are for sissies.

Become not only a perfectionist, but set impossible standards. And either beat yourself up, feel guilty, depressed, discouraged, and/or inadequate when you don't meet those standards.

The Stop Start Syndrome does not affect you.

6. Lose touch with reality

Never think philosophically. You do not have to live in the real world. Who wants to anyway these days?

7. Get rid of your social support system

For the few friends who are willing to tolerate you, let them know friendship is for when you have time, and you never have time. If a few people persist in trying to be your friend, avoid them. Hate pets and animals.

8. Believe that you will stay young forever

Even if I don't, I'll live a long time and get away with not having to change my lifestyle. Aren't they developing pills that will take care of it?

9. Be cavalier about your safety

Drive as fast as you can. Don't wear seat belts. Do lots of sun baking. Live in the fast lane. Trust everybody. Even if you have been taught to be cautious, ignore it.

10. Believe money is the route to all evil

What will be will be... besides I'm sure I'll win the lottery one of these days. If I don't, the government will look after me. Let's live... and tomorrow will take care of itself.

Looking to the future

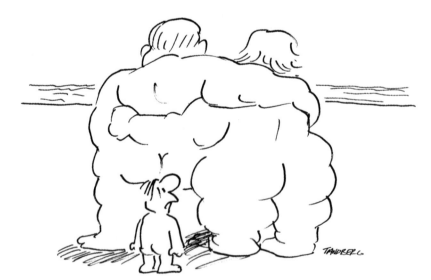

LOOKING INTO THE FUTURE...WHAT DO YOU SEE?

Whether Polar Bear or Humming Bird, unless you get out of your comfort zone regularly, you will not be healthy. You need to experience and control **POD** - the Pain of Deprivation and **POEx** - the Pain of Exercise.

Our metabolism needs "discomfort" to stay in good shape.

If you are a Polar Bear you will get **GOFES** - the Genetic Over Fat Environmental Syndrome. You are simply born that way. You must create your *own* **DES** - a Demand, Effort and Supply regime to suit your individual metabolism.

Adopt the principles of this book and you will be starting something very meaningful in your life - something that that will have a dramatic and positive influence on the rest of your life. Or there is an alternative...

These two case histories from my patient files illustrate these outcomes.

Silvana

Silvana, a 28 year old, consulted me in company with her husband. Rick was quite concerned about the amount of weight Silvana had gained in the six years since their marriage. She also had a fertility problem.

"Sweetie," he said, "tell the doctor that I promised you I will take you overseas to visit the relatives if you lose weight. You know we don't have much money, but I will find it somehow."

Silvana started the program with great enthusiasm. Her excess fat just melted away. When she had lost 52kg (115lb), Rick came in with her again. He was very appreciative of his "new wife" and he produced an envelope: "Here are the tickets, Sweetie, we are off to Europe to visit the relatives."

They stayed away quite a long time and Silvana send me entertaining postcards on an almost weekly basis. When they came back she presented me with a hand painted porcelain statue of a doctor writing a prescription. I felt embarrassed knowing they could ill afford it. I took it home and it is in a prominent place in my study.

I thanked her profusely and at the same time congratulated her for doing so well with her GOFES, particularly during their long stay in Europe. Like I always do at this point, I reminded her of the ongoing need to control her weight and reminded her that GOFES is an incurable disease that can only be controlled.

Silvana missed her follow-up appointments for two years and when she had returned she had not only regained the lost 52kg, but added another 38kg. She was 90kg (198lb) heavier than the last time I saw her. She looked grotesque. For a few moments I stood speechless as she waddled into the consulting room.

Her marriage was in ruins. She looked miserable and I put her back on the program and tried my best to motivate her, but she had lost all enthusiasm. She lost a little weight, but very slowly, and eventually we lost touch.

Joan

Joan came to see me in tears. She was very distraught about her weight gain. As she told me her story, I suddenly realised who she was.

Joan was 28 and her husband was 46. He was a local celebrity, a well-known businessman and a good public speaker. He was handsome and women sought his attention. Husband and wife had very compatible personalities and a well-matched relationship. In years past they adorned the social pages and gossip columns as a couple. In recent years Joan had disappeared from public life.

Joan gained a moderate amount of weight during her first pregnancy, but then she had twins and gained a tremendous amount of weight and her husband would shun her in public. He would phone from the office: "Darling, I know I promised to take you to tonight's function, but I am caught up at the office and I can't pick you up."

Joan knew he was lying and that he didn't want to be seen with her in public.

Seeing Joan distressed and in tears I tried to cheer her up and said: "It looks to me that you just have to lose weight - let's start."

Joan got onto the program very enthusiastically. I was surprised at her commitment and compliance.

Joan had lost 44kg (90lb) when I measured her fat percentage and said: "Congratulations, you are in the normal fat percentage range and ready for maintenance - you're looking great."

I will never forget the shocked look on her face. She slumped in the chair and started crying. "Why are you crying?" I asked. "Aren't you happy that you've lost all this weight?"

"That is exactly why I am crying - I am so happy," she said. "Since losing the fat my husband has taken a new interest in me. He's now organising parties especially to show me off."

That was years ago and we still stay in touch. Joan has kept off her excess fat, the children are teenagers and she is very happily married.

I have often seen how a person can not only change their own life, but also impact those around them. You too will be very pleased with the results if you stick to this health program. Never lose sight of the alternative - hopefully it will spur you to strive for success.

Enjoy your journey - you will never regret it if you do it well.